MENTAL HEALTH
POLICY FOR NURSES

SAGE has been part of the global academic community since 1965, supporting high quality research and learning that transforms society and our understanding of individuals, groups, and cultures. SAGE is the independent, innovative, natural home for authors, editors and societies who share our commitment and passion for the social sciences.

Find out more at: **www.sagepublications.com**

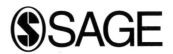

MENTAL HEALTH POLICY FOR NURSES

Edited by
IAN HULATT

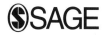

Los Angeles | London | New Delhi
Singapore | Washington DC

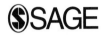

Los Angeles | London | New Delhi
Singapore | Washington DC

SAGE Publications Ltd
1 Oliver's Yard
55 City Road
London EC1Y 1SP

SAGE Publications Inc.
2455 Teller Road
Thousand Oaks, California 91320

SAGE Publications India Pvt Ltd
B 1/I 1 Mohan Cooperative Industrial Area
Mathura Road
New Delhi 110 044

SAGE Publications Asia-Pacific Pte Ltd
3 Church Street
#10-04 Samsung Hub
Singapore 049483

Editor: Becky Taylor
Associate editor: Emma Milman
Production editor: Katie Forsythe
Copyeditor: Audrey Scriven
Proofreader: Bryan Campbell
Indexer: David Rudeforth
Marketing manager: Tamara Navaratnam
Cover design: Naomi Robinson
Typeset by: C&M Digitals (P) Ltd, Chennai, India
Printed and bound by CPI Group (UK) Ltd,
Croydon, CR0 4YY

Introduction and editorial arrangement © Ian Hulatt 2014
Chapter 1 © Peter Nolan 2014
Chapter 2 © Neil Brimblecombe 2014
Chapter 3 © Ben Hannigan 2014
Chapter 4 © Norman Young 2014
Chapter 5 © Elizabeth Collier and Catherine McQuarrie 2014
Chapter 6 © Trevor Adams 2014
Chapter 7 © Karen M. Wright 2014
Chapter 8 © Mick McKeown and Fiona Jones 2014
Chapter 9 © Ann Jackson and Lindsey Ambrose 2014
Chapter 10 © Tim McDougall 2014
Chapter 11 © Cheryl Kipping 2014
Chapter 12 © Cris Allen 2014

First published 2014

Library of Congress Control Number: 2013951477

British Library Cataloguing in Publication data

A catalogue record for this book is available from
the British Library

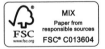

MIX
Paper from
responsible sources
FSC
www.fsc.org   FSC® C013604

ISBN 978-1-4462-5250-5
ISBN 978-1-4462-5251-2 (pbk)

CONTENTS

ABOUT THE EDITOR AND CONTRIBUTORS

Trevor Adams is a consultant in dementia care and presently is developing work on personalisation with dementia and the creation of dementia friendly communities. He holds a PhD in dementia care and has written extensively on dementia and contributed to conferences in the UK, Australia, Japan and Europe.

Cris Allen has been a nurse in mental health and learning disability for 34 years. He has occupied a range of positions in practice and management, was for several years the Mental Health Adviser at the Royal College of Nursing of the United Kingdom and now works independently. Cris has written widely in the nursing and health press, often on policy issues, and has been the Consultant Editor of the journal *Mental Health Practice* for over a decade. He has always been interested in health and nursing policy, a subject that has caused him elation and frustration in equal measure.

Lindsey Ambrose is a qualified lawyer and guidance professional, currently Equality, Diversity and Human Rights Lead at leading mental healthcare charity, St Andrew's, specialising in improving patient experience. In 2013 and 2014 Lindsey has led St Andrew's participation in the Stonewall UK Healthcare Equality Index, leading to 'top performer' rankings (3rd in 2014, 4th in 2013). Previously Lindsey's work at Northampton Borough Council (2004 to 2012) led to recognition including a National Diversity Award, through HRH Prince Charles's Mosaic Awards, praise from the Head of the Equality and Human Rights Commission, a special award from the Anne Frank Trust UK and awards from the Northants Children and Young People's Partnership. Lindsey has helped multi-million pound organisations improve the inclusivity and accessibility of their services and user experience. Born in the UK, Lindsey's interests in equality, diversity and human rights were particularly informed through childhood experience of horrific violence in Sri Lanka at the start of its civil war and being a young carer.

Elizabeth Collier is a Registered Mental Health Nurse who is employed as a lecturer in mental health at the University of Salford in Greater Manchester. She has worked with older people in various clinical settings during her career and has particular interest in age discrimination and in people who have aged with on-going functional mental health problems. Her PhD focused on the life experiences of people who had aged to older age with mental health problems and how this had affected their achievements. Her academic and research interests also include dementia, being a member of the Higher Education Dementia Network and also the International

Dementia Design network hosted at Salford university. She is involved in a European project, POSADEM to develop a pan-European Masters degree in dementia. She is an active member of the university service user and carer forum as well as being an honorary associate of blueSCI, a social, cultural and inclusion service in Trafford which operates within contemporary mental health recovery values.

Ben Hannigan is a Reader in Mental Health Nursing in the School of Healthcare Sciences at Cardiff University. In his research into mental health systems he has addressed these interrelated areas: policy; service organisation and delivery; work, roles and values; the characteristics and wellbeing of the workforce; practitioner education; and the experiences of users. He has published widely in these areas in nursing, health and social scientific journals and in books. He blogs at http://benhannigan.com

Ian Hulatt has been the mental health adviser in the nursing department at the Royal College of Nursing since 2004. Prior to this role he spent 20 years as a teacher of nurses at both undergraduate and post graduate levels. He undertook Thorn training at the Institute of Psychiatry and has maintained a keen interest in this area of practice ever since. His role at the RCN requires him to advise on mental health nursing policy and practice across the UK and whilst based in Wales he continues to travel the country in his work. Ian has engaged in many regional, national and international policy initiatives for the RCN and continues to be a passionate advocate for what he describes as the "craft" of mental health nursing.

Ann Jackson's clinical background is in acute in-patient mental health care. She has 20 years' experience working in practice development and research; working with teams as external facilitator to systematically review practice and integrate with best evidence and policy. From 1998, she was at the Royal College of Nursing and gained a wealth of experience working across national policy, research and practice agendas, primarily in mental health and social inclusion. Secondments to the Department of Health (Offender Health) and Leicestershire Partnership NHS Trust from 2005-2010 led to specific policy making and practice around women's mental health in the criminal justice system. From February 2012, she has been the Director of Nursing at St.Andrew's Healthcare, the largest UK charitable provider of specialist mental health services. She has particular interest in violence against women and mental health and equalities.

Fiona Jones has lengthy experience of using mental health services and has latterly volunteered with EmPowerMe (formerly Lancashire Advocacy) a service user-led voluntary sector organisation. Recently she has taken up the position of research assistant working alongside colleagues at the University of Central Lancashire. Fiona is also active in the university's community engagement and service user involvement initiative, Comensus, making a significant contribution to teaching and learning. On the research front, she has helped plan and deliver a number of projects that have benefited enormously from her lived experience and unique skills. This work has included a study of involvement in secure services across Yorkshire and an appreciative inquiry project to develop recovery orientated practices with mental health inpatient teams on Merseyside. Current studies focus on recovery and involvement practices in a high secure setting and the experiences of relatives of forensic patients in Scotland.

Cheryl Kipping began her career as a general nurse at Guy's Hospital before going on to train in mental health at the Maudsley. She has held clinical and managerial posts in the statutory and voluntary sectors, in mental health and addictions. Cheryl completed a social psychology degree at the London School of Economics, and a PhD at King's College, London. She has worked as a consultant nurse in dual diagnosis for 12 years. Cheryl has provided dual diagnosis expertise to a range of national advisory groups including the Department of Health and NICE. She has given conference presentations nationally and internationally, and published about dual diagnosis. Cheryl is a member of PROGRESS, the national consortium for consultant nurses in dual diagnosis.

Tim McDougall is Nurse Consultant and Clinical Director for Tier 4 CAMHS and Trust-wide CAMHS at the Cheshire & Wirral NHS Foundation Trust. Tim has worked in a range of CAMHS settings including community child mental health teams, adolescent in-patient services and secure adolescent forensic services. With a National profile in CAMHS and, with over 100 book and journal publications, Tim has spoken at National and European conferences about the mental health of children and adolescents. Tim was formerly Nurse Advisor for CAMHS at the Department of Health in England and was a member of the National Advisory Council for Children's Mental Health and Psychological Wellbeing. Tim is currently Chair of the UK Nurse Consultants in CAMHS Forum and the Quality Network for Inpatient CAMHS (QNIC) Executive Committee. He has been involved in the development of NICE guidelines on Psychosis and Schizophrenia in Children and Young People and Bipolar Disorder in Children, Young People and Adults.

Mick McKeown is a mental health nursing researcher in the School of Health at the University of Central Lancashire. He instigated the Comensus service user and carer involvement initiative at the university which has a growing reputation for extensiveness and authenticity of involvement practices. Recent research has explored service user and staff alliances for involvement in secure services and appreciative inquiry with inpatient mental health teams. Mick edited the book *Forensic mental health care: a case study approach* (Churchill Livingstone) and co-ordinated the production of the collectively written text: *Service user and carer involvement in education for health and social care* (Wiley-Blackwell). Mick is a Unison activist and interested in democratic alliances with mental health service user/survivor movements. This intersects with efforts to ensure universities become assets in their local communities, to this end Mick supports an international network of scholars committed to 'Mad Activism in the Academy'.

Catherine McQuarrie has been a lecturer in mental health nursing at the University of Salford since 2006. Prior to this, she was a lecturer/practitioner, working as a Clinical Nurse Specialist with the Manchester, Bolton, Salford and Trafford Substance Misuse Directorate. She has worked in the field of substance misuse (alcohol and drug services) since 1995 and completed an MSc in Drug Use and Addictions in 2003 and an MSc in Public Health and Society in 2010. She has a strong interest in promoting mental health and social inclusion. Cath was jointly responsible for 'A synthesis of grey literature around public health interventions and programmes' for NHS North West taking editorial responsibility for mental health and well being. She has recently developed and delivered training to the Being Well Coaches in Salford, a new initiative in relation to working with people in relation to behaviour change.

Peter Nolan was born in the West of Ireland and undertook mental health and general nurse training in London in the 1960s. He spent time in various posts including working as an Occupational Health Nurse in the Sahara Desert, as a journalist for the North African Radio Service based in Tripoli, Broadmoor Special Hospital, and subsequently as a Professor of Mental Health Nursing at the universities of Birmingham and Staffordshire. His research interests have included the changing face of mental health provision in the UK, Ireland, Sweden and the USA. He has had a long-standing interest in the relationship between spirituality and mental health and the extent to which some service users experience a 'crisis of meaning' in the modern world. He has published widely in the field of the history of mental health policies, institutions, interventions and the origins of various mental health disciplines. He is currently working on community care prior to the establishment of asylums.

Karen M. Wright is a mental health nurse and academic. She is the principal lecturer and lead for mental health within the School of Health at the University of Central Lancashire (UCLan). Karen designed and delivered the first MSc in Personality Disorder in the UK and continues, as part of the course team, to deliver this programme to a range of healthcare professionals at UCLan.

Karen originally trained as an RGN, specialising in cardio-thoracic surgery before moving to mental health in 1986. Since then she has worked in a range of clinical practice areas including acute in-patient services, community mental health, crisis intervention services and forensic services. She still works clinically within an in-patient service, on a weekly basis and sees this as vital to her role as an academic and researcher. Her most recent research activities have focussed on the therapeutic relationship, attitudes to violence and aggression, and service user involvement in forensic services.

Norman Young became interested in mental health after studying biochemistry and psychology at Keele University. After graduating he moved to Cardiff and qualified as a mental health nurse in 1994. Norman soon wished to follow a clinical academic career focusing on psychosis. After gaining therapy skills in congnitive and behavioural psychotherapy he set up, with Ian Hulatt, the first Thorn course in Wales. After this he developed an educational programme in acute care and collaborated in setting up the national accreditation of inpatient services. He subsequently led quality improvement initiatives in inpatient care and patient safety. Norman currently works as a Nurse Consultant with Cardiff and Vale University Health Board and Cardiff University.

Norman's current research interests are in organisational approaches to safety in mental health. Norman continues to provide care and treatment to people with psychosis and in involved in local and national improvement projects. Norman was a member of the NICE guideline development group for schizophrenia and psychosis in 2014.

LIST OF ACRONYMS

AC	Approved Clinician
ADHD	Attention Deficit Hyperactivity Disorder
AIMS	Accreditation of Acute Inpatient Mental Health Services
AMHP	approved mental health professional
ANARP	Alcohol Needs Assessment Research Project
ANP	Advanced Nurse Practitioner
BBC	British Broadcasting Corporation
BME	Black and Minority Ethnic
BPS	British Psychological Society
CAB	Citizen's Advice Bureau
CAMHS	Child and Adolescent Mental Health Services
CAS	Citizen's Advice Scotland
CBT	Cognitive Behavioural Therapy
CHC	Community Health Councils
CHI	Commission for Health Improvement
CMHNs	Community Mental Health Nurses
CMHT	Community Mental Health Centres and Teams
CRHT	Crisis Resolution and Home Treatment Teams
COHSE	Confederation of Health Service Employers
CPA	Care Programme Approach
CQC	Care Quality Commission
CQUIN	Commissioning for Quality and Innovation
CSIP	Care Services Improvement Partnership
CRHT	Crisis Resolution/Home Treatment
CRU	Civil Resettlement Units
CTO	Community Treatment Order
DAT	Drug Action Team
DH	Department of Health
DHSS	Department of Health and Social Services
DHSSPS	Department of Health, Social Services and Public Safety
DoH	Department of Health
DRE	Delivering Race Equality
DSM	Diagnostic and Statistical Manual of Mental Disorders
DSPD	Dangerous with Severe Personality Disorder
DUCIE	Developers of User and Carer Involvement in Education
DWP	Department for Work and Pensions
EC	European Commission
EDHR	Equalities, Diversity and Human Rights

EHRC	Equality and Human Rights Commission
EU	European Union
GP	General Practitioner
HAS	Health Advisory Service
HEI	Higher Education Institution
HIV	Human Immunodeficiency Virus
HMSO	Her Majesty's Stationery Office
IAPT	Improving Access to Psychological Therapies
ICD	International Classification of Diseases
IPS	Individual Placement and Support
LIT	Local Implementation Team
LGBTQ	Lesbian, Gay, Bisexual, Transgender and Questioning
LSE	London School of Economics
MAPPA	Multi-Agency Public Protection Arrangements
MHA	Mental Health Act
MHA	Mental Health Alliance
MHAC	Mental Health Act Commission
MHHE	Mental Health in Higher Education Network
MHP	Mental Health Practice
MoC	Models of Care
MoCAM	Models of Care for the Treatment of Alcohol Misuse
MSc	Master of Science
NCSS	National CAMHS Support Service
NCI	National Confidential Inquiry
NCISH	National Confidential Inquiry Reports into Suicide and Homicide by People with Mental Illness
NDTi	National Development Team for Inclusion
NHS	National Health Service
NHSE	National Health Service Executive
NHSLA	National Health Service Litigation Authority
NICE	National Institute for Clinical Excellence
NIMHE	National Institute of Mental Health for England
NMHDU	National Mental Health Development Unit
NPSA	National Patient Safety Agency
NHS	National Service Framework
NSF-MH	National Service Framework for Mental Health
OCTET	Oxford Community Treatment Order Evaluation Trial
ONS	Office for National Statistics
PALS	Patient Advice and Liaison Service
PD	Personality Disorder
PMS	Psychiatric Morbidity Survey
PPI	Patient and Public Involvement
QNIC	Quality Network for Inpatient CAMHS
RCN	Royal College of Nursing
RCP	Royal College of Psychiatrists

RGN	Registered General Nurse
RMA	Risk Management Authority
SCIE	Social Care Institute for Excellence
SCMH	Sainsbury Centre for Mental Health
SEAL	Social and Emotional Aspects of Learning
SHC	Scottish Health Council
SNAP	Scottish Needs Assessment Programme
SRI	Scottish Recovery Indicator
STR	Support, Time, Recovery
SURGE	Service Users in Research Group, England
UCLAN	University of Central Lancashire
UK	United Kingdom
UKCC	United Kingdom Central Council for Nursing, Midwifery and Health Visiting
USA	United States of America
WAG	Welsh Assembly Government
WAT	Workforce Action Team
WHO	World Health Organization

INTRODUCTION

Welcome to this edited volume of chapters addressing the issue of mental health policy and how it impacts and indeed determines your practice as a nurse. You will see from the chapter topics that they contain a broad range of practice areas and will touch on most areas of contemporary mental health nursing practice. If you have come to this topic with a question such as 'What has policy got to do with me?', then I trust you will leave the book with at least that question answered.

It is the basic premise of this book that policy determines much of what nurses actually do on a daily basis. It will be argued that in all areas of practice the actual process and means and indeed nature of services that mental health nurses work in are shaped by the influence of policy.

Policy itself is a complex issue with many determining factors. As we all know, at present in Britain the influence of the wider economic/political agenda impacts in a real way upon the delivery of health care. It may be that like many readers of this book you will have had to undergo yet another re-organisation of the service you work in order to address the diminished resources that are available for health care. Whilst economic determinants may seem obvious and indeed painful there are other more subtle and yet profound influencing factors that shape policy.

The whole ethos of the delivery of mental health services has been greatly shaped by the influence of the society it is delivered in. It is the current views of society and contemporary culture that have greatly influenced the way mental health care is delivered. Just as public health had its big leap forward in the realm of clean water, hygiene and housing, mental health made huge changes in ways that may now seem archaic. Our almost universal ambivalence to the asylum era makes us quickly forget the huge investment in both resources and energies that was required in addressing the scandals of private 'madhouses' and the inhumane conditions these provided for people in distress. The huge building programme that was compelled by law was part of an era of social change and the gradual dawning of an air of optimism that had never been present before. That change – built upon revulsion at the cruelties exposed by various Royal Commissions – was later mirrored by further public disquiet at the warehousing and 'therapeutic nihilism' that eventually characterised the end of the asylum era. It could be argued that this mood of disquiet was harnessed by those who were keen to promote a community-focused model of care.

Social policy underpinned by political leverage has produced much change, not only in the physical estate in which services are delivered but also and obviously in the resources available to provide these. This reaches far back into the education and training of the professionals available to deliver them and the resources allocated to the research and development of new modes of care and treatment. We have seen how central directions of a policy nature have shaped (if not actually required) the ways services are provided. Who will not recall the huge expansion of different forms of service models that have been centrally required? The growth in models of care has given rise to many new forms of service. The list probably appears bewildering at times as professionals and service users attempt to differentiate between Assertive Outreach, Home Treatment, Early Intervention, First Episode, Reablement, Recovery and Peer Led. This list will of course continue to grow as new models are developed and introduced.

As has been argued, policy has to respond to the public mood as well and not purely in ways that seem to be in the interests of individuals alone. Policy has also had to respond to public concern when a strict utilitarian concern has arisen that the needs of the wider society should outweigh (or must be balanced against) those that are purely of the individual. Such public concern in the late 1990s initiated a long and expensive revision of the 1983 Mental Health Act – and indeed, will probably prove a strong disincentive to the legislation being addressed again for many years to come! Yet that change of legislation saw requirements not only in the way that service delivery had to change but also in the legal requirements that could be placed upon how individuals had to behave. This was best evidenced through developments such as community treatment orders.

It is of course tempting as mental health nurses to argue that we practise in a manner that is devoid of others' influence, and that we make assessments, decide on programmes of care and monitor their implementation with a detached air of professional autonomy. However, this book will clearly discuss the many and varied influences which shape the policy that drives and determines the way we work. It has become an accepted truism that 'culture devours strategy': I would like you to think carefully as you read through the following chapters about how social policy determines the culture of the profession you belong to and practise in.

Each chapter will begin with a brief introduction from me and this will contain a number of questions that you can refer to after you have completed the chapter. I hope that these will stimulate you to consider why you do what you do and how you have decided to do it. You may also wish to discuss these questions in the context of a group of colleagues, perhaps in an educational setting. Wherever you do so I trust they will enable you to reflect not only on the chapters you have read, but also (and more importantly) upon the service you provide for those service users, carers and families you care for.

HOW THE BOOK IS ORGANISED

Chapter 1 – The history of mental health policy in the United Kingdom

Chapter 1 sets the scene for the entire book by placing the current developments in an historical context. You will see how the evolution of policy has attempted to deal with issues of social concern in a variety of ways and how current concerns can also be of a longstanding nature.

Chapter 2 – The European context

This chapter places the way we deliver mental health services in the UK in the context of fellow European countries. You will be able to recognise how mental health nursing is not a European-wide practice as we know it here in the UK. In addition, there is an opportunity to ask why mental health nursing has developed in such divergent ways from familiar and shared practices in the past.

Chapter 3 – Community services

Transitions that form institutional models of care to community-delivered services show a wide divergence across Europe, yet here in the UK these have proven to be the most radical transformation (though yet to be completed) of service provision. The chapter will explore this policy 'triumph' here in the UK, with all its attendant concerns and successes

Chapter 4 – Psychosis

Individuals who have been labelled with psychosis have traditionally provoked the most austere policy responses, yet it has been the case that this area of practice has seen wide and far-reaching changes in service provision. The chapter will explore this area and offer a commentary on service providers' concerns and achievements.

Chapter 5 – Older people

With the growth in effective treatments for previously life-limiting conditions older people are now present in more and more services. The need to reconsider images and perceptions of aging will be explored together with the various implications for policy and service.

Chapter 6 – Dementia

Dementia was perhaps one of the reasons for the very creation of the asylum system, and whilst poorly understood it challenged earlier generations to provide a humane service response. The chapter will express the progress and challenges that remain for mental health nurses in providing services for clients in a group considered as destined to grow exponentially in number.

Chapter 7 – Personality disorder

People with a diagnosis of personality disorder possess a label that retains professional, public and political anxiety. Poorly understood and loaded with therapeutic nihilism it remains contentious, and this chapter discusses the challenges in the policy response.

Chapter 8 – Service user involvement

Perhaps next to the actual location of services this has been the biggest transformation in the culture of mental health services. The journey from patient to co-producer – and indeed peer support worker – has transformed many services and lives. This chapter unpacks the agendas and actions that achieved this change.

Chapter 9 – Equalities in mental health nursing

While it may be tempting to consider mental health services as hermetically sealed against the broader society this clearly isn't the case. The broader social agenda regarding equalities resonates clearly with some service users' experiences and the chapter discusses the challenge that nurses (amongst others) face.

Chapter 10 – Child mental health policy in the UK

Children and young people are not 'little adults' and their needs in the context of mental health services are far from being just a smaller version. Thus, the chapter places children's and young people's policy in the wider context of social perspectives on children and their needs. The clear transition from being ignored to having a legitimate and assertive voice is demonstrated in the policy responses provided.

Chapter 11 – Dual diagnosis

The interaction between mental health and substance use is fraught with many complex balances. The picture of therapeutic interactions is further complicated by its proximity to the criminal justice system. The chapter demonstrates how policy makers have tried to ensure that such a fine balancing of priorities remains secondary to client need.

Chapter 12 – Policy into action?

The challenge for a long time has been to try and ensure that policy becomes practice. Common terms today – such as 'nudge', 'policy levers', and even 'traction'– all try to describe how this can be achieved. This final chapter takes a wry look at just how difficult this process can prove to be.

1 THE HISTORY OF MENTAL HEALTH POLICY IN THE UNITED KINGDOM

Peter Nolan

Chapter Overview

In this introductory chapter to the book Professor Nolan provides an overview of mental health policy in the UK. Like any book there is a very good chance that by the time this is read there will have been further developments and occurrences of note, however, he has provided you the reader with an opportunity to see the development of policy in a broad historical sweep and with reference to social events that may well have informed the policy development. As alluded to in the introduction to this volume, policy does not occur in a vacuum.

So as you will see here there are wider social and political events and movements that can be said to have shaped the world within which you now practise. The history of policy has certain pivotal moments and in this chapter you can clearly recognise the influence of those who we would now describe as reformers: individuals who possessed a vision of how care and treatment could be improved and delivered in a more humane way. This perhaps reached its peak with the de-institutionalisation programme of the 1980s from which in some senses we are still emerging. The water towers are now few and those that remain in the midst of housing estates do so as 'listed' reminders of a past age.

(Continued)

(Continued)

As this book was nearing completion the NHS was still undergoing close scrutiny and this was exemplified by the Francis Report (2013) which investigated the failings of care in Mid Staffordshire. It is possible that mental health services had their 'Francis moment' many years ago, but there is still a need to be vigilant and also aware that the current service models provide for those in our society who number amongst the most vulnerable.

INTRODUCTION

In the second decade of the twenty-first century, policy has assumed a much greater degree of importance in the design, delivery and direction of mental health services than was previously the case. Health is now seen as a fundamental human right that is indispensable for the exercise of other human rights and every human being is entitled to attain a standard of health conducive to living a dignified life (Andersen et al., 2006; Penhale and Parker, 2007). But there are other reasons also, including an ageing population, increasing demands on mental health services, advances in medical technology, efficiency savings in the NHS, and heightened expectations on the part of patients and service users. If those responsible for the provision of health care become so preoccupied with administrative minutiae then it is possible that health-care provision could become deeply embedded in routine and unable to respond to need, with the result that it becomes little more than a mechanism for perpetuating the social, economic, and political order of an inegalitarian society (Sullivan, 1987; Goodwin et al., 1999). Addressing all of these issues requires understanding and consideration of the varying perspectives of providers, consumers and the general public. In addition, health policy must currently confront a challenging economic climate in which uncertainty is all pervading. Governments faced with rising health-care costs must seek ways of achieving higher quality and productivity without increasing expenditure (Propper, 2011). In the UK and elsewhere, policy makers are challenged by numerous questions: does competition or collaboration produce better healthcare; how can closer working relationships be brought about between providers; what should be the roles of the private and voluntary sectors; how can a strong consumer voice exist alongside, but distinct from, the regulators (Dixon, 2011).

It is apparent that, given such complex circumstances, a systematic development of mental health services and sustained improvement are unlikely to occur without a clear mental health policy. While the boundaries of health policy are regularly contested and redefined, four objectives seem to remain constant:

- Devising services which can be accessed early and easily.
- Ensuring that services are diverse and appropriate.

- Training health-care workers so they are appropriately skilled to deliver services.
- Putting in place suitable support for people recovering from mental health problems in ways that can be seen as constituting '*recovery capital*'.

This chapter offers a succinct overview of the evolution of mental health policy in the UK, briefly examining why certain policies were introduced at certain times and concluding with a discussion of the challenges that both confront those who formulate policy and those who are charged with implementing it. Although mental health policy throughout the UK is largely similar differences do occur, both with respect to content and focus, and these will be highlighted and briefly discussed towards the end of the chapter. Although few mental health nurses will be directly involved in formulating policies, all nurses – irrespective of their position or grade – have a responsibility to be informed about these and active in their implementation. The seeming indifference of nurses towards mental health policy has been due in previous decades to a perceived lack of professional autonomy that arose from an anachronistic, 'handmaiden' relationship with psychiatric medicine (Barker, 1989). Until recently, the work of nurses was poorly defined and largely shaped by the culture of medically-dominated institutions and the preferences of psychiatrists and managers for specific therapeutic approaches. It was inconceivable to the majority of nurses that centralised policies might impact directly on their work.

Analysts have noted that mental health-care policy has not only lagged behind other areas of health care, but also that it is one of the most neglected facets of health care worldwide. However, it would be inaccurate to assert that policies in other branches of health care always determine interventions or are always implemented homogeneously; *theory is not always made incarnate* (Weiss, 1995). On the contrary, argue Greenhalgh et al. (2011), most interventions – including those in mental health – are driven by hypotheses, hunches and aspirations. While policies are directed at populations, services are provided for individuals in circumstances which vary considerably. However, it is generally agreed among policy commentators that without the spur of policy to direct practice, some people with mental health problems have been poorly treated while others have received no treatment at all, and as a result, these individuals have experienced disrupted relationships, unemployment, social exclusion, and increased exposure to the criminal justice system.

Public attitudes towards mental health services have fuelled policy neglect, with attitudes based on the belief (held even by some of those who provide mental health care) that people with mental health problems could get well 'if they really wanted to'. Ignorance impedes the development of services: mental health problems are poorly understood both by the general public and by practitioners; researchers have not illuminated sufficiently the causes of mental illness; treatments are idiosyncratic and conjectural; and few in public life champion those who suffer with mental health problems (Koffman & Fulop, 1999; Pilgrim & Rogers, 2001).

However, when prominent people have supported improvements in the quality of services they have effected change, even if not to the extent that they would have hoped for (Pilgrim & Rogers, 2001). In the 1950s in the UK, Donald Macintosh, a Conservative MP, doctor and ex-psychiatric patient, used his influence as a parliamentarian to get mental health care onto the political agenda. He highlighted the poor conditions in which the mentally ill were cared for in comparison to patients in other branches of medicine and the lack of access to effective treatments. Similarly, in the 1990s Ian McCartney, a Labour MP, spearheaded a policy review of conditions and practices in mental health, while Tessa Jowell, in the same decade, sponsored a number of private members' bills relating to aftercare provision for service users (the latter drew on her extensive previous experience in mental health care as the Training and Education Director for MIND). Equally dedicated was former Tory Minister of Health, Virginia Bottomley, an ex-psychiatric social worker who regularly participated in debates on mental health policy and services. While the work of these few is admirable, it is also remarkable by virtue of the fact that it is confined to such a small number, given that one in five of the 650 MPs in the House of Commons has admitted to having experienced a mental health problem at some point in their lives (MIND, 2008). This almost unanimous failure on the part of MPs to advocate for the mentally ill has seriously impeded the development of services and their availability and accessibility. The UK has seen very little of the courage demonstrated by the Norwegian Prime Minister, Kjell Magne Bondevik, who developed a mental illness while in office, disclosed it, and acknowledged that it prevented him from carrying out his duties as Premier. His honesty stimulated an outpouring of sympathy and understanding from all sectors of society, and his candour was rewarded by his being re-elected with an increased majority (Knapp et al., 2007). This incident has much to say about how political leadership can be instrumental in increasing public awareness, interest and commitment.

REMIT OF MENTAL HEALTH POLICY

Carpenter (2000) states that the student of health policy should commence by focusing on the process of policy making rather than undertaking an exploration of what it was that specific policies were designed to achieve. He contends that policy is an umbrella term encompassing legislation, research, economics and politics, all of which are distilled to yield an indication of what can realistically be provided and achieved. Policy, he continues, should take into account the culture of public services and the variety of ways in which mental health services can be made available to people from a variety of cultural and social backgrounds. Mental health policy has to be to be viewed from multiple standpoints. How has policy evolved? How is it presented and what language is used to express it? What implications does it have for resources? How is it to be implemented? What recommendations, if any, are there for how it is to be evaluated? And most importantly, what are the limitations of a specific policy and to what extent does it conflict or overlap with other policies?

All policies – regardless of their intentions – constitute a discourse between the individual and the state, and although there is disagreement about the precise definition of policy it is generally agreed that it provides a vision of how a particular society would wish things to be (Andrews, 2001). Policies are essentially declarations of an intended direction of travel, and of necessity these will change over time in accordance with changing social circumstances: they are not absolute edicts meant to be adhered to regardless of circumstances, and should not appear to be unrealistically utopian in their aspirations. In contrast to the law which is mandatory, public policy is expressed in the regulations, decisions and actions of government: it does not only refer to the actions of government, but also to the intentions that determine those actions. In short, public policy consists of the political decisions that are taken in implementing programmes to achieve societal goals (McCool, 1995). Explaining why policies are necessary, Grayling (2006) states that these support human societies to evolve in a reasoned, compassionate and civilised way, while Osbourne (2008) suggests that policies should attempt to define health and highlight tried and tested strategies for its maintenance: it is thus the function of policy to state unequivocally what people should expect by way of state provision in order to be healthy. Osbourne considers that without transparency and candour, health-care providers are liable to interpret directives in different ways, giving rise to postcode lotteries which can result in both apparent and real injustices with respect to the availability of services and treatments. Mental health policy should paint a vision of what the future should look like and act as a declaration of the level of wellbeing that a government seeks to attain for the population it serves.

Osbourne also contends that in a state-run health service it is incumbent on the government to explain the political and economic ideologies that gave rise to its policies, to provide evidence of public need, and give an assurance that what is being proposed is deliverable and affordable. As the NHS is a tax-funded system and the chief means by which people take care of each other, it is – of necessity – an intensely political institution. Good health service governance requires the commitment of three key stakeholders if its implementation is to be successful, namely users, funders and workers. In formulating and implementing policy, government seeks to foster a dialogue and build consensus between professionals, service users and the public. Differences in the social and cultural context of health care in different countries or regions of the same country, in the personnel involved in delivering it, in costs, in perceived consequences for the community as a whole, and in people's expectations inevitably result in health-care policy that is constantly changing. Providers and professionals will therefore not universally comply with policies, and these may be seen as unstable and as externally-imposed constraints which threaten professionals' self-interest (Pilgrim & Rogers, 2001).

Behavioural economists will frequently invoke 'nudge theory' in examining the importance of policy, the essence of which is to persuade people of the rightness of what is being suggested (Thaler & Sunstein, 2009). Closely aligned to this is *libertarian paternalism*, which holds that state involvement in the welfare of citizens does not have to compromise or ignore individual autonomy. People's choices can be steered in directions that will improve their welfare but without the coercive proscription of certain courses of action. Andrews (2001) argues that all policies, regardless of their theoretical assumptions, are no more than navigational aids and do not provide clear explanations as to how they should be implemented. While policies must be persuasive, intelligible and credible, they must also appear to be pragmatic and achievable – and above all, clearly capable of contributing to the improvement of people's lives. To attain a high level of agreement on policy between state and public, Andrews (2001) posits certain *a priori* conditions: there must exist an educated population capable of critical thinking and reflection; there must also be debate and discussion that include all sections of society; and time must be set aside to allow people to explore the meaning and implications of certain courses of actions. People must be sufficiently public-spirited to see what is in the best interest of others as well as themselves. These conditions are especially relevant as those managing and delivering services come under increasing pressure to cut costs, to be more transparent, and to include members of the public in exploring how improvements could be initiated and sustained.

EVOLUTION OF MENTAL HEALTH POLICY

In his history of psychiatry, Shorter (1997) asserts that mental health policy can be related to three phases in the development of mental health services: the establishment of the asylum system; the beginnings of community care; and finally, the expansion and consolidation of community services. In the nineteenth century, the principal concern of policy makers was to manage a social problem by confining the insane and removing them from the public gaze. At the end of the following century the objective was to create a system whereby support for people with mental health problems would be derived within the communities in which they lived. Porritt (2005) concludes that while both sets of policies impacted on where and how services were provided, their main outcome was to redefine individuals' relationship with the state and their immediate environments. Communities are not just places where people live – they comprise a set of mediating agencies between individuals and their mental health and wellbeing. It is perhaps surprising that some of the fiercest opponents of community care have been mental health professionals who seemed unhappy to confer the rights of full citizenship on people whose personhood they considered to be severely limited, as evidenced by their need for ongoing monitoring by psychiatric personnel (Porritt, 2005).

Writings by social philosophers in the eighteenth and nineteenth centuries were highly influential in the development of social philosophies that encompassed the weak and the vulnerable, and which eventually influenced the setting up of institutional mental health services in the mid-nineteenth century. Much consideration was given to the relationship that should exist between the public and those in power, and particularly to how the disenfranchised should be treated. French and English Enlightenment writers such as Rousseau, Voltaire, Hobbes, Locke and Mill examined political and ecclesiastical powers and speculated about how the church and the state acquired their power and then maintained it, appearing to place their own survival foremost. In societies where church and state wielded considerable power, these writers felt that injustice abounded and inequalities in access to resources and assistance were not challenged. Rousseau and Hobbes referred to the theory of *possessive individualism* to explain how individuals who held power were driven by primitive urges of self-interest and avarice, often at the expense of others and especially the poor whose lives, as Hobbes remarked, were so often 'nasty, brutish and short' (Malcolm, 2002). Mill, however, contended that the social order was negotiable and did not have to be either unjust or unkind (Capaldi, 2004). A civilised society would allow the sovereignty of the people to be supreme and ensure that political power was in service to the people. Good political governance would restrain the excesses of the strong, empower the weak, make justice available to all, and strive to achieve the greatest happiness of the greatest number of people. For the people to be able to participate in their own governance, they had to have access to education, be able to make judgements, exercise freedom of thought, and have the autonomy to make choices in their own best interests. Laws and policies should be judged not by their intentions but by their effects.

In terms of mental health legislation and policy making, many of today's issues would have been familiar to our predecessors in the eighteenth century. How is it possible to balance caring for people suffering from mental distress and controlling them, or to respect individual liberties and personal autonomy? What amount of public funding should be allocated to addressing the causes of mental ill health and alleviating its effects? What should governments do about public attitudes towards the mentally ill? What role should they play in trying to reduce stigmatisation? What can health services and professionals realistically achieve?

The origins of mental health policy in the UK, where the state intervenes directly in the lives of people, can be traced back to the Vagrancy Act of 1744, which enabled those who were considered a threat to civil order to be securely detained. While the act sought to reassure the public that they were safe from possible threats to life and limb posed by the mentally ill, it reinforced the association between mental illness, poverty and dangerousness in the public mind. As no extra resources were provided to implement the act, local officials had little choice but to make use of existing facilities such as prisons, workhouses and Houses of Correction in order to confine people. This exacerbated the overcrowding that already existed, led to a deterioration in standards of care, and in many instances, added to the burden of the physical and mental ill health of inmates (Porter, 1987). By the beginning of the nineteenth century, the need to remove the mentally ill from public places had been replaced by anxiety relating to what should be done with them once they were securely confined.

At the end of the eighteenth century, a number of events served to increase public awareness of mental illness and to stimulate interest in what types of treatments or interventions could be provided to remedy the anguish that mentally ill people had to endure. These events included the madness of the monarch, King George III, the opening of the York Retreat in 1796, the founding of Ticehurst House in 1797, and the trial of James Hadfield in 1800 (who had attempted to assassinate the king but was found to be of unsound mind and so not accountable for his actions). These events not only enlightened public opinion, but also prompted those in authority to seek ways of managing the mentally ill while at the same time alleviating the effects of mental illness. The nineteenth century brought new stimuli for the state to increase its involvement in health care, education and welfare provision in which until this time – as Karl Marx noted – it had taken little interest (McLellan, 2006). Rapid urbanisation saw epidemics of diseases such as cholera which affected people regardless of class. The Eugenics movement raised concerns about the breeding stock of the nation, and in Germany Bismarck's domestic policies (1871–1890) which entailed the state taking responsibility for health and education appeared to have contributed to the country's strong economy (Farmer & Stiles, 2007). Social ills and political theories, coupled with the perceived threat of the growing numbers of mentally ill people, gave rise to the passing of Acts of Parliament which affected the whole nation. Prior to the nineteenth century these acts usually related only to particular counties, cities or towns.

Between 1801 and 1807 no fewer than 71 bills, reports from select committees and inquiries relating to mental health were published. The County Asylums Act of 1808 required asylums to be built in 'airy and healthy' locations and to admit patients who were too 'dangerous to be at large'. Few counties however in fact responded and little additional provision was made available for the mentally ill. A humanitarian emphasis on protecting 'lunatics' against abuse led to the 1828 Madhouses Act which required all asylums and private hospitals to have a medical officer. Patients who had recovered were to be discharged by Justices of the Peace. In 1845, the Lunatics Act strengthened the 1808 County Asylum Act and made it compulsory for each county to have specialist provision for the mentally ill: it also established an inspection system to be overseen by the Lunacy Commission. Pilgrim and Rogers (2001) see this act as a triumph of confinement and a sop to those who wanted the threat of moral contagion posed by the mentally ill to be removed from civilised society. The new asylums were designed with magnificent facades but these often disguised the fact that those working inside were preoccupied with security and control (Busfield, 1986). Nursing staff, called attendants, were poorly paid and poorly treated, and were probably not highly motivated to improve the lot of inmates confined to 'refractory wards' who were restrained in padded cells and sedated at night. Medical staff spent most of their time on administrative and supervisory duties, but were becoming increasingly powerful inside the asylums as the General Medical Registration Act (1858) decreed that only those with training in biological disorders could oversee the management and treatment of the insane.

By the time the Lunacy Act (1890) was passed, over 100 asylums had been built across the country. The act allowed for Justices of the Peace to oversee and certify the admission of patients, while at the same time increasing the status and power of the medical superintendent and psychiatry. However, the hoped-for medical cures and outcomes were not forthcoming. Some superintendants expressed regret that owing to their poor quality attendants were ill-equipped to play their part in achieving the therapeutic aspirations of medical staff. In 1885 a training course became available for asylum doctors, and in the same year the *Handbook for the Instruction of Attendants of the Insane* was published. Rayner (1884) saw training as the chief means of invigorating the work of mental health personnel by conferring professional credibility and satisfying the lunacy commissioners that more effective ways of managing and treating the mentally ill were being pursued. A few enthusiastic doctors went on to devise a national training scheme for attendants: the course took three years and the first qualified asylum nurses received their certificates in 1893.

The First World War made unprecedented demands on the asylums with over 100,000 soldiers requiring treatment for various psychiatric conditions, principally in what is now termed post-traumatic stress disorder. This demand impelled a new interest in psychiatry in approaches to treating the mentally ill. The British Psychological Society was founded in 1919, strongly influenced by Freudian theories, and a year later, the Tavistock Clinic opened to provide psychoanalytic treatment for outpatients. *The Royal Commission Report* (HMSO, 1926) significantly stated that mental and physical illnesses were not distinct and its recommendations were restated in the Mental Treatment Act (1930) which further strengthened the power of doctors by permitting forced treatments. As a result medical interventions such as, hydrotherapy, insulin, narcosis and electrical therapies became more widespread.

During the Second World War, psychiatrists and psychiatric nurses were recruited into the armed forces in the belief that providing an immediate on-site response for shell-shocked soldiers was preferable – both therapeutically and financially – to removing them from the battlefield and treating them elsewhere (Harrison & Clarke, 1992). As is often the case, war had focused government policy in a way that peace time conditions had not. It was as a direct result of the experience of treating large numbers of military personnel that therapeutic communities, group therapies and Civil Resettlement Units (CRU) for ex-prisoners of war were established (Newton, 1988). The main focus of the CRUs was to help ex-POWs reintegrate into society and reclaim their previous work skills. Vocational guidance and help in finding work aimed to rebuild confidence and develop resilience. Families were also encouraged to be involved in soldiers' rehabilitation. This approach was quickly adopted into mainstream psychiatry and became a foundation for the community-based services that were subsequently to emerge.

The post-war period was one of optimism. Following the inauguration of the NHS in 1948, there was unlimited access to free health care and this heralded state intervention on a much larger scale than ever before. The state had now replaced private charities as the main provider of personal and social services. Keynes (Sullivan, 1987) argued that state intervention in healthcare should only aim to provide those services which people cannot provide for themselves. However, such was the range of services provided that financial problems soon began to emerge. It became apparent that 75% of NHS beds were being occupied by psychiatric patients. Once the responsibility for admitting patients was handed over to doctors admissions escalated, with the result that there were 150,000 people in mental hospitals by 1954. By 1956, 2000 more beds had been made available and there were 1000 more psychiatric nurses and 77 more consultants (Rogers & Pilgrim, 2001). This expansion took place without adequate planning and the country could not afford it. The Percy Commission was convened to address this serious situation, and its 1957 Report underpinned the Mental Health Act (1959) which introduced the voluntary admission of patients and recommended short stays in hospital.

Government policies of the time acknowledged that institutionalising the mentally ill could lead to their degradation as persons and the corruption of care: institutions designed to look after very vulnerable people ended up betraying the trust placed in them (Martin, 1984). The Department for Health and Social Security commissioned a development project in Worcester in 1968 which demonstrated that a large psychiatric hospital could be replaced by community-based facilities (Hall, 1992). However, community alternatives to institutional care – although attractive in theory – did not yet appear to be a feasible option.

POLICY-DRIVEN DEINSTITUTIONALISATION

Clare (1976) described the 1960s as the 'decade of rhetoric'. Enoch Powell announced the government's intention to begin shifting hospital-based psychiatric services into the community (Powell, 1961). This was a time of severe staff shortages, particularly in nursing, and many hospitals were forced – albeit reluctantly – to accept unsuitable recruits with a subsequent impact on standards of care. It quickly became apparent that it had been easier to establish institutional services than disestablish them. However, the government pressed on and the publication of *Better Services for the Mentally Ill* (DHSS, 1975) accelerated the running-down of psychiatric hospitals and the provision of more treatments and support in community settings. This was the first attempt at pulling back state control in the field of health care, an attempt that was to be accelerated under the first Thatcher government in 1979. While the idea of community care found acceptance among health-care practitioners, they were given little guidance in how to implement it nor any information about how it was to be monitored. Community care represented a denunciation of the past and hopeful vision for the future which amounted to no more than hypothetical conjecture. Finch and Groves (1980) predicted that as community care evolved, greater responsibilities would fall on relatives and carers, and especially on women, as they would have to pick up where the statutory services left off.

From the early 1980s there was more direction from central government about the shape and content of community services. The Mental Health Act (1983) addressed the sensitivity needed to distinguish between people who wanted to be left alone and those who wanted treatment in the community. It reflected on how human rights should be incorporated into mental health services and under what circumstances someone should be forcibly taken into a psychiatric facility. There was also consideration given to what constituted a duty of care in relation to discharged patients. The rise of service-user movements increased the sense of urgency in relation to the reorganisation of mental health care. In a climate of liberal thinking, the scientific basis of psychiatry was questioned. The process of reaching a diagnosis by means of clinical investigation was seen as part of a now denigrated institutional culture. Johnstone (1992) argued that as long as problem identification remained the focus of doctors, scant progress could be made in understanding the causes of mental health problems and how to help people once treatment ceased. Growing insecurity and uncertainty at the heart of psychiatry affected the work of planners, commissioners and providers who were initially ambivalent about committing to primary mental care initiatives, inter-agency working and shared funding arrangements.

Further assistance in the form of policy arrived with the introduction of the Care Programme Approach (CPA) (DH, 1990) as a form of case management, with the aim of improving community care for people with severe mental illness. Its adoption implied that despite the rolling back of state power the state had a duty of care to individuals, and that professionals could not necessarily be relied on to deliver policy-directed care. While at one level state control of health was waning, at another it appeared that the state was engaging in the micro-management of individual care. The CPA represented a new direction, signifying the direct involvement of government in how services should be delivered. Simpson et al. (2003) concluded that it was a flawed policy that had been introduced inappropriately in an inhospitable socio-political and financial context, thereby exacerbating clinicians' resistance to political and managerial interference and raising new objections to the bureaucratisation of care. The CPA also presumed levels of community resources and inter-professional team working that were patently absent. Nevertheless, today it remains central to the care of people with severe mental health problems in the community and is used as a tool in the allocation of scarce resources.

Towards the end of the decade the White Paper, *Safe, Sound and Supportive* (DH, 1998b), signalled a major modernisation agenda in healthcare. In the following year the *National Service Framework for Mental Health* (DH, 1999) was published, which stated that service delivery should aim to achieve seven standards over a ten-year period. These tackled five areas: health promotion and stigma; primary care and access to specialist services; the needs of those with severe and enduring mental illness; carers' needs; and suicide reduction.

- **Standard one:** addressed mental health promotion and strategies to combat discrimination.
- **Standards two and three:** set out how primary care should work, including onward referrals, access to round-the-clock care and NHS Direct.
- **Standards four and five:** described effective services for those with severe and enduring mental illness, including crisis plans, round-the-clock access, in-patient treatment and rehabilitation care.
- **Standard six:** established annual checks for carers of those with severe and enduring mental illness, and written and implemented care plans.
- **Standard seven:** was a composite of standards one to six, with additional guidelines to ensure staff could assess the suicide risk, learn lessons from local suicide audits and be supported to prevent prisoner suicide.

Delivering the standards called for much closer cooperation between NHS staff and those employed by local authorities working in social care. In order to meet those standards and achieve a better integration of services, the necessity of improved education and training – as well as the recruitment of new staff and their retention – was recognised.

This was followed by the *NHS Plan* (DH, 2000) which set out specific targets for the establishment of 220 assertive outreach and 335 crisis resolution teams by 2004. To assist in creating a robust culture and structure for the coordination and implementation of policy and practice, a National Institute of Mental Health for England (NIMHE) was suggested, based on a model from the USA. NIMHE's role was to bring together research and legislation and then disseminate good practice so that effective partnerships could be developed between agencies, service users, carers, professionals and managers.

NIMHE's mission was to improve the quality of life for people of all ages experiencing mental distress. At the outset it identified conceptual vagueness as a major impediment to planning preventive services, with multiple definitions of primary, secondary and tertiary prevention being used. Research lacked coherence and often failed to inform policy, while policy initiatives were found to have a patchy impact on practice rather than being adopted in a widespread manner. The quality of services varied nationally as did the quality of education and the training of mental health personnel. Medical practitioners had a vested interest in the diagnosis of disorders and their treatment as opposed to the creation of conditions in which problems could be prevented or minimised. With the intention of bringing about closer collaboration between services NIMHE was given responsibility to coordinate the whole of mental health services – that is, of all services for people of all ages including primary, secondary and tertiary care.

Improving community care and focusing on health promotion were central to *Our Healthier Nation* (DH, 1998a) and to WHO (2003b). These documents stated that mental health promotion should be informed by a different set of assumptions from those that informed the treatment of the mentally ill, and should enshrine the belief that services users have rights of citizenship and should have access to all facilities that could be regarded as recovery capital. These ideas were further developed in the Helsinki Agreement (WHO, 2005) in which it was stated that the following priorities should be adopted by EU countries:

- Promoting individual and societal mental wellbeing.
- Tackling stigma, discrimination and social exclusion.
- Preventing the causes of mental health problems.
- Providing comprehensive and effective interventions for people with mental health problems whilst offering involvement and choice.
- Rehabilitating and including in society people who have experienced serious mental health problems.

WHO (2010) declared that there was 'No Health Without Mental Health' and that mental health was pivotal to individual and community wellbeing. It recommended that societies should endeavour to minimise the distress-inducing effects of rapid social change, poor working conditions, gender discrimination, social exclusion, unhealthy lifestyles, and human rights violations. In policy terms, a theme was emerging that the factors that would make a difference to people with mental health problems were not associated with psychiatrists, nurses or psychologists, they were instead good housing, supportive social relationships and safe communities. *No Health Without Mental Health* (DH, 2011) states that the role of government is to assist citizens to have more control over their lives and build more capable communities, although it remains conjectural as to how that will be achieved across the country. Responsibility for mental health is not the responsibility of one department, but rather a cross-department responsibility of all government divisions. Citizenship now encompasses the obligation to take responsibility for one's own mental health and that of others, and to challenge all forms of stigma and discrimination which could adversely affect human flourishing.

In order to make mental health everyone's business, *No Health Without Mental Health* called on organisations and government departments to work together on key shared objectives:

- More people will have good mental health.
- More people with mental health problems will recover.
- More people with mental health problems will have good physical health.
- More people will have a positive experience of care and support.
- Fewer people will suffer avoidable harm.
- Fewer people will experience stigma and discrimination.

MENTAL HEALTH POLICY AND DEVOLUTION

It is undoubtedly the case that mental health policy within the UK has tended to be anglocentric, although since devolution this is no longer so. *No Health Without Mental Health* (DH, 2011) refers specifically to England but notes that many of the problems confronting mental health services are similar to those presenting to other UK administrations. However, while the challenges may be similar, England, Wales, Scotland and Northern Ireland each adopts its own strategies for helping people with mental health problems. In England, the strategy devised by the coalition government is based on principles of freedom, fairness and responsibility, principles that are highly dependent on the financial and human resources for their implementation. Government policy presents itself as less directive and more facilitative than has been the custom. The responsibility for improvements in mental health is devolved to local authorities and agencies on the understanding that they are best placed to confront health inequalities, reduce stigma, and foster better mental well-being in their communities. Action at a local level will lead to whole population outcomes, including improved life expectancy, better educational achievement, reduced health risks behaviour and anti-social behaviour, higher levels of social interaction and participation, and greater happiness and fulfilment.

In Northern Ireland the public are invited to become actively involved in shaping policy, identifying deficits in health care, and suggesting areas for development (Priorities for Action, 2010). This approach focuses on how policies are formulated and to what extent they are capable of bringing about change in how services are delivered. Its review captured the experiences of people with mental health needs and learning disabilities as well as those of their families and carers, and explored people's priorities for effective health and social care services. When the responses were collated they provided fascinating insights into how people viewed services:

- More rapid access to care and treatment was urgently requested.
- People were not convinced that community care was effective and questioned its planning, delivery and availability.
- Service users and carers wanted to be more involved in their care and to have care plans which they could hold in their own homes.
- Young carers' needs were not being prioritised.
- Services must be available for all, regardless of age, gender, creed and location, and the standards applied equally to all groups.
- Better communication between health and social care staff at all levels was needed – people wanted to have greater continuity of care and not to see different people at every appointment.

Rather than rewriting the current policy framework, Wales by contrast sought to strengthen the existing Mental Health Act (1983) by introducing a number of measures to assist individuals in the receipt of services and involved in recovery programmes following contact with services. There is a strong understanding that mental health services should mean more than simply identifying and treating conditions, but should also help people to resume their normal social, domestic and occupational lives. The Mental Health (Wales) Measure (2010) drew on evidence that advocacy could lead to an improved experience for the service user by providing independent support for decision making around appropriate interventions, engagement with services and desired outcomes. The measure has been focused both at the macro policy level inhabited by planners and service managers and at the micro level where individuals are concerned about their daily lives, housing, benefits and ongoing support. Closer collaboration between primary and secondary services, health boards and local authorities is suggested, with GP services at the centre.

The measure also adopted an admirably realistic approach to its implementation by being phased in gradually during 2012 so as not to over-burden those with responsibility for overseeing it. The rationale for this was to address criticism of the kind of multiple level reorganisation that education and health have been required to engage in during recent years. The measure has four aims:

1. To assess and treat a person's mental health within primary care across all of Wales.
2. To create statutory requirements around treatment planning and care coordination for people in secondary services.
3. To ensure that secondary mental health services can provide a timely assessment for previous service users.
4. To ensure that all patients receiving care and treatment, be they detained under the act or not, have access to an independent and specialist mental health advocacy service.

Scottish mental health policy considers culture and values as central to the improvement and maintenance of good quality mental health care (Rights, Relationships and Recovery, 2011). Policy aims to ensure that recovery from mental illness goes hand in hand with social inclusion and citizenship. Services should endeavour as far as possible to provide support without resorting to the use of compulsory powers. At the micro level, carers who provide support on an informal basis should receive appropriate information and advice and have their views and needs taken into account. Mental health nurses are seen as fundamental to the development of therapeutic relationships with service users, families and carers, and to ensuring that the cultural change which is needed at every level of health care is brought about.

In order to enable mental health nurses to play the part for which their role equips them so well, training and education in values-based practice should be a feature of all pre-registration programmes, and all nurses – regardless of status – should have access to post-basic training. Training should be multidisciplinary and involve service users and carers. Nurses are encouraged to have *personal development plans* and to access good quality clinical supervision, as the evidence suggests that these give rise to a higher quality of care giving.

REFLECTIONS ON MENTAL HEALTH POLICY

The history of modern mental health policy is closely allied to the history of mental health nursing. Without the contribution of nurses, little of any substance would have been achieved in mental health services. Treatments have in the past been delivered by nurses and, to a large extent, continue to be so. The Munich Declaration (WHO, 2000) recommends that nurses be central to mental health services because they are in a position to tackle public health challenges and are manifestly cost effective. The WHO (2003a) singled out mental health nurses as primary agents in combating psychiatric morbidity and the impact of stigma. However, the potential of nursing remains limited owing to its subordinate relationship to medicine, a relationship that is sometimes enshrined in law, and frequently described in protocols and procedures. Other factors constraining nurses include limited time for face-to-face-contact with service users and their carers, increasing administrative demands, a lack of quality training courses, and decreasing opportunities for career advancement.

In recent years, mental health policy has directed mental health services and shaped the content of what is being delivered. The quality of some services has improved, but high quality care is not consistent across the country, and access to services is inequitable. It would be foolhardy to conclude that policy has achieved all that it set out to do. As Webster (1998) remarked, only about a third of all policy is implemented in the way intended, and some is never considered for implementation. Policy has consistently failed to acknowledge that mental health problems are far more complex than diagnostics, research and therapeutics would imply. Burnside (2010) is critical of the simplistic approach adopted by policy makers and points to the deep spiritual malaise that underlies the country's mental health problems. We live in an age of anxiety in which many people feel trapped in a meaningless existence and are intellectually, culturally and spiritually paralysed. Porritt (2005) talks of a time of cognitive dissonance when it is difficult to understand how to achieve objectives for people who have multiple and conflicting interests. There are limits to economic growth, and limits to human resources, and neither government nor individuals may be the free agents they would like to think themselves to be.

There is also growing distrust of large-scale institutions such as churches, banks, schools, universities and healthcare organisations which are seen to promise more than they are capable of delivering. The post-modern world invites people to be critical of public services, and to make themselves the final arbiters of the quality of services (Seldon, 2009). They are persuaded that how they live and behave is a matter of individual choice. It is not surprising, therefore, that in such an ethical and social climate there is little enthusiasm for the democratic process, for undertaking civic duties, and assuming responsibility for one's own health and that of others (McKnight, 1995).

In comparison to what has been achieved in cancer and cardiovascular care and infectious diseases, mental health care has been far less successful. Many policies verge on the utopian and in reality amount to little more than 'window dressing' (Burnside, 2010). Adopting a policy-first approach as a means of transforming services fails to take account of the political, economic and social differences that exist nationwide, many of which are the direct causes of social and health inequalities (Marmot, 2005; Dowding, 2008). Without an understanding of, and willingness to address, the social determinants of poor health, mental health policy cannot lead to effective action (Lewis, 2008).

Starfield and Shi (2002) found little evidence that the quality of health care was linked to policy. They concluded that the most significant factors affecting the health status of a population were the structure, location and delivery of health services. In short, people's perceptions of health services were dependent on where services were located and the types of people who worked in them. Countries which have achieved overall good levels of health enjoy an equitable distribution of resources, public financial accountability and comprehensive family-orientated services. In the UK policy makers have failed to take into account the context in which their policies must be implemented (Chinitz, 2006). Out-of-date practices and entrenched organisational cultures stifle policies. Policies are frequently poorly explained to health-care professionals working in clinical practice, and too few opportunities are provided for them to participate in health improvement plans. Without an enlightened and motivated workforce that can initiate and sustain change, it will not be possible to achieve quality health outcomes with limited resources.

Else (2011) contends that too many policies focus on individuals and are simplistic. The origins of mental health problems are to be found not in individuals, but in the social environments in which people live – the gap that exists between the rich and the poor which affects life expectancy, levels of crime and violence, and the prevalence of mental illness. Being trapped in poverty exacerbates the emotional pain and isolation associated with divorce, ill health and unemployment.

This viewpoint is supported by Stuckler et al. (2009) who state that conditions in workplaces are not generally supportive of people with mental health problems. Many feel obliged to keep their mental illness hidden from their employers and colleagues for fear of being ridiculed or sacked (Shaw Trust, 2010). Fifty per cent of managers in the Shaw Trust study revealed that they would not employ a person with mental health problems for fear of how other employees might respond, yet the report also revealed that some industries, most notably supermarkets, found that employees with mental health problems were more reliable, enthusiastic, better able to communicate with the public, and less prone to time-wasting and absenteeism than other staff.

There is much assistance that can be given to people to help them safeguard their own wellbeing, such as providing facilities and encouragement for them to be physically active, engage in lifelong learning, and volunteer in their local communities so as to connect with family and neighbours (The Foresight Project, 2009). Much may been learned from the voluntary sector about how people can look after themselves if adequately supported and given information in a form they can understand and utilise (Goddard, 2001). By contrast, mental health services remain wedded to the diagnosis and treatment of severe forms of mental illness, such as the psychoses and major affective disorders, at the expense of developing services that can educate people, enable self-help and promote individual responsibility. Mental illness remains a taboo subject and people with mental health problems still feel marginalised and discriminated against. There are too few opportunities for them to attain a better future outside the health-care arena. Failing to acknowledge and confront prejudice renders governments complicit in its persistence. Frequent changes of government, short-termism, the fact the health departments are spending ministries rather than wealth-creation ones, and that not all government departments have understood the importance of mental health in the way suggested in various White Papers (DH, 2011) are further obstacles to effective policy implementation. Changing public attitudes is a slow process, but striving to create a culture in which mental health is accepted as everybody's responsibility must nonetheless be the aim.

Reflective Exercises

1. Can you identify any contemporary social or political influences upon mental health policy in the UK today?
2. To what degree do you think that any institutional response to individual issues is out of step with a society based upon the needs and rights of individuals?
3. If mental health services truly had their 'Francis moment' years ago with the worst excesses of institutional care, then what are the protective factors to ensure safe and effective services now?
4. What do you consider will drive change in the future? Will it be economic factors or the promise of treatment breakthroughs driven by emerging science?

BIBLIOGRAPHY

Andersen, R., Grabb, E., & Curtis, J. (2006) Trends in civic association activity in four democracies: the special case of women in the United States, *American Sociological Review,* 71: 376–400.

Andrews, B. (2001) *Political Machines: Governing a Technological Society*. London and New York: Athlone.

Barker, P. (1989) Reflections on the philosophy of caring in mental health, *International Journal of Nursing Studies,* 26(2): 131–141.

Burnside, J. (2010) A healthy nudge? No, shock us to our souls, *The Guardian*, 1 December.

Busfield, J. (1986) *Managing Madness: Changing Ideas and Practice*. London: Hutchinson.

Capaldi, N. (2004) *John Stuart Mill: A Biography*. Cambridge: Cambridge University Press.

Carpenter, M. (2000) 'It's a small world': mental health policy under welfare capitalism since 1945, *Sociology of Health and Illness*, 22(5): 602–620.

Chinitz, D. (2006) *Realistic Entrepreneurialism in Healthcare, Hospital Healthcare Europe 2006/7*. London: Camden.

Clare, A. (1976) *Psychiatry in Dissent*. London: Tavistock.

Department of Health (1990) *Caring for People: The Care Programme Approach for People with a Mental Illness Referred to Specialist Mental Health Services* (Joint Health/Social Services Circular, C(90)23/LASSL(90)11). London: DH.

Department of Health (1998a) *Our Healthier Nation*. London: HMSO.

Department of Health (1998b) *Modernising Mental Health Services: Safe, Sound and Supportive*. London: HMSO.

Department of Health (1999) *National Service Framework for Mental Health: Modern Standards and Service Models*. London: HMSO.

Department of Health (2000) *The NHS Plan: A Plan for Investment, A Plan for Reform, cmd. 4818-1*. London: HMSO.

Department of Health (2011) *No Health Without Mental Health*. London: DH.

DHSS (1975) *Better Services for the Mentally Ill*. London: DHSS.

Dixon, A. (2011) What other regulators can teach Monitor, *New Statesman*, 15 December, pp. 14–15.

Dowding, K. (2008) Model or metaphor? A critical review of the policy network approach, *Political Studies*, 43, Issue Supplement 1: 136–158.

Else, L. (2011) The happiness agenda, *New Scientist*, 16 April, pp. 46–47.

Farmer, A. & Stiles, A. (2007) *Bismarck's Domestic Policy 1871–90: The Unification of Germany 1815–1919*, 3rd edition. London: Hodder Education. pp. 114–124.

Finch, J. & Groves, D. (1980) Community care and the family: a case for equal opportunities, *Journal of Social Policy*, 9: 4.

Foresight Project on Mental Capital and Wellbeing (2009) *Mental Capital and Wellbeing: Making the Most of Ourselves in the 21st Century – Final Project Report*. London: Government Office for Science.

Goddard, M. (2001) Equity of access to health care services: theory and evidence from the UK, *Social Science & Medicine*, 53: 1149–1162.

Goodwin, I., Holmes, G., Newnes, C. & Waltho, D. (1999) A qualitative analysis of the view of in-patient mental health service users, *Journal of Mental Health*, 8: 43–54.

Grayling, A.C. (2006) *The Heart of Things: Applying Philosophy to the 21st Century*. London: Phoenix.

Greenhalgh, T., Wong, G., Westhorp, G. & Pawson, R. (2011) Protocol – realist and meta-narrative evidence synthesis: evolving Standards (RAMESES), BioMed Central Medical Research Methodology (www.biomedcentral.com/1471-2288/11/115) (last accessed August 2012).

Hall, P. (1992) The current literature – Worcester Development Project, *British Journal of Psychiatry,* 160: 871–872.

Harrison, T. & Clarke, D. (1992) 'The Northfield experiments', *British Journal of Psychiatry,* 160: 698–708.

HMSO (1926) *Royal Commission Report on Lunacy and Mental Disorder.* London: HMSO.

Johnstone, L. (1992) *Users and Abusers of Psychiatry.* London: Routledge.

Knapp, M., McDaid, D., Mossialos, E. & Thornicroft, G. (2007) *Mental Health Policy and Practice Across Europe.* Milton Keynes: Open University Press.

Koffman, J. & Fulop, N. (1999) Homelessness and the use of acute psychiatric beds, *Health and Social Care in the Community,* 7: 140–147.

Lewis, J. (2008) *Cultural Studies,* 2nd edition. London: Sage.

Malcolm, N. (2002) *Aspects of Hobbes.* New York: Oxford University Press.

Marmot, M. (2005) Social determinants of health inequalities, *The Lancet,* 365 (9464): 1099–1104.

Martin, J.P. (1984) *Hospitals in Trouble.* Oxford: Blackwell.

McCool, D. (1995) *Public Policy Theories, Models, and Concepts: An Anthology.* Englewood Cliffs, NJ: Prentice-Hall.

McKnight, J. (1995) *The Careless Society.* New York: Basic.

McLellan, D. (2006) *Karl Marx: A Biography,* 4th edition. London: Palgrave Macmillan.

McLeroy, K., Bibeau, D., Steckler, A. & Glanz, K. (1988) An ecological perspective on health promotion programs, *Health Education and Behaviour,* 15: 351–377.

Mental Health (Wales) Measure (2010), Welsh Assembly Government (www.cymru.gov.uk) (last accessed September 2010).

MIND (2008) *Mental Health in Parliament,* www.mind.org.uk/assets/10000/0105/m (last accessed June, 2012).

Newton, J. (1988) *Preventing Mental Illness.* London: Routledge.

Osbourne, T. (2008) *The Structure of Modern Cultural Theory.* Manchester: Manchester University Press.

Penhale, B. & Parker, J. (2007) *Working with Vulnerable Adults.* London: Routledge.

Pilgrim, D. & Rogers, A. (2001) *Mental Health Policy.* London: Palgrave.

Porritt, J. (2005) *Capitalism, as if the World Matters.* London: Earthscan.

Porter, R. (1987) *Mind-Forg'd Manacles.* London: Athlone.

Powell, J.E. (1961) Speech by the Minister of Health. London: Report of the Annual Conference of the Association for Mental Health.

Priorities for Action (2010) *Patient and Client Council – Your Voice in Health and Social Care – Report on Public Engagement, Department of Health, Social Services and Public Safety in Northern Ireland* (www.patientclientcouncil.hscni.net/bamford-monitoring-group) (last accessed September 2012).

Propper, C. (2011) The price of competition, *New Statesman,* 15 December, pp. 11–13.

Rayner, H. (1884) Presidential Address to the Medico-Psychological Association, *Journal of Mental Science,* 30: 352.

Rights, Relationships and Recovery (2011) *The Report of the National Review of Mental Health Nursing,* www.scotland.gov.uk/Topics/Health/health/mental/RRRmentalhealth (last accessed September 2012).

Seldon, A. (2009) *The Question of Trust at the Heart of Politics.* London: Biteback.

Shorter, E. (1997) *A History of Psychiatry: From the Era of the Asylum to the Age of Prozac*. New York and London: Wiley.

Simpson, A., Miller, C. & Bowers, L. (2003) The history of the Care Programme Approach in England: Where did it go wrong?, *Journal of Mental Health Care*, 12(5): 489–504.

Starfield, B. & Shi, L. (2002) Policy relevant determinants of health: an international perspective, *Health Policy*, 60: 201–218.

Stuckler, D., Basu, S., Suhrcke, M., Coutts, A. & McKee, M. (2009) The public health effect of economic crises and alternative policy responses in Europe: an empirical analysis, *The Lancet*, 374 (9686): 315–323.

Sullivan, M. (1987) *Sociology and Social Welfare*. London: Allen and Unwin.

Thaler, R. & Sunstein, C. (2009) *Nudge: Improving Decisions about Health, Wealth and Happiness*. London and New York: Yale University Press.

The Shaw Trust Report (2010) *Mental Health: Still the Last Workplace Taboo*. London: The Shaw Trust. (Accessed at www.shaw-trust.org.uk)

Webster, C. (1998) *The National Health Service: A Political History*. Oxford: Oxford University Press.

Weiss, C. (1995) 'Nothing as practical as a good theory: exploring theory-based evaluation for comprehensive community initiatives for children and families'. In J. Connell (ed.), *Evaluating Community Initiatives: Concepts, Methods, and Contexts*. Washington, DC: Aspen Institute.

World Health Organization (2000) *Munich Declaration: Nurses and Midwives: A Force for Health*. Geneva: WHO.

World Health Organization (2003a) *WHO Europe Mental Health Nursing Curriculum: WHO European Strategy for Continuing Education for Nurses and Midwives*. Copenhagen: WHO.

World Health Organization (2003b) Quality Improvement for Mental Health. www.who.int/mental_health/resources/en/Quality.pdf. (last accessed 16 April 2011).

World Health Organization (2005) *Report on the European Ministerial Conference on Mental Health*. Helsinki: WHO.

World Health Organization (2010) *Mental Health: Strengthening Our Response. Fact sheet N°220*. www.who.int/mediacentre/factsheets/fs220/en/ (last accessed 10 April 2012).

2 THE EUROPEAN CONTEXT

Neil Brimblecombe

Chapter Overview

Whilst it is an oft-quoted quip that 'Europe begins at Calais', this chapter should disabuse the reader of any such notion. The author has placed mental health nursing squarely in a European context and draws your attention to the differences and common features across the continent of Europe. He helpfully describes not only the variance but also the factors that may drive and explain the differences observed.

However, there is much in common as the majority of interventions herald the successful transfer and growth of a predominantly bio-medical model of causation and treatment for mental disorders/illness. It is within that context of the dominance of psychiatry that the mental health nurses of Europe practise. You will note that there are areas of Europe where the nurses are educated in a generic manner and where also any specialisation in the area of mental health will predominantly occur after initial registration. The UK remains one of only a few European countries where there is a specific registration/qualification offered to practice as a mental health nurse.

Similarly there is a wide range of ways that mental health nursing is practised in relation to issues such as autonomy and development of the role to include the adoption and integration of practices such as psychological therapies and the independent prescribing of medication.

INTRODUCTION

This chapter provides an overview of the development of policy and services across Europe. Its purpose is not only to place UK policy and practice in a context but also to illustrate how different services are across Europe. The impact of policy is described on nursing, for example in terms of the status and range of nursing roles, interprofessional relationships and the nature of the services which nurses may work in. The clinical work of nurses is especially affected by legal frameworks used in inpatient care, for example in terms of the use of tranquilisation and mechanical restraint. Differences in approach to education are also described.

The European Union today

The population of the European Union (EU), encompassing 28 countries, is currently over 500 million. Population density varies widely, for example, ranging from 16 people per square kilometre in Finland to 393 in Holland. Within the EU are found many languages and ethnicities, including significant populations of recent immigrants from Africa, Asia and South America. Commonality is found in the fact that all EU countries are governed by democratic processes, although the detail of political structures does vary, including constitutional monarchies and republics, and highly centralised and federalised states. The population size of countries in the EU ranges from just 417,000 in Malta to Germany with over 81 million (Europa, 2012).

Nursing is by far the largest profession working in mental health services across Europe, and approximately half a million people are employed in the EU alone (WHO, 2011). Nursing has played a major role in the development of mental health services in most European countries, particularly during the asylum period and also during the transition to community care, and continues to do so (Brimblecombe & Nolan, 2012). The work of nurses in mental health services is affected by a whole range of national policies, concerning the role of nursing specifically, the type and character of the organisations that actually provide health care, the availability of funding to employ nurses, and prioritisation as to which types of services and which health interventions are actually provided.

Mental health need

Trying to identify the level and nature of mental health need in a particular country, or across Europe, is a challenge. There are issues concerning

- the availability of data;
- the reliability and comparability of that data;
- the 'meaning of data', i.e. how these should be interpreted.

Nevertheless, conclusions have been drawn that suggest very high levels of need. The World Health Organization suggests that mental health disorders are among the ten most common health conditions in all EU countries, typically ranking first or second (WHO Regional Office for Europe, 2005). Such disorders also make up by far the largest single category of chronic conditions affecting the population, accounting for 39.7% of the total burden (WHO, 2008).

Although there are wide variations in the extent of mental health services across different countries in Europe (see below), all of these ultimately have the similar challenge of an imbalance between the estimated needs of people with mental health problems and the availability of services to meet them. Even in countries with well-developed mental health systems, it is estimated that over 90% of people suffering alcohol abuse and dependence receive no effective treatment, and nor do around 60% of those with anxiety disorders, almost 50% of those with panic disorders, 45% of those with major depression, 40% of those with bipolar affective disorder, 25% of those with obsessive compulsive disorder, and 18% of those with schizophrenia and non-affective psychosis (Kohn et al., 2004). In reality, the inevitably limited availability of mental health services is responsible for only part of the treatment gap, as even when services are available many of those who suffer from mental health problems will avoid or delay treatment and choose not to engage or maintain contact with mental health services and adhere to treatment.

It is also apparent that the extensiveness or otherwise of mental health services does not always correlate with clinical outcomes. For example, Greece has a relatively low expenditure on mental health services, yet has one of the lowest suicide rates in Europe (cultural and social factors presumably being more important than service structures). There is a general lack of evidence to demonstrate that those states which spend more on mental health have a mentally healthier population, although this may simply be a consequence of the impossibility of controlling for other factors.

It is also important to note the criticisms that exist of the very high estimates for prevalence of mental health problems within various societies. Doubts have been raised that such calculations reflect a medicalisation of the normal range of human experience and the confusion of common unhappiness with pathological conditions. It is alleged that data concerning the prevalence of mental health problems are often exaggerated and the methodologies deployed in gathering these lack rigour (Wootton, 2007), as well as suggesting that high rates for mental health problems may be due to the diagnostic practices deployed (Richter et al., 2008).

However, if such high figures are accepted as, at least, rough reflections of a reality and that all such cases needed treatment, then the implications would make the design and provision of services simply impossible, in terms of the sheer size, cost and manpower. If only 10% of people with alcohol problems currently receive effective treatment for alcohol problems (Kohn et al., 2004), then does this suggest that we need ten times the volume of capacity to treat alcohol problems in the future? Such figures are clearly alarming when taken to their logical conclusion. The nature and use of data are important factors in attempting to understand the development of mental health policies across Europe and in individual countries. Figures that show high levels of need can be helpful politically in providing a lever to apply pressure on governments to better fund mental health services.

Mental health problems certainly create a significant financial burden for countries. Data from countries where information is available show that mental health problems account for as much as 44.4% of social welfare benefits or disability pensions in Denmark, 43% in Finland and in Scotland, and 37% in Romania. Even in Moldova, one of Europe's poorest countries, mental disabilities account for 25% of all social welfare benefits or disability pensions afforded by the government (Petrea, 2012).

Funding

The most common means of funding for mental health services across Europe are

- *central taxation* – being the predominant form in the United Kingdom;
- *compulsory employee healthcare insurance* – either payable to the government or to insurance companies, as in Germany, Holland and Luxembourg;
- *voluntary healthcare insurance* – an important addition to central national funding in Ireland, and part of a range of payment sources in Greece;
- *direct patient payments* – found as a 'top up' for specific services in many countries: for example prescription charges in England, payment for visits to general practitioners in Ireland, and a fixed charge for examinations and treatment in the Czech Republic.

Undoubtedly, the commonest picture is one of a mixture of funding sources. In many countries, individuals who are unable to work have access to health care.

The amount spent on mental health services in any country depends on a number of factors (Brimblecombe & Nolan, 2012), including

- the economic strength of a country;
- the political attitude to public spending;
- the relative priority given to different aspects of health.

Undoubtedly, the recent and continuing economic downturn in Europe has affected the ability to deliver pre-existing health policies. Even in Germany, which has made a major economic recovery, the level of spending on public health services has been affected. In the UK, social care services have been cut in many areas and health spending is severely constrained. In Ireland, cuts have led to an embargo on recruitment across the public sector including health services; public sector salary reductions of up to 30% along with an increase in pension payments; and an extensive programme of early retirement from the public sector with the majority exiting from health services, as well as a reduction in student numbers.

There are major differences across Europe about the amount spent on health, which tends to correlate with the wealth of countries. However, differences between countries in relation to their policies on and attitudes towards mental health are more sharply illustrated by examining the *proportion* of total health spend that goes on mental health (although caution is required as to the accuracy of these estimates). The range of spending goes from 2% in Bulgaria up to 13% in parts of the United Kingdom (Petrea & Muijen, 2008). Mental health spend in Ireland, although above the European average, is now markedly less than is the case in the United Kingdom, having reduced in real terms from 13% of the health budget in 1986 to 5.4% in 2010. The median percentage of health spend applied to mental health in Europe is actually only 5% (WHO, 2011).

History

In order to understand current policy it is important to understand the historical context in which it has developed. The generally held view is that mental health services across Europe have followed a common developmental pathway, with the establishment of large institutions in the nineteenth and early twentieth century, and towards the end of the twentieth century these being gradually replaced, at least theoretically, by community-based services (Priebe, 2006). When trying to compare the historical development of mental health services in detail across countries, an undoubted challenge is the variability in quality and availability of secondary source material (Gijswift-Hoftra & Oosterhuis, 2005), however the picture that does emerge from national histories is remarkably consistent in general features, although greatly variable in terms of exact timing and local circumstance (Brimblecombe & Nolan, 2012).

Asylums, providing institutionally-based care for the mentally ill, were developed in the majority of European countries in the nineteenth century (Brimblecombe & Nolan, 2012), with only a few exceptions, such as in Hungary (Shorter, 2007). In some countries, specific institutions for the mentally ill or 'insane' were available prior to that date: for example, in Portugal there were specialised wards for 'patients who lost their minds' in the sixteenth century; in Finland institutions specifically for the purpose of housing the mentally ill were available from the late eighteenth century; and the Bethlem Hospital ('Bedlam') in London had admitted the insane from the fourteenth century. The church certainly played a major role in many countries, with monastic orders providing care framed within a religious understanding of mental illness.

There is also evidence from some countries of early attempts to encourage the care of the mentally ill by families and community. In Ireland, the Brehon Laws originated in pre-Christian Ireland and continued until the Elizabethan period. These attempted to ensure the provision of care for the insane person by their family or the community, featuring various penalties for failing to care for the insane person. However, most commonly – prior to the establishment of specific asylums for the mentally ill – the mentally ill would be likely to wander the country or be contained in other institutions, such as, for example, in prisons or workhouses

The policies leading to the near universal growth of asylums in the nineteenth century seem to relate to a number of factors, including

- the growth of central power in nation states;
- the wish for such states to typically both better control and better care for their populations;
- evidence produced at the time that seemed to demonstrate the beneficial effects of compassionate care in asylums;
- the strengthening of the medical profession and its attempt to take authority over the field of mental illness, which was best done in the controlled environment of the asylum.

Once established, the number of beds in institutions typically rose well beyond initial expectations, limiting the asylums' ability to provide therapeutic care and consequently ending up with the warehousing of large numbers of people. The latter reframing of asylums as 'hospitals' and the further emphasising of the medical nature of mental illness did little to improve conditions, treatment or outcome, with the exception of such demonstrably biologically-based illnesses as General Paralysis of the Insane, caused by syphilis.

Changes towards a more community-focused approach to care have been linked with a post-war public rejection of institutional care, with mounting evidence of the potentially harmful effects of such care (e.g. Barton, 1959; Goffman, 1961) and following numerous public exposures of poor and abusive practice in asylums. An important facilitator of change was the introduction of antipsychotic medication from the mid-1950s onward, enabling people with psychosis to be managed and cared for in less restrictive environments However, it does seem likely that this effect has been overstated, as in some countries, such as the United Kingdom, significant bed reductions had taken place prior to the common use of chlorpromazine.

The exact point at which there was a policy shift towards providing more community-focused care varied across Europe. In Portugal it was not until the end of 1970 that an attempt was made to regionalise and decentralise mental health services so that a greater emphasis was given to the creation of community-based support structures. Similarly, in Germany it took until the mid-1970s for the psychiatric landscape to change, when in a general climate of social and political reform the country turned towards community-based mental health care. The high point for bed numbers in both Ireland and Finland was reached in the 1970s. These were in contrast to England when bed occupancy was at its highest in the mid-1950s.

Finnane (2009: 6) rightly points out that 'More than other modern medical institutions, mental hospitals labour under the burdens of their histories'. The stigma associated with mental illness undoubtedly remains strong across Europe. For example, in Luxembourg the modern psychiatric hospital is reported as still being closely associated with the Ettelbruck asylum, seen by the population as 'a dark place to which mad people are sent for lengthy periods of time' (Besenius, 2012). Stigma remains one of the greatest obstacles in all countries to improving community care facilities and continues to be a priority if mental health improvement is to become a reality.

Political commitment to mental health care

Undoubtedly the last twenty-five years have seen much greater attention placed on mental health by governments in Europe (Petrea, 2012), at least in terms of their public pronouncements. European governments have stated that they recognise the size and complexity of the challenges produced by mental ill health and have publicly committed themselves to protecting the rights of people with mental health problems, tackling discrimination against mental health service users, and ensuring 'appropriate' treatment and care. Typically, broad commitments have been made by countries as member states of the United Nations (UN), the World Health Organization (a specialised agency of the UN), the Council of Europe, and the European Commission (EC).

The United Nations

European states have signed up to a range of United Nations' documents which refer specifically to people with mental health problems. The 1991 *Resolution on the Principles for the Protection of Persons with Mental Illness and the Improvement of Mental Health Care* remains a reference document for national mental health legislation (United Nations, 1991). This identifies rights to which service users are entitled, including the right to access mental health facilities equivalent to the access provided to any other health facility for any other illness, the right to treatment and care that meet the same standards as for people with other illnesses, and the right of persons admitted to mental health facilities to the same level of resources as in any other health establishment.

The 1993 *UN Standard Rules on the Equalization of Opportunities for Persons with Disabilities* (United Nations, 1993) required governments to guarantee persons with disabilities (including mental disabilities) the same level of medical care within the same system as other members of society, and to develop national programmes for all groups of persons with disabilities based on the actual needs of the persons with disabilities and on the principle of full participation and equality.

For people with mental health problems, probably the single most important UN document remains the *Convention on the Rights of Persons with Disabilities* (United Nations General Assembly, 2007). The convention lays out the legal obligations of states to promote and protect the rights of persons with disabilities, including those with mental health problems. The 2006 convention conceptualises people with disabilities as 'subjects' with rights who are entitled to 'physical and mental integrity on an equal basis with others' (Article 17), and are capable of making decisions for their lives based on their free and informed consent. They are no longer to be viewed merely as objects of charity, medical treatment or social protection. The convention also reiterates disabled people's civil rights, such as the freedom to choose a place of residence, and rights to personal mobility, to property, to enter into contracts, to manage one's own financial affairs, to marry, work and retain custody of one's children, and to participate in political and public life. It prohibits discrimination against people with disabilities in health insurance, employment and education, and requires member states to prevent discriminatory practices in the delivery of health care.

In 2001, the WHO published the World Health Report, entitled 'Mental Health: New Understanding, New Hope'. Member states were urged to improve care for people with mental health problems. Importantly, the report emphasised that 'Effective solutions for mental disorders are available' (WHO, 2001:109) and reiterated that governments were as responsible for the mental health as for the physical health of their citizens and should ensure that mental health policies were developed and implemented. The report called for member countries to provide universal access to appropriate and cost-effective services for people with mental health problems, the provision of adequate care for service users, and the protection of human rights for people with mental health problems. In all it included ten recommendations for member states that asked them to do the following:

1. Provide treatment in primary care.
2. Make psychotropic drugs available.
3. Give care in the community.
4. Educate the public.
5. Involve communities, families and consumers.
6. Establish national policies, programmes and legislation.
7. Develop human resources.
8. Link with other sectors.
9. Monitor community mental health.
10. Support more research.

By adopting the report governments committed themselves to implementing its recommendations, but significantly, each country's approach was to be tailored to the resources available in that particular state.

European-wide initiatives

Global initiatives by the WHO and UN strongly influenced work subsequently carried out in regions around the world. In Europe two important policy documents were developed, namely the Mental Health Declaration and the Action Plan for Europe (WHO Regional Office for Europe, 2005). Both documents were subsequently endorsed by European health ministers in January 2005, at the first European Ministerial Conference on Mental Health, held in Finland.

The Helsinki Agreement (WHO, 2005) stated the commitment of all EU member states to improve mental health care and echoed many of the recommendations from earlier reports. It recognised the need for comprehensive, evidence-based mental health policies and sustainable means of implementing them. A number of priority areas were identified:

- Promoting individual and societal mental wellbeing.
- Tackling stigma, discrimination and social exclusion.
- Preventing the causes of mental health problems.
- Providing comprehensive and effective interventions for people with mental health problems whilst offering involvement and choice.
- Rehabilitating and including in society people who had experienced serious mental health problems.

As with previous policy statements, the Helsinki Agreement aimed to improve the general mental health and wellbeing of individuals, families and local communities.

Mental health services should aim to enhance the wellbeing of people, build up their resourcefulness and resilience, and enable them to enjoy a meaningful and productive life (WHO, 2005). The Ministerial Conference was, at least theoretically, a major breakthrough in terms of a public commitment from all EU countries, both to prioritising mental health and adopting policies that were not solely and narrowly focused on the treatment of established mental illness. Priebe (2006) comments that, although ultimately the work of the conference may not be seen as seminal, it does illustrate important challenges to mental healthcare at the beginning of this century and highlights key issues that might change the direction in the future.

Role of different bodies

Petrea (2012) points out that the impact at a national level of these various declarations by international organisations depends on those organisations' status and mandate, political influence and financial power. The United Nations and its specialised health agency (i.e. the World Health Organization) are intergovernmental membership organisations aiming to promote cooperation between countries. Legally binding international agreements relevant to mental health have been adopted in the framework of the United Nations and the UN conventions have certainly been influential, particularly in the area of disability.

The WHO focuses on health-related policies, while the EC concentrates on its established areas of competence (namely types of services, key personnel and effective treatments). The World Health Organization's role is to support member states in all areas of health, including mental health, and in particular by bringing countries together to address critical health issues. In fact, the WHO was relatively uninvolved with respect to mental health until near the end of the last century (Petrea, 2012) and the European Commission was also not very active in this area until the late 1990s. Current EC mental health policy documents remain at the level of consultation papers or loose agreements, with no binding commitments from the EU member states (Petrea & Muijen, 2008). Despite these limitations, the EC can still influence policy making in mental health and support changes in countries (and has indeed done so in some cases).

Even though EC mental health policies indicate directions of travel and what the aims of good mental health services should be, no prescription is provided as to which structures and services would ensure their implementation, and neither is there any mention of how services should be measured, monitored or reviewed. The interpretation and implementation of policies are largely left to the discretion of each member country, utilising and revising their existing systems and structures as they see fit (Lavikainen et al., 2000). On endorsing international policies, all countries are then expected to reflect on how these will impact on their own national policies.

National policies

The development of national policies is influenced by both internal and external political factors. International organisations, such as the WHO, do provide technical support to the process of drafting national policies, building on international declarations of support such as the Helsinki Agreement. Typically, countries with more complex and better funded health-care systems are those that most actively promote and develop (and deliver) internationally supported policies.

Countries with less 'advanced' policies and practices (i.e. typically those with low levels of resources largely invested in institutional care) do also endorse these international policies, although in practice policies are not always the real drivers of change in these countries and are also not always real indicators of a genuine willingness to induce change. A number of factors create this situation. International pressure can be strong, and professing support for initiatives makes for good public relations. Governments can use the adoption of these policies as a way of, at least temporarily, satisfying strong local requests for action from national champions, even if they have no real intent to implement planned actions. Internationally, the adoption of legislation that complies with international requirements brings about financial support in the form of international funding for these countries, as well as political support and acceptance amongst powerful countries. Even where the motives of politicians are noble, where policies are not rooted in local processes they consequently do not have sufficient ownership from key stakeholders and decision makers.

Petrea (2012) describes the typical characteristics of policy development in countries where they have only recently started to move from a historically institutional focus. In this situation, national mental health policies and legislation are often developed using international policies and recommendations as a guide. Political commitment may also be prompted by international pressure due to reports of human rights violations. The subsequent laws and policies often set ambitious goals and cover a wide range of areas, from mental health promotion to deinstitutionalisation and human rights – however, they often lack specific targets to be achieved within a determined time-frame, the means by which any progress towards these targets will be measured, clearly established funding mechanisms, and funding sources for the implementation of policy and achievement targets. Thus what is created is aspirational rather than achievable.

It is notable that, even in Western Europe, there are many countries where the development of national mental health strategies and policies has simply not delivered what was promised (Sheridan, 2012). Machiavelli rightly pointed out, several centuries ago, that drawing up laws and policies without having the means of enforcing them is futile (Fischer, 2000). For example, Santos et al. (2012) comment that 'Portugal considers the production of policies, guidelines and directives to be important, but, by themselves they are insufficient'. Schulz (2012) takes a more forgiving view when commenting on the slow progress made in Germany to creating change: '... progress in German mental health services is slow and deliberate and perhaps attempting to speed up the process might result in confusion and failure'.

Beyond giving at least lip-service to the principles laid out in international policies, such as the Helsinki Agreement and other WHO-influenced policies, there are numerous other factors that can influence an individual country's approach to how it tackles the principles for mental health policy (see Box 2.1).

> **Box 2.1   Factors potentially influencing mental health policy**
>
> | Population factors | e.g. size, age, ethnicity, density, accessibility, mental health needs |
> |---|---|
> | Attitudinal/cultural factors | e.g. attitudes towards mental illness, attitudes to state funding |
> | Financial factors | e.g. relative wealth, public spending budgets, availability and cost of health insurance |
> | Political factors | e.g. party political approaches to spending and prioritisation, lobbying power of professions |

Development of national policies

The WHO (2001) reported that, at that time, one third of European countries did not have specific mental health policies, suggesting that policies were a major driver of change and improvement. However, since that time there appears to have been steady growth in policies across Europe: for example, the Czech Republic is currently developing a strategy for dementia after previously totally lacking any central mental health strategy or clear policy (Novotná & Petr, 2012).

The responsibility for the planning of health care lies between national and local governments, with the degree to which the responsibility is divided varying from country to country. As discussed above, the English National Service Framework (DH, 1999) is a good example of centralised planning whereby central government devised a detailed policy and plans that were then expected to be provided locally, with a range of financial and other penalties and incentives to support the required action being taken. Somewhat differently, in Finland the Ministry for Social Affairs and Health administers the overall functioning of health and social care services, but the municipalities are responsible for the local organisation and planning of health services. In federal states, such as Germany, planning typically lies at a state level, potentially leading to variations in the availability of services across a country as a whole.

Are services changing?

Despite evidence that national policies often do not fully deliver what they set out to do, a WHO study monitoring the mental health status in 42 countries – as compared to commitments made in the Helsinki documents – showed that while the quality and provision of mental health care varied greatly across Europe, the vast majority of countries had made significant progress over recent years (Petrea &

Muijen, 2008). However, many countries also reported that services such as crisis care, home treatment, assertive outreach and early intervention were only available to a small proportion of the population. Only Germany, Luxembourg and the United Kingdom (England and Wales) reported that all or almost all people with mental disorders had access to home treatment and early intervention. In eight countries home treatment was unavailable, while eleven countries reported that early intervention services are virtually absent. The United Kingdom (England and Wales) alone reported that all or almost all people with mental disorders had access to assertive outreach. Conversely, sixteen countries reported that they did not provide these services at all (Petrea & Muijen, 2008).

Despite the focus on more community-based services in policy, there is actually some evidence showing that reinstitutionalisation is, in some ways, on the increase (Priebe et al., 2008). This is expressed through, for example, the replacement of large institutions with smaller ones (e.g. health service-managed group homes) and an increased number of forensic beds. Although community care facilities have generally increased, factors such as social support and risk management strategies have played some part in the increase in beds (Priebe et al., 2008).

It is of note here that progress is measured by the WHO and most national governments in terms of the range of services available (i.e. system inputs), rather than the outcomes for people with mental health problems. Certainly the challenge of trying to agree what data would be most meaningful in this context and then being able to gather these is problematic. In England (a country which has invested more than most in mental health, and is typically seen elsewhere in Europe as being 'ahead of the game') it is interesting to note the recent changes in mental health policy, from a heavy focus on *inputs* – namely, the existence of particular services such as crisis resolution and early intervention in psychosis – to one that is more concerned with *outcomes,* and that those outcomes relate to social as well as symptomatic factors (DH, 2011).

A significant issue that mental health policies have not yet resolved in many countries is the uneven distribution of resources. It is apparent that when new resources are committed these often build on existing services and not in locations where the need is greatest. The challenge of a geographical inequity of resources is found in Portugal (Santos et al., 2012) and Greece (Koukia, 2012) where – although all residents are entitled to health services – the availability is often limited in some areas, and especially on the many Greek islands. In the Czech Republic there is also an unbalanced distribution of resources, with inadequacies outside of large cities (Novotná & Petr, 2012).

Most national plans/strategies in the recent past have tended to place the greatest emphasis on planning the move away from large psychiatric hospitals towards general hospitals and on increasing community-based services. Little prominence appears to have been attached to increasing mental health promotion activities or devising methods for preventing mental health problems (WHO, 2005). Even where the need for such action is specifically cited, such as in the *English National Service Framework for Mental Health* (DH, 1999), the reality is that this particular objective has not been realised. This is largely due to the fact that resources would have to be diverted from services that currently provide treatment to those that deliver health promotion – always a challenging prospect politically.

Stigma and policy

Stigma against people with mental health problems remains endemic across Europe (Brimblecombe & Nolan, 2012). This affects both the way that mental health policy is developed and more significantly the way it is delivered. An important consideration in attempting to implement policies that aim at the provision of more care away from institutional settings, in the community, is the willingness or otherwise of the community itself and health and social care professionals, not specifically working in the mental health field, to accept this and share some of the responsibility for, at least tolerating, people with evident mental health problems being in their midst. The Helsinki Declaration recognises the importance of stigma and urges action to fight it (WHO, 2005). Although many countries have localised schemes that fight stigma in a number of ways, national schemes are rarer (Brimblecombe & Nolan, 2012).

Not only does the risk to the development of community-based care come from those who, arguably, may simply be influenced by the weight of historical and cultural stigma, but as Porritt (2005) notes some of the most vociferous opponents of community care are actually mental health professionals who fail to see any therapeutic advantages.

Nurses and mental health care

The WHO has repeatedly highlighted the potential importance of the contribution to be made by nurses in the mental health arena. The Munich Declaration (WHO, 2000) advised that nurses should be central to mental health services because they could tackle public health challenges and were manifestly cost-effective, whilst in 2003 (WHO, 2003) mental health nurses were again characterised as a primary means of combating psychiatric morbidity. Despite this advocacy for nursing, there is great variability in the availability of qualified nursing staff in EU mental health services and in the work they do: Finland, for instance, has approximately 163 nurses per 100,000 population, while in Greece there are only three nurses per 100,000 (Petrea, 2012).

Differences and similarities in nursing

It is clear that policy has resulted in significant differences across Europe in the way that nurses are employed and trained and how they practise in mental health settings. These differences are typically enshrined in law (and hence 'policy'), however, on close examination some appear to be as linked to the local/national health-care culture as specific policy intentions.

Education

Striking differences exist across Europe in terms of approaches to the education of nurses working in mental health services, and in terms of the nature and focus of the training received and the academic level at which it is taught (Nolan & Brimblecombe, 2007). Two basic approaches to obtaining an initial qualification for nurses who work in mental health settings exist. The first has a specialist qualification designed specifically for psychiatric/mental health nurses (which typically does not allow such nurses to work in other specialities) and one which is based on a 'general' training which allows qualified nurses to work across the entire range of health care. The more specialised training is now only found in the UK, Ireland and Malta, although this was formerly more widespread (for example, in Germany). A critique of this model is that such a training can fail to equip nurses with sufficient physical health-care skills to care for people with severe mental health problems and who may suffer from markedly high levels of morbidity (Thornicroft, 2011).

The second and most common approach to training is for nurses to initially qualify as 'general nurses', with an emphasis on physical illnesses and healthcare. The majority of countries who follow this model, including Germany, espouse further post-registration specialist training in mental health if practising in that area. However, in Germany (and other countries) the reality is that the proportion of nurses working in mental health with a postgraduate qualification is low, and is often only achieved after many years spent working in mental health settings (Schulz, 2012). The critique for such less specialised training is that it does not provide sufficient focus on psychological and psychiatric aspects (especially where postgraduate training fails to compensate for this) (Simons et al., 1998).

The academic level for qualifying courses in nursing is predominantly – but not exclusively – at graduate level, for example in Germany and Ireland, and in 2013 this will be mandated in England. However, the relatively recently introduced nature of graduate training means that some countries still have a majority of nurses working with other level qualifications: for example, in the Netherlands 60% of mental health nurses are educated to diploma level and the remaining 40% are prepared to Bachelor's or Master's level (Van de Sande & Hellendoorn, 2012).

Some hospitals in Eastern Europe have taken the initiative of offering training to their staff in priority areas (e.g. violence management, human rights, cognitive behavioural therapy, the identification of mental disorders), utilising either internal or external training modules. However, one of the problems faced by managers in these countries is that returns from staff training are low as the best trained staff members are most likely to emigrate (Petrea, 2012).

Clinical approaches and national 'policy'

There are very little comparative data to understand if there are significant differences in the clinical approach of nurses across Europe. Arguably, if such differences exist then they may do so because of national differences in the clinical view and culture as opposed to the effects of policy. However, policy does influence the shape of services (e.g. in terms of whether specialist teams such as Crisis Resolution or Assertive Outreach exist), and hence may affect the work nurses do.

Another way in which policy appears to affect nursing differentially in different states is in the area of the control and response to disturbed or challenging behaviour in inpatient settings, as differences will typically lie within legal frameworks. Bowers and colleagues have described differences of approach towards disturbed/challenging behaviour in inpatient care areas in the United Kingdom, Italy and Greece (Bowers et al., 2005), and differences certainly also exist as to the legal framework and culture in other countries. For example, 'mechanical restraint' is common in many countries (e.g. Germany) but is very rare in the UK (where it has been considered undesirable since the early 1800s) and Ireland (where the use of mechanical restraint was made illegal by the 1945 Mental Treatment Act). Legalities also limit the use of tranquilising medication in some countries, such as the Netherlands (Van de Sande & Hellendoorn, 2012), more than in others, such as the UK. Conversely, the use of seclusion and the number of seclusion rooms available appear markedly higher in the Netherlands compared to the UK for example. These differences affect the training of nurses and how they would respond to situations on a day-to-day basis.

Nursing roles and inter-professional issues

The combined workings of policy, history, culture and established practice have led to there being differences in the roles and responsibilities of nurses across Europe. Key to understanding this is knowledge of inter-disciplinary relationships within countries and across Europe, particularly between nursing and psychiatry. Many disciplines working in mental health have grown in numbers and academic strength across Europe, and exist in what is normally termed the 'multi-disciplinary team' – however, this is contextualised by the reality of the current power structure. The historical context of this relationship across Europe is that psychiatric nursing was born in a managerially subservient position to the fledgling psychiatric profession in the asylums of the nineteenth century (Brimblecombe, 2005), and while nursing in most countries has increasingly professionalised and is typically a graduate profession, in most countries psychiatrists still define the work that nurses can do with individual patients.

The range of nursing roles and the levels of responsibility attached to them remain significantly limited in many countries, particularly in Central and Eastern Europe (Petrea, 2012): for example, where nurses are not permitted to take on some of the tasks of psychiatrists, tasks which are usually delegated to nurses in countries with 'modern' mental health services (e.g. care coordination, the assessment of patient needs, consultation with other health professionals to establish and provide an individualised care plan, the provision of high-level support to service users and their families).

Petrea (2012) is critical of the fact that nurses working in some areas of Central and Eastern European inpatient units also frequently delegate to auxiliary staff many tasks that in other European countries would be considered core nursing tasks (e.g. carrying out assessments, administering medication, and delivering psycho-educational programmes). The issue of the distribution of tasks between nurses and auxiliary staff is rarely addressed. Such auxiliary staff will rarely have any training in providing care nor experience in nursing people with mental health problems. However, these personnel can be preferred by hospital managers since auxiliary staff cost less than nurses and they are readily available, as they are usually recruited from local communities within the surroundings of mental hospitals. According to Petrea, under these circumstances the quality of nursing care received by service users is uncertain and sometimes substandard.

The reality is that across almost all of Europe, auxiliary staff – known, for example, as nursing assistants or support workers – certainly *do* provide a significant role in providing part of the inpatient nursing workforce. The degree of training for such staff varies from virtually nothing to formal training programmes lasting over a year or more. Finland is rare indeed in having an inpatient nursing workforce that is entirely composed of registered nurses (Ellilä et al., 2012).

It is also certainly not only in countries with institutionally-focused mental health-care systems where severe limitations are placed on the scope of nursing. In Germany the hierarchical relationship is clear: nurses are expected, by law, to carry out the prescribed care of medical staff, even where working in community settings (Schulz, 2012). This situation is a source of frustration to many German nurses but change seems unlikely in the short term.

Policy and practice elsewhere are different. In the United Kingdom psychiatrists are typically the clinical lead for the care in inpatient settings, but nurses must make clinical decisions based on their own view of what is in the patient's best interests and the instructions of a psychiatrist cannot make them act in a way that they believe is not in such interests. Interestingly, a recent change in mental health law in England theoretically allows nurses (following recognition as having the right experience and abilities) to become the lead clinician in multi-disciplinary teams for individual inpatients. It is even more interesting that this opportunity has, as yet, been rarely taken up, suggesting that one hundred and fifty years of tradition are hard to change.

Nurses' role in Finland is also seen as independent and they are responsible for the decisions they make in daily nursing care (Ellilä et al., 2012). In Ireland the position is similar, although with the added complexity that – regardless of the emphasis placed on individual professional accountability – the reality of the authority of psychiatrists is embedded in law, with mental health services being defined in the Mental Health Act (2001) as 'services which provide care and treatment to persons suffering from mental illness or a mental disorder under the clinical direction of a consultant psychiatrist' (Sheridan, 2012).

Extended roles

A further area in which differences in national nursing policy and approach affect is that of extended roles, varying from none at all to a great diversity of such. Some have no national training requirements whereas others have a formal academic pathway. For example, in the Netherlands a two-year Master's degree in advanced nursing practice in mental health care is available. At present, those who have completed this degree (including pharmacotherapy and physical examination) are allowed on the national health care specialist register. The Master's degree allows nurses to undertake specific medical and psychiatric assessments and prescribe medication. However, in reality there are a variety of definitions as to what constitutes the extended roles for those specialist nurses.

In Ireland psychiatric nurses function across a range of diverse practice settings, and in 2011 a total of 568 clinical nurse specialists (CNS) and 20 advanced nurse practitioner (ANP) posts undertook work in a wide range of specialty roles, such as counselling and psychotherapy, eating disorders, dementia care and liaison services. Similarly, in the United Kingdom there exists a wide range of nurse specialist roles and nurse consultants. The nurse consultant role was introduced in 1999 and all nurse consultants are expected to spend a minimum of 50% of their time working directly with patients, ensuring that people using the NHS continue to benefit from those with the very best nursing skills. In addition, the nurse consultants are responsible for developing personal practice, being involved in research and evaluation, and contributing to education, training and development. In 2010, there were 153 consultant nurses working in mental health in England (The Information Centre for Health and Social Care, 2011). Although individual nurse consultant roles have had considerable success and become authoritative figures, the role is not always well embedded and frequently incumbents are not replaced when they decide to move on.

Elsewhere in Europe the availability of specialty nursing roles varies considerably. In Finland nurses frequently work as psychotherapists, and in Germany – although historically the roles have been relatively narrow – there are signs of change, for example with the first professor of mental health nursing being appointed. In Eastern Europe specialist posts remain very rare.

Nurse prescribing is a particularly interesting example where law and policy and professional cultures come together. A recent literature review has identified the existence of just a small number of countries in Western Europe where there is legal authority for nurses to prescribe with specific qualifications, namely the United Kingdom, Ireland and Sweden (Kroezen et al., 2011). However, there is some evidence of planned growth in other countries, specifically the Netherlands, Spain and Finland. There are no such plans in Germany. The United Kingdom has well-established nurse prescribing, although its growth in mental health settings has been slow and variable from area to area (Dobel-Ober et al., 2010). In Ireland significant numbers of nurses are now prescribing in mental health settings. In both countries this development has taken place despite objections from many medical groups.

CONCLUSION

European policy affecting mental health issues has received increasing attention over the last few years, with initiatives by the World Health Organization and the European Union establishing it as – at least theoretically – a major health priority. The focus has increasingly moved to providing care in non-hospital settings, promoting positive mental health, fighting stigma, and delivering care through multi-disciplinary teams. However, the reality shows that despite a plethora of policies across the EU in many countries these have been slow to deliver real change and the current financial climate makes further delays likely. Whatever the policy of individual countries, nurses are key to the delivery of mental health services, being numerically the greatest resource within all services. However, local policies (and, importantly, culture) often limit the ability of nurses to develop new roles or strengthen old ones so that they can meet their full potential. Even in the UK, with the potential for nursing to legally take on a wide range of new roles and respond to the policy agenda, the profession has not typically responded as quickly as it could have done, perhaps indicating once again the importance of culture as well as policy.

Reflective Exercises

1. Why have so few countries developed a specific educational preparation for mental health nursing?
2. Does the dominance of psychiatry directly correlate to a nursing role that is subservient to medical instruction?
3. Can mental health nursing assert an advanced role more clearly as it grows in professional strength?
4. Can we untangle mental health nursing's role from gender politics in the countries considered?

BIBLIOGRAPHY

Barton, R. (1959) *Institutional Neurosis*. Bristol: Wright & Son.
Besenius, C. (2012) 'Mental health services in Luxembourg'. In N. Brimblecombe and P. Nolan (eds). *Mental Health Services in Europe: Provision and Practice*. London: Radcliffe.
Bowers, L., Douzenis, A., Galeazzi, G.M., Forghieri, M., Tsopelas, C., Simpson, A. & Allan, T. (2005) Disruptive and dangerous behaviour by patients on acute psychiatric wards in three European centres, *Social Psychiatry and Psychiatric Epidemiology*, 40 (10): 822–828.
Brimblecombe, N. (2005) The changing relationship between mental health nurses and psychiatrists in the United Kingdom, *Journal of Advanced Nursing*, 49 (4): 344–353.
Brimblecombe, N. and Nolan, P. (eds) (2012) *Mental Health Services in Europe: Provision and Practice*. London: Radcliffe.
Department of Health (1999) *National Service Framework for Mental Health: Modern Standards and Service Models*. London: DH.
Department of Health (2011) *No Health Without Mental Health: A Cross-government Mental Health Outcomes Strategy for People of All Ages*. Available at www.dh.gov.uk/prod_consum_dh/groups/dh_digitalassets/documents/digitalasset/dh_124058.pdf (last accessed 8 April 2011).

Dobel-Ober, D., Brimblecombe, N. & Bradley, E. (2010) 'Nurse prescribing in mental health: national survey', *Journal of Psychiatric and Mental Health Nursing*, 17: 487–93.

Ellilä, H., Välimäki, M., Kuosmanen, L. & Hätönen, H. (2013) 'Mental health services in Finland'. In N. Brimblecombe and P. Nolan (eds) *Mental Health Services in Europe: Provision and Practice*. London: Routledge. pp. 73–96.

Europa (2012) *Living in the EU*. Available at http://europa.eu/about-eu/facts-figures/living/index_en.htm (last accessed 10 July 2012).

Finnane, M. (2009) 'Australian asylums and their histories: introduction', *Health and History*, 11: 6–8.

Fischer, M. (2000) *Well-Ordered License: On the Unity of Machiavelli's Thought*. New York: Lexington.

Gijswift-Hoftra, M. & Oosterhuis, H. (2005) 'Introduction: comparing national cultures of psychiatry'. In M. Gijswift-Hoftra, H. Oosterhuis, J. Vijselaar et al. (eds), *Psychiatric Cultures Compared*. Amsterdam: Amsterdam University Press. pp. 9–28.

Goffman, E. (1961) *Asylums: Essays on the Social Situation of Mental Patients and Other Inmates*. New York: Doubleday Anchor.

The Information Centre for Health and Social Care (2011) *NHS Hospital and Community Health Service Non Medical workforce Census 2010*. Available at www.ic.nhs.uk/webfiles/publications/010_Workforce/nhsstaff0010/Non-medical/Non-Medical_Detailed_Results_Tables_2010_v2.xls (last accessed 4 January 2012).

Kohn, R., Saxena, S., Levav, I. & Saraceno, B. (2004) The treatment gap in mental health care, *Bull World Health Organ*, 82: 858–866.

Koukia, E. (2012) 'Mental health services in Greece'. In N. Brimblecombe and P. Nolan (eds), *Mental Health Services in Europe: Provision and Practice*. London: Radcliffe.

Kroezen, M., van Dijk, L., Groenewegen, P.P. & Francke, A.L. (2011) Nurse prescribing systematic review of the literature, *BMC Health Services Research*, 11. Available at www.biomedcentral.com/1472-6963/11/127 (last accessed 10 January 2012).

Lavikainen, J., Lahtinen, E. & Lehtinen, V. (eds) (2000) *Public Health Approach on Mental Health in Europe, National Research and Developmental Centre for Welfare and Health* (STAKES). Gummerus: Saarijarvi.

Nolan, P. and Brimblecombe, N. (2007) A survey of the education of nurses working in mental health settings in twelve European countries, *International Journal of Nursing Studies*, 444: 407–414.

Novotná, B. and Petr, T. (2012) 'Mental health services in the Czech Republic'. In N. Brimblecombe and P. Nolan (eds), *Mental Health Services in Europe: Provision and Practice*. London: Radcliffe.

Petrea, I. (2012) 'Mental health need in Europe'. In P. Brimblecombe and P. Nolan (eds), *Mental Health Services in Europe: Provision and Practice*. London: Radcliffe.

Petrea, I. & Muijen, M. (2008) *Policies and Practices for Mental Health in Europe: Meeting the Challenges*. Copenhagen: WHO Regional Office for Europe.

Porritt, S. (2005) *Capitalism, as if the World Matters*. London: Earthscan.

Priebe, S. (2006) Sign of progress or confusion? A commentary on the European Commission Green Paper on mental health, *Psychiatric Bulletin*, 30: 281–282.

Priebe, S., Frottier, P., Gaddini, A. et al. (2008) Mental health care institutions in nine European countries, 2002 to 2006, *Psychiatric Services*, 59: 570–573.

Richter, D., Berger, K. & Reker, T. (2008) Are mental disorders on the increase? A systematic review, *Psychiatric Praxis*, 35 (7): 321–330.

Santos, J., Loureiro, C. & Mendes, A. (2012) 'Mental health services in Portugal'. In N. Brimblecombe and P. Nolan (eds), *Mental Health Services in Europe: Provision and Practice*. London: Radcliffe. pp. 235–270.

Schulz, M. (2012) 'Mental health services in Germany'. In N. Brimblecombe and P. Nolan (eds), *Mental Health Services in Europe: Provision and Practice*. London: Radcliffe.

Sheridan, A. (2012) 'Mental health services in Ireland'. In N. Brimblecombe and P. Nolan (eds), *Mental Health Services in Europe: Provision and Practice*. London: Radcliffe.

Shorter, E. (2007) Historical development of mental health services. In M. Knapp, D. McDaid, E. Mossialos and G. Thornicroft (eds), *Mental Health Policy and Practice Across Europe*. Berkshire: Open University Press. pp. 15–33.

Simons, H., Clarke, L., Gobbi, M. & Long, G. (1998) *Nurse Education and Training Evaluation in Ireland. Independent External Evaluation. Final Report*. Southampton: University of Southampton.

Thornicroft, G. (2011) Physical health disparities and mental illness: the scandal of premature mortality, *British Journal of Psychiatry*, 199: 441–442.

United Nations (1991) *Principles for the Protection of Persons with Mental Illness and the Improvement of Mental Health Care*. UN General Assembly (Resolution 46/119). Available at www2.ohchr.org/english/law/principles.htm (last accessed 20 June 2010).

United Nations (1993) *UN Standard Rules on the Equalization of Opportunities for Persons with Disabilities*. UN General Assembly (Resolution 48/96). Available at www.un.org/esa/socdev/enable/dissre00.htm (last accessed 20 June 2010).

United Nations General Assembly (2007) *Convention on the Rights of Persons with Disabilities: resolution / adopted by the General Assembly*, 24 January 2007, A/RES/61/106. Available at www.unhcr.org/refworld/docid/45f973632.html (last accessed 12 July 2012).

Van de Sande, R. & Hellendoorn, E. (2012) 'Mental health services in the Netherlands'. In N. Brimblecombe and P. Nolan (eds), *Mental Health Services in Europe: Provision and Practice*. London: Radcliffe.

WHO Regional Office for Europe (2005) *Mental Health Action Plan for Europe. Facing the Challenges, Building Solutions*. Copenhagen: WHO Regional Office for Europe.

Wootton, D. (2007) *Bad Medicine: Doctors Doing Harm Since Hippocrates*. Oxford: Oxford University Press.

World Health Organization (2000) *Munich Declaration. Nurses and Midwives: A Force for Health*. Geneva: WHO.

World Health Organization (2001) *Mental Health: New Understanding, New Hope*. Geneva: WHO. Available at www.who.int/whr/2001/en/whr01_en.pdf (last accessed 20 June 2010).

World Health Organization (2003) *Mental Health Declaration for Europe: Facing the Challenges, Building Solutions*. Available at www.euro.who.int/__data/assets/pdf_file/0008/88595/E85445.pdf (last accessed 4 January 2012).

World Health Organization (2005) *Report on the European Ministerial Conference on Mental Health*. Helsinki: WHO.

World Health Organization (2008) *The Global Burden of Disease: 2004 Update*. Geneva: WHO. Available at www.who.int/evidence/bod (last accessed 20 June 2010).

World Health Organization (2011) *Mental Health Atlas 2011*. Available at http://whqlibdoc.who.int/publications/2011/9799241564359_eng.pdf (last accessed 14 October 2011).

3 COMMUNITY SERVICES

Ben Hannigan

Chapter Overview

At the time of writing there is much discussion about models of care in the Acute Sector (physical health). There seems an agreed ambition to bring health services much closer to people's homes and indeed to see admission to hospital as very much a last resort. It is argued in particular with reference to long-term conditions (or remitting illnesses) that people should be supported to self manage and only require treatment in hospital when all community options have been exhausted.

As such a radical change is being considered and one often hears in policy circles that mental health services provide an example of how this may be achieved. Partially this argument is somewhat disingenuous as many residents of institutional care were not actually in need of care and treatment but were left behind as actually disabled by the service that attempted to help them. Therefore the wholesale closure programme of large institutions (yet to be completed) was in part a reprovision of care in more appropriate settings, and not an actual relocation to a health setting. Yet in many ways the model holds true, with mental health beds only available now for those who meet a high threshold of need and for whom community services have failed. In this chapter the author details how such a transformation occurred in mental health services, and in particular identifies the drivers for this huge change in service provision.

INTRODUCTION

In his broad scene-setting chapter which appears earlier in this book, Peter Nolan writes of the journey by which the UK's mental health system transformed from being largely hospital-centred into providing most of its care in the community. I now continue this story here. In order to properly contextualise my analysis I begin with a brief account of developments taking place in the years immediately following the end of the Second World War. This preamble is important, because it was in the 1950s that the seeds of the (global) policy of community mental health care were sown. As the story chronologically unfolds I touch on the emergence and spread of the inter-professional community mental health team throughout the 1970s and 1980s, and the simultaneous rise of community mental health nursing. The 1990s I describe as having started as a decade of crisis and challenge, characterised by policy makers becoming increasingly concerned with the apparent failures of community care and practitioners growing evermore frustrated at the underfunding of services. With all of this as essential background, for the greater part of the chapter I concentrate on policy and service developments from the late 1990s onwards. This has been an era of large-scale strategies and national service frameworks, of evidence-based policy and practice, and of new types of team and new roles for practitioners. It is in this most recent period that ideas of recovery from mental ill-health, and of personalised care, have moved centre stage – for policymakers, professionals, and service users alike. More recently this has become the age of policy for the promotion of 'wellbeing', and in the context of a devolved UK an era in which strategies developed across England, Wales, Scotland and Northern Ireland increasingly diverge. This is also the age of global and national economic collapse, and of public services operating in conditions of austerity.

THE EARLY DECADES

Driven by complex forces the UK's mental health system began its turn towards the community in the 1950s (Hannigan & Allen, 2006). Lester and Glasby (2010) draw attention to the conclusions of the Percy Commission, which reporting in 1957 urged the development of an infrastructure to support the expansion of community health and social care for people who might otherwise remain resident inside the psychiatric hospitals. In 1961, Minister of Health Enoch Powell made his landmark 'watertower speech' at the annual conference of the organisation now known as Mind (Rogers & Pilgrim, 2001). Powell spoke of the unsuitability of the Victorian asylums, an idea which lay at the heart of the government's Hospital Plan that appeared in the following year. This envisaged a system in which mental health care would be provided through the district general hospitals and via a new network of services to be set up in the community.

During the process of deinstitutionalisation which followed the number of people in psychiatric hospitals steadily declined. Similar processes happened in other parts of the industrialised world. In his detailed comparative analysis of mental health policy in Europe and North America, Goodwin (1997) reviews the combination of forces that made this historic development possible. These included advances in treatments, including the synthesis of the first anti-psychotic medications. Ideological changes were also taking place within the mental health professions, including the appearance of social psychiatry which placed a renewed emphasis on the importance of the environment and relationships. For governments, community care appealed as a means of reducing the costs of looking after people in expensive institutions. Goodwin (1997) adds that community care may also have been helped by a growing public tolerance of people with mental health difficulties, and in the 1960s by the emergence of civil rights and other social movements lobbying for change.

For students of mental health nursing specifically a parallel story is how emerging policy for community care helped in the development of the profession. The first mental health nurses to spend time caring for people in their own homes appeared in the early part of the 1950s, from bases in Warlingham Park Hospital in Surrey and in Moorhaven Hospital in Devon (Hunter, 1974). Over a period of decades a series of surveys of the workforce produced evidence of a remarkable expansion thereafter in community mental health nursing numbers. Hunter (1974) cites a Royal College of Nursing survey from 1966 which reported 42 hospitals employing 199 qualified mental health nurses working full- or part-time in the community. Further growth in numbers was driven by the loss of specialist social work expertise in the years following the passing of the Local Authorities Act in 1970, which pulled psychiatric social workers into new, generic, social services departments (Sheppard, 1991). Community mental health nurses (CMHNs) were perfectly placed to fill the vacancy, as they were not only able to visit patients in their own homes but were also able to administer medication (Godin, 1996).

Community mental health policy took a further, distinct, turn with the appearance in 1975 of the government White Paper *Better Services for the Mentally Ill* (DHSS, 1975). This was important not least for its endorsement of a multidisciplinary approach to care, and the idea that in any given geographical locality services might be best provided by a team comprising psychiatrists, nurses, social workers and others. Services of this type first emerged from this period, with the numbers of community mental health centres (as they were then called) doubling every two years throughout the latter part of that decade (Sayce et al., 1991). As new ways of organising teams and services took root the numbers of CMHNs continued to grow. In one of the first major textbooks for community mental health nurses, Simmons and Brooker (1986) reported from a further national survey, completed in 1980, which found 1,667 qualified CMHNs in post. By 1985 this number had risen to 2,758, with many describing themselves as 'specialists' in some way (Brooker, 1987).

CRISIS AND CHALLENGE

By the beginning of the 1990s an active policy of supporting community mental health care had been in place for over thirty years. Hundreds of nurses had taken up posts in community teams, and many thousands of people who would otherwise have remained in hospital had been discharged. For some nurses the shift into the community had also opened up new opportunities to work with colleagues in primary care, and to provide help for people who might otherwise have had no dedicated mental health care at all (Hannigan, 1997).

The mental health system was also entering a period of crisis and challenge. At the start of the decade, the passing of the NHS and Community Care Act 1990 had succeeded in fragmenting mental health care and obscuring the responsibilities of health and social care agencies (Hannigan, 1999). Whilst policy continued to endorse the inter-professional community mental health team (CMHT) as the preferred means of organising local services (DH, 1995), some commentators had come to see this model as a flawed one, arguing that it encouraged an unhelpful blurring of professional roles (Galvin & McCarthy, 1994). Many involved in providing day-to-day care were frustrated at what they saw as the meagre resources available to them. This observation was supported by the findings of an external review of mental health services for adults, which pointed to the general under-funding of community care (Audit Commission, 1994).

Firmly propelling the system under the policy making and public spotlight during this period were tragedies involving people in contact with community mental health services, and the findings of the independent inquiries which usually followed. The most widely reported of these addressed the care and treatment of Christopher Clunis, a man with a long history of mental health problems who had killed a stranger at a London tube station (Ritchie et al., 1994). Reports of this type were significant in forcing policy makers, managers and professionals to reconsider how 'risk' should be assessed and addressed, and to think about how care should be best provided to vulnerable people living in the community and to those causing concern. The care programme approach (CPA) had been introduced in England in the early part of the 1990s, with the aim of ensuring that needs were met and care properly provided and coordinated (DH, 1990). To this was added, in England, an additional requirement for the closer monitoring of some people (DH, 1994), and in both England and Wales the passing of an amendment to the law (the Mental Health (Patients in the Community) Act) which in certain circumstances allowed users of services to be subjected to supervised discharge in the community.

Community mental health nurses, whose numbers across the UK had reached 5,000 by 1990 (White, 1993) and closer to 7,000 in England and Wales alone by 1996 (Brooker & White, 1997), were also subjected to new scrutiny during this time. In a context in which policy makers were becoming increasingly concerned to make sure that services were more carefully targeted (DH, 1995), the argument was made that the closer alignment of CMHNs to primary care had led to nurses neglecting the group which needed their services the most – namely, people with severe and long-term mental health problems (Gournay, 1994). New, skills-oriented, education programmes for nurses and other mental health practitioners appeared at this time, designed to better equip workers for the task of safely supporting people with severe mental health problems living in the community (Young & Hulatt, 2003).

Policy for mental health services continued to occupy the Conservative government right up to the general election of 1997, with one of its final actions being the publication of a Green Paper with suggestions for improving health and social care collaboration (DH, 1997). In the event, this election delivered a resounding victory for New Labour, and in so doing this paved the way for the formation of a government with clear ideas for the reshaping of public services. In a way which caught many in the field off-guard, mental health quickly emerged as an area for specific policy-making action. It is to this most recent period that I now turn.

NEW LABOUR, NEW POLICIES

Most people working within the mental health system in the mid-1990s had become used to thinking of their field of practice as being something of a neglected one. The immediate attention paid by New Labour to policy and services for mental health therefore came as a surprise. As Boardman and Parsonage (2007) observed, many embraced this as welcome evidence that the new government was, finally, preparing to give the mental health system the time and resources it needed.

Underpinned by complex systems thinking and by the idea that, in some fields, the challenges facing policy makers and service developers were exquisitely tricky to solve (Rittel & Webber, 1973), Hannigan and Coffey (2011) identified a series of broad, overlapping, sequences of mental health policy making from the late 1990s onwards. In the first phase New Labour took issue with services, before moving on to perceived shortcomings with the professions, and then on to the fundamental problem of mental ill-health *per se*. In the first of these periods identified, policy for mental health care was clearly informed by the idea that the system of services in the community had broken down (Pilgrim & Ramon, 2009). This formulation was evident in the government's first major published policy document in this area, *Modernising Mental Health Services* (DH, 1998). In this the direct claim was made that community mental health care had failed, and that urgent action was now needed to rectify the deficiencies. Contained within the broad prescription for improving services was a plan to amend mental health law for England and Wales, in order that people with mental health problems could – in some circumstances – be compelled to accept community treatment. In *Modernising Mental Health Services* the idea was also outlined to tackle service shortcomings through the establishment of a raft of new types of community team. Subsequent policy implementation guidance was to specify, in detail, how assertive outreach, crisis resolution/home treatment and early intervention teams should be set up and operated (DH, 2001).

Following the publication of the *Modernising Mental Health Services* White Paper in 1998 there came the *National Service Framework for Mental Health* (the NSF-MH) (DH, 1999). This was an important publication for everyone with a stake in mental health care in England, as contained within it were details of a projected decade of service development. National Service Frameworks were a New Labour innovation, designed to concentrate on a particular client group or area of care delivery and to set out large-scale evidence-based standards for future provision. As blueprints for change with anticipated lifespans of many years, national service frameworks were also expected to provide good practice examples for others to follow, and to include clear measures by which progress might be assessed. England's NSF-MH was one of the first National Service Frameworks to be commissioned, and was produced in consultation with representatives drawn from across the mental health field in a process chaired by the Institute of Psychiatry's Professor Graham Thornicroft. Published in September 1999, the NSF-MH contained seven standards linked to five areas: mental health promotion and action to tackle discrimination; primary mental health care and specialist services; care for people with severe mental health difficulties; services for carers; and suicide reduction. As Lester and Glasby (2010) point out, one of the most interesting and indeed distinctive features of the NSF-MH as a policy document was its explicit use of evidence to inform the standards it contained. Standards four and five, for example, dealt with services for people with severe mental illness. These standards set out requirements for all people whose care was organised using the CPA to have copies of their care plans, for these plans to include the action to be taken in the event of crisis, and for care to be regularly reviewed by a designated care coordinator. This part of the NSF-MH also included a section on the importance of providing services close to home, and in the least restrictive environment possible. Underpinning these standards was a description of helpful interventions and ways of organising services, with direct references made throughout to the supporting evidence base and the quality of this.

The NSF-MH ran for ten years, over which period it exerted (as its architects had intended) a profound effect on services in England. It raised the profile of mental health and of services in this area, and contributed to a dramatic reshaping of the system as new standards came into play. It put the spotlight on care for people with severe mental illnesses, and simultaneously on the provision of services through primary health care. Its impact is also best considered alongside that of other policy initiatives launched during its lifetime. Less than a year following the release of the NSF-MH the *NHS Plan* appeared (DH, 2000a). This confirmed mental health as a priority area for England, and pledged an increase in resources to support an expansion of the workforce and the commissioning of large numbers of new types of community team. Targets were set to fast forward the goals of the NSF-MH, with specific plans set out to expand assertive outreach, crisis resolution/home treatment (CRHT) and early intervention teams, and to invest in primary mental health care. Community-based CRHT teams, for example, were subsequently commissioned in large numbers across England (National Audit Office, 2007), and were given the task of providing short-term intensive care and treatment to people with acute mental health problems as an alternative to inpatient admission.

Further reflecting the elevation of mental health to a government priority status, the newly created National Institute for Clinical Excellence (NICE, since renamed the National Institute for Health and Clinical Excellence, and following the passing of new legislation in 2012, as the National Institute for Health and Care Excellence) chose schizophrenia as the topic for its first ever set of clinical guidelines. These appeared in 2002, and contained detailed and evidence-based guidance on the core interventions to be provided across both primary and secondary care settings

(NICE, 2002). One of the consistent goals of NICE has been to regularly review and update its publications. A second version of its guidelines on services for people with schizophrenia appeared in 2009 (NICE, 2009a), with (at the time of writing in summer 2012) work ongoing on the creation of a further iteration. In the period since its establishment, NICE has also gone on to produce and revise clinical guidelines for other mental health conditions affecting people across the lifespan. Original guidelines on depression and anxiety, for example, are both now in revised versions (NICE, 2009b, 2011).

Since their first release, these NICE guidelines on depression and anxiety have recommended cognitive behavioural therapy (CBT) as an intervention of choice. CBT moved firmly into the policy arena when a team at the London School of Economics and Political Science (the LSE), led by Lord Layard – a distinguished professor of economics – produced a report in 2006 which made the economic as well as the human case for the expansion of psychological therapies (Centre for Economic Performance's Mental Health Policy Group, 2006). *The Depression Report*, as this was called, was influential in informing national-level action to improve the treatment of common mental health problems across England, including the commissioning of the Improving Access to Psychological Therapies (IAPT) initiative (Clark, 2011). Through this specific development, a programme of 'low intensity' and 'high intensity' services became available to large numbers of people living in the community who might otherwise have been denied dedicated mental health care of any type.

Running alongside these multiple developments (the NSF-MH, the *NHS Plan*, the development of national evidence-based clinical guidelines, and the expansion of psychological therapies) was a stream of work reflecting New Labour's post-1997 election commitment to review mental health law for England and Wales. In the event this initiative proved both contentious and protracted. Pilgrim (2007) traces the history of this strand of policy activity, showing how it began with the establishment of an independent committee chaired by the legal expert Professor Genevra Richardson, the publication of this committee's report, and the simultaneous appearance of a government Green Paper. Later came the publication of a White Paper, two draft Bills, and a critical report by a parliamentary scrutiny committee. Throughout this process the government faced concerted opposition led by the umbrella organisation the Mental Health Alliance, a group bringing together representatives of professional, service user, carer and campaigning organisations. In 2007, a full ten years after the initial announcement that England and Wales' Mental Health Act 1983 would be 'modernised', work finally concluded with the passing of an amendment to the existing legislation.

In the context of community care the outcome of this legal review process was significant for a number of reasons. The amendments to the 1983 Mental Health Act passed in 2007 changed the legal definition of 'mental disorder', and altered the circumstances in which people could be detained. Contentiously, it also made provision for supervised community treatment. This meant that, under certain conditions, people previously detained in hospital could be discharged subject to a community treatment order (CTO) (DH, 2008). The imposition of a CTO gave professionals the legal authority to require adherence to treatment and care, with a provision to recall patients to hospital (Macpherson et al., 2010). In other parts of the act policy makers took the opportunity afforded them to refashion the responsibilities of different groups of professionals. This, in Hannigan and Coffey's (2011) analysis, reflected a further policy-making reformulation of 'the problem' within the system as now being one of professional practice rather than with the organisation or funding of services.

New Labour's interest in using its review of legislation to realign practitioner responsibilities reflected the government's wider motivation to erode the boundaries between different groups of health and social care professionals. These divisions it saw as a hindrance to the provision of integrated services. Through documents like *A Health Service of all the Talents* (DH, 2000b), policy makers advocated the breaking down of inter-occupational demarcations and greater flexibility in workplace roles across the entire NHS. The mental health field emerged as a particular focus for action in this area (Hannigan & Allen, 2011), with a number of initiatives being brought together under the banner of 'new ways of working' (DH, 2007). The review of the mental health legislative framework for England and Wales provided the UK government with a clear opportunity to reshape statutory roles and responsibilities. Competency, rather than occupational background, was to become key in determining the suitability of professionals to participate formally in Mental Health Act decision making. Social workers, on completion of a post-qualifying course, had previously had the exclusive authority to fulfil the 'approved' role and make applications for the use of compulsory orders (Evans et al., 2005). With the passing of the Mental Health Act 2007 this work opened up to other groups of professionals (nurses included) via the introduction of the approved mental health professional (Coffrey & Hannigan, 2013). The exclusive authority of psychiatrists to act as responsible medical officers was also modified in favour of the new cross-professional position of approved clinician (AC).

CURRENT AND EMERGING STRATEGY

The NSF-MH for England formally ended in 2009. Towards the end of its lifetime important new themes came to the fore, including an emphasis on the promotion of recovery, and more recently on personalisation. Drawing on transatlantic ideas (Anthony, 1993) the recovery agenda resonated with many in the mental health field, including nurses, who shared concerns to develop more user-centred styles of care provision (see, for example, *England's Chief Nursing Officer's Review*: DH, 2006). Personalisation emphasises the value of providing collaborative and integrated health and social care which is tailored to individual needs in highly flexible ways (Duffy, 2010).

As these ideas were emerging and beginning to influence policy frameworks, and shortly before losing office in the year which followed, New Labour proposed a replacement for the NSF-MH in England called *New Horizons* (HM

Government, 2009). In Hannigan and Coffey's (2011) analysis this represented a further reframing of 'the problem' to which policy should be directed, this time in favour of a cross-government cross-sector approach aimed at improving 'well-being' across the lifespan. In the event, with a coalition Conservative/Liberal Democrat UK government installed in 2010 *New Horizons* was consigned to the archive, to be replaced in 2011 by a new cross-government strategy for England entitled *No Health Without Mental Health* (DH, 2011). In significant respects this demonstrated a continuation of the ideas set out in *New Horizons*, in that it emphasised the importance of 'wellness' and of making sure that mental health became everybody's business, rather than the responsibility of the NHS and other statutory care providers alone. England's *No Health Without Mental Health* contained a 'call to action', setting out the goal of achieving six outcome-oriented objectives. Reproduced word-for-word here, these stated that more people will have good mental health, more people with mental health problems will recover, more people with mental health problems will have good physical health, more people will have a positive experience of care and support, fewer people will suffer avoidable harm, and fewer people will experience stigma and discrimination. In terms of actions to be taken, whilst the document committed to the continued expansion of psychological therapies the detail of the work to be done to achieve this, as the NHS Confederation noted (NHS Confederation, 2011), was to be left to the discretion of decision makers at a local level. Where New Labour's NSF-MH exerted a centralising force, by creating national standards to uniformly drive up quality throughout the whole of England, this now-current strategy looks to be a far more decentralising one.

THE IMPACT OF DEVOLUTION

Differences in health care policy and provision have long existed across the territories of the UK, though the commitment to devolved government initiated whilst New Labour was in office has created conditions favouring increased diversity (Greer, 2005). How far post-devolution policy for the health service has truly diverged across England, Wales, Scotland and Northern Ireland is still debated (Smith & Hellowell, 2012), but in the mental health field differences in emphasis can certainly be detected.

Whilst England was pressing ahead with its centrally-driven NSF-MH and its associated implementation guidance in the early part of the new century, in Wales post-devolution policy makers were taking a far less interventionist stance. Clear standards for the setting up of new types of community team in England were, at first, not mirrored in Wales where the strategy instead focused on clarifying the values which should underpin care, and where policy makers restated their continued support for the locality CMHT as the principal means of organising local services (National Assembly for Wales, 2001). Two iterations of a National Service Framework for adults with mental health difficulties have since been produced in Wales (Welsh Assembly Government, 2002, 2005), but it is only relatively recently that (for example) significant numbers of assertive outreach and crisis resolution/ home treatment services have appeared (Jones & Robinson, 2008). Wales also offers a particularly good example of recent, post-devolution, policy difference with the case of the Mental Health (Wales) Measure (2010) (Welsh Assembly Government, 2011). This is being implemented as part of the legal framework in Wales, and places statutory obligations on providers in a number of important areas: the provision of primary mental health services; the planning and coordination of care; advocacy; and accessing secondary services. Wales's National Assembly election held in 2011 delivered a Labour government, with consultation on a new whole-lifespan mental health strategy for the country (*Together for Mental Health*) opening in the year following (Welsh Government, 2012). Themes of promoting wellbeing, listening and responding to service users and creating a more integrated system of services featured strongly in this.

Unlike in England and Wales, Scotland's review of mental health law and the subsequent passing of the Mental Health (Care and Treatment) (Scotland) Act 2003 was accomplished in a relatively straightforward and consensual fashion (Cairney, 2009). In this part of the UK important post-devolution innovations have included the development of the Scottish Recovery Indicator (SRI), now in its second version, which is designed to support practitioners promote recovery in their day-to-day work (for more information, see www.sri2.net). Consultation on a proposed new mental health strategy for Scotland closed in early 2012 – a document in which the further development of psychological therapies, community care and alternatives to hospital admission are prominent goals (Scottish Government, 2011). In Northern Ireland, a detailed service framework designed to improve mental health and wellbeing, and to develop services, was launched in 2011 (DH, Social Services and Public Safety, 2011). Noting the high rates of mental ill health in the region, and its history of civil conflict, this document laid out 58 detailed standards for improving services and promoting mental health. Underpinning this Service Framework was the earlier work of the Bamford Review. This had been established in 2002 (under the chairmanship, until his death, of Professor David Bamford of Ulster University) with the responsibility to conduct a detailed and independent review of Northern Ireland's law, policy and provision for people with mental health needs or learning disabilities (for more information, see www.dhsspsni.gov.uk/bamford.htm). One of the review body's recommendations lay specifically in the area of the legal framework, and consultation has since taken place on the construction of new mental health and capacity law (see, for example, DH, Social Services and Public Safety, 2009).

FUTURE DIRECTIONS?

It is impossible to write about health care in the UK in the middle of 2012 without saying something about the economic conditions prevailing. The rise to policy-making prominence of the mental health field, and the associated investment in new services from the last part of the twentieth century, has yielded now to an era of retraction in conditions of austerity. Public services, including health care, are under intense pressure as funds are reined in. Whilst the case is being made for the continued prioritisation of mental health services, and for the ongoing importance of promoting wellbeing, it is clear that the global and national economic collapse represents a major threat at a time when the demand for care is likely to increase (Royal College of Psychiatrists et al., 2009). At a national level in England, a supporting document to *No Health Without Mental Health* was devoted to outlining areas where efficiency might be improved (DH, 2011). Observers speculated how the demand for cost reductions could trigger a mental health services' reorganisation, and promote new and less people-intensive ways of providing help and support (McDaid & Knapp, 2010).

As austerity bites, evidence accumulates of accelerating differences in health policy across the countries of the UK. In England – in the face of concerted opposition from professionals, trades unionists and campaigning organisations – the newly elected coalition government in Westminster pressed ahead from 2011 onwards with plans for a radical restructuring of the NHS. This process culminated in the passing of the Health and Social Care Act 2012. This introduced GP-led clinical commissioning groups (which have responsibility for overseeing the greater part of England's NHS budget), and explicitly promoted competition in the provision of health services. Monitor (the organisation originally set up to regulate NHS foundation trusts in England) is expanding its role to take on new functions in this area. It will regulate NHS prices, license health care providers, and be required to act to prevent 'anti-competitive behaviour'. Competition and the fragmentation of commissioning, introduced via the NHS and Community Care Act 1990, have not served community mental health services well in the past (Hannigan, 1999). During the period leading up to the passing of the 2012 Act, leading organisations in the mental health field made clear their concerns at the risks the proposed legislation posed (Centre for Mental Health et al., 2011). Specific campaigning was also needed at this time to protect the rights of people previously detained under treatment sections of the Mental Health Act to continue to receive statutory, integrated, aftercare, the provision of which was threatened by the planned new legislation.

CONCLUSION

Inevitably, in a single policy-oriented chapter of this type significant gaps in coverage will remain. Apologies are offered to readers hoping to learn something of the specific development of community mental health services for children and young people, or for older adults. Both are vitally important areas, but space prevents a detailed account of either. The reader is also referred to Tim McDougal's and Trevor Adams' contributions to this volume. What this chapter has done is to have accessibly laid out, in a broad chronological fashion, key moments in the UK's journey towards a system of mental health services which has at its centre the provision of care in the community. The idea that mental health care should, wherever possible, be provided in the community rather than in hospitals is one that the UK's policy makers have now pursued for almost six decades. This chapter has shown how the system of services which has grown up to support the realisation of this idea remains complex and dynamic. It has continued to shift in response to new policy imperatives and other forces. Nurses and others with stakes in the community mental health field can expect more of the same in the future.

Reflective Exercises

1. What factors promoted the emergence of community mental health nursing?
2. What are your views and experiences of inter-professional team working in mental health?
3. To what degree have debates emerging in the 1990s over the identification and management of risk continued to shape mental health policy and everyday practice into the present?
4. What differences have assertive outreach, crisis resolution/home treatment and early intervention services made in the lives of people with long-term mental health difficulties?

BIBLIOGRAPHY

Anthony, W.A. (1993) Recovery from mental illness: the guiding vision of the mental health service system in the 1990s, *Psychiatric Rehabilitation Journal*, 16 (4): 11–23.

Audit Commission (1994) *Finding a Place: A Review of Mental Health Services for Adults.* London: HMSO.

Boardman, J. & Parsonage, M. (2007) *Delivering the Government's Mental Health Policies.* London: Sainsbury Centre for Mental Health.

Brooker, C. (1987) An investigation into the factors influencing variation in the growth of community psychiatric nursing services, *Journal of Advanced Nursing*, 12 (3): 367–375.

Brooker, C. and White, E. (1997) *The Fourth Quinquennial National Community Mental Health Nursing Census of England and Wales.* Manchester and Keele: Universities of Manchester and Keele.

Cairney, P. (2009) The 'British policy style' and mental health: beyond the headlines, *Journal of Social Policy*, 38 (4): 671–688.

Centre for Economic Performance's Mental Health Policy Group (2006) *The Depression Report: A New Deal for Depression and Anxiety Disorders.* London: London School of Economics and Political Science.

Centre for Mental Health, Mental Health Foundation, Mind, Rethink and Royal College of Psychiatrists (2011) *Health and Social Care Bill: Briefing.* Available at www.mind.org.uk/assets/0001/1513/Health_and_Social_Care_Bill_second_reading_mental_health_briefing.pdf

Clark, D.M. (2011) Implementing NICE guidelines for the psychological treatment of depression and anxiety disorders: the IAPT experience, *International Review of Psychiatry*, 23 (4): 318–327.

Coffey, M. & Hannigan, B. (2013) New roles for nurses as approved mental health professionals in England and Wales: a discussion paper, *International Journal of Nursing Studies*, 50 (10): 1423–1430.

Department of Health (1990) *The Care Programme Approach for People with a Mental Illness Referred to the Specialist Psychiatric Services; HC(90)23/LASSL(90)11*. London: DH.

Department of Health (1994) *Introduction of Supervision Registers for Mentally Ill People from 1st April 1994: HSG(94)51*. London: DH.

Department of Health (1995) *Building Bridges: A Guide to Arrangements for Interagency Working for the Care and Protection of Severely Mentally Ill People*. London: DH.

Department of Health (1997) *Developing Partnerships in Mental Health*. London: The Stationery Office.

Department of Health (1998) *Modernising Mental Health Services: Safe, Sound and Supportive*. London: DH.

Department of Health (1999) *A National Service Framework for Mental Health*. London: DH.

Department of Health (2000a) *The NHS Plan: A Plan for Investment, A Plan for Reform*. London: DH.

Department of Health (2000b) *A Health Service of all the Talents: Developing the NHS Workforce. Consultation Document on the Review of Workforce Planning*. London: DH.

Department of Health (2001) *The Mental Health Policy Implementation Guide*. London: DH.

Department of Health (2006) *From Values to Action: The Chief Nursing Officer's Review of Mental Health Nursing*. London: DH.

Department of Health (2007) *Mental Health: New Ways of Working for Everyone. Developing and Sustaining A Capable and Flexible Workforce*. London: DH.

Department of Health (2008) *Mental Health Act 1983: Code of Practice*. London: The Stationery Office.

Department of Health (2011) *No Health Without Mental Health: A Cross-Government Mental Health Outcomes Strategy for People of All Ages. Supporting Document: The Economic Case for Improving Efficiency and Quality in Mental Health*. London: DH.

Department of Health, Social Services and Public Safety (2009) *Legislative Framework for Mental Capacity and Mental Health Legislation in Northern Ireland: A Policy Consultation Document*. Belfast: Department of Health Social Services and Public Safety.

Department of Health, Social Services and Public Safety (2011) *Service Framework for Mental Health and Wellbeing*. Belfast: Department of Health, Social Services and Public Safety.

DHSS (1975) *Better Services for the Mentally Ill*. London: HMSO.

Duffy, S. (2010) *Personalisation in Mental Health*. Sheffield: Centre for Welfare Reform.

Evans, S., Huxley, P., Webber, M., Katona, C., Gateley, C., Mears, A., Medina, J., Pajak, S. & Kendall, T. (2005) The impact of 'statutory duties' on mental health social workers in the UK, *Health and Social Care in the Community*, 13 (2): 145–154.

Galvin, S.W. & McCarthy, S. (1994) Multi-disciplinary community teams: clinging to the wreckage, *Journal of Mental Health*, 3 (2): 157–166.

Godin, P. (1996) The development of community psychiatric nursing: a professional project?, *Journal of Advanced Nursing*, 23 (5): 925–934.

Goodwin, S. (1997) *Comparative Mental Health Policy: From Institutional to Community Care*. London: Sage.

Gournay, K. (1994) Redirecting the emphasis to serious mental illness, *Nursing Times*, 90 (25): 40–41.

Greer, S.L. (2005) The territorial bases of health policymaking in the UK after devolution, *Regional and Federal Studies*, 15 (4): 501–518.

Hannigan, B. (1997) A challenge for community psychiatric nursing: is there a future in primary health care?, *Journal of Advanced Nursing*, 26 (4): 251–257.

Hannigan, B. (1999) Joint working in community mental health: prospects and challenges, *Health and Social Care in the Community*, 7 (1): 25–31.

Hannigan, B. & Allen, D. (2006) Complexity and change in the United Kingdom's system of mental health care, *Social Theory & Health*, 4 (3): 244–263.

Hannigan, B. & Allen, D. (2011) Giving a fig about roles: policy, context and work in community mental health care, *Journal of Psychiatric and Mental Health Nursing*, 18 (1): 1–8.

Hannigan, B. & Coffey, M. (2011) Where the wicked problems are: the case of mental health, *Health Policy*, 101 (3): 220–227.

HM Government (2009) *New Horizons: A Shared Vision for Mental Health*. London: HM Government.

Hunter, P. (1974) Community psychiatric nursing in Britain: an historical review, *International Journal of Nursing Studies*, 11 (4): 223–233.

Jones, R. & Robinson, B. (2008) *A National Survey of Crisis Resolution Home Treatment Teams in Wales*, All Wales Crisis Resolution Home Treatment Network.

Lester, H. & Glasby, J. (2010) *Mental Health Policy and Practice,* 2nd edition. Basingstoke: Palgrave Macmillan.

Macpherson, R., Molodynski, A., Freeth, R., Uppal, A., Steer, H., Buckle, D. & Jones, A. (2010) Supervised community treatment: guidance for clinicians, *Advances in Psychiatric Treatment*, 16 (4): 253–259.

McDaid, D. & Knapp, M. (2010) Black-skies planning? Prioritising mental health services in times of austerity, *British Journal of Psychiatry*, 196 (6): 423–424.

Mental Health (Wales) Measure (2010), Welsh Assembly Government (www.cymru.gov.uk) (last accessed September 2010).

National Assembly for Wales (2001) *Adult Mental Health Services for Wales: Equity, Empowerment, Effectiveness, Efficiency.* Cardiff: National Assembly for Wales.

National Audit Office (2007) *Helping People through Mental Health Crisis: The Role of Crisis Resolution and Home Treatment Services*. London: The Stationery Office.

National Institute for Clinical Excellence (NICE) (2002) *Schizophrenia: Core Interventions in the Treatment and Management of Schizophrenia in Primary and Secondary Care*. London: National Institute for Clinical Excellence.

National Institute for Health and Clinical Excellence (NICE) (2009a) *Schizophrenia: Core Interventions in the Treatment and Management of Schizophrenia in Primary and Secondary Care (Update)*. London: National Institute for Health and Clinical Excellence.

National Institute for Health and Clinical Excellence (NICE) (2009b) *Depression: the Treatment and Management of Depression in Adults (Update)*. London: National Institute for Health and Clinical Excellence.

National Institute for Health and Clinical Excellence (NICE) (2011) *Generalised Anxiety Disorder and Panic Disorder (with or without Agoraphobia) in Adults*. London: National Institute for Health and Clinical Excellence.

NHS Confederation (2011) *No Health Without Mental Health: The New Strategy for Mental Health in England*. London: NHS Confederation.

Pilgrim, D. (2007) New 'mental health' legislation for England and Wales: some aspects of consensus and conflict, *Journal of Social Policy*, 36 (1): 79–95.

Pilgrim, D. & Ramon, S. (2009) English mental health policy under New Labour, *Policy & Politics*, 37 (2): 271–288.

Ritchie, J.H., Dick, D. & Lingham, R. (1994) *The Report of the Inquiry into the Care and Treatment of Christopher Clunis*. London: HMSO.

Rittel, H.W.J. & Webber, M.W. (1973) Dilemmas in a general theory of planning, *Policy Sciences*, 4 (2): 155–169.

Rogers, A. & Pilgrim, D. (2001) *Mental Health Policy in Britain* (2nd edition). Basingstoke: Palgrave.

Royal College of Psychiatrists, Mental Health Network NHS Confederation and The London School of Economics and Political Science (2009) *Mental Health and the Economic Downturn: National Priorities and NHS Solutions*. London: Royal College of Psychiatrists, NHS Confederation, LSE.

Sayce, L., Craig, T.K.J. & Boardman, A.P. (1991) The development of community mental health centres in the UK, *Social Psychiatry and Psychiatric Epidemiology*, 26 (1): 14–20.

Scottish Government (2011) *Mental Health Strategy for Scotland 2011–15: A Consultation*. Edinburgh: Scottish Government.

Sheppard, M. (1991) *Mental Health Work in the Community: Theory and Practice in Social Work and Community Psychiatric Nursing*. London: Falmer.

Simmons, S. & Brooker, C. (1986) *Community Psychiatric Nursing: A Social Perspective*. Oxford: Butterworth-Heinemann.

Smith, K. & Hellowell, H. (2012) Beyond rhetorical differences: a cohesive account of post-devolution developments in the UK, *Social Policy & Administration*, 46 (2): 178–198.

Welsh Assembly Government (2002) *Adult Mental Health Services: A National Service Framework for Wales*. Cardiff: Welsh Assembly Government.

Welsh Assembly Government (2005) *Raising the Standard: The Revised Adult Mental Health National Service Framework and an Action Plan for Wales*. Cardiff: Welsh Assembly Government.

Welsh Assembly Government (2011) *Implementing the Mental Health (Wales) Measure 2010: Guidance for Local Health Boards and Local Authorities*. Cardiff: Welsh Assembly Government.

Welsh Government (2012) *Together for Mental Health: A Cross-Government Strategy for Mental Health and Wellbeing in Wales. Consultation Document*. Cardiff: Welsh Government.

White, E. (1993) 'Community psychiatric nursing 1980 to 1990: a review of organization, education and practice'. In C. Brooker and E. White (eds), *Community Psychiatric Nursing: A Research Perspective, volume 2*. London: Chapman and Hall.

Young, N. & Hulatt, I. (2003) 'Developing courses in psychosocial interventions'. In B. Hannigan and M. Coffey (eds), *The Handbook of Community Mental Health Nursing*. London: Routledge.

4 PSYCHOSIS

Norman Young

Chapter Overview

Providing care for the most ill, unwell, vulnerable, challenged by poor mental health (the choice of term is yours) remains an area of not only contested language but also choice of social response. In this chapter the author commences with an event that seemed to define a moment when society became disturbed about the welfare of individuals labelled with severe mental illness. There seemed to be a rapid descent into a narrative that community care had failed (endorsed by senior politicians) and something needed to be done. There was also justifiable concern that the welfare of the most vulnerable had been ignored in the rapid pursuit of service provision in the community. This chapter describes what that 'something' was and to an extent remains.

The events and debates (again) gave rise to a fundamental change in how services were/are delivered, and also precipitated a review of mental health legislation which in England and Wales took seven years to be completed. However, it also heralded unparalleled investment and innovation in service delivery models. Critics decried the emphasis on the most unwell, describing it as a movement to a National Psychosis Service. Advocates for the reformed service models saw it as a justified redress of provision. It is also worth mentioning that there was much campaigning from the perspective of carers who felt to a certain extent abandoned to provide care in the absence of services. Their activism and concern – sometimes highlighted by the tragic occurrence of service 'failures' – maintained a profile that energised policy makers to act. Increasingly the concern was not exclusively voiced by carer groups but by service users themselves who felt services were inaccessible until moments of extremis, and again through the work of service user charities strongly advocated for better services and in particular access at times of crisis.

Providing services for people with psychosis remains an area of controversy. There are debates about the needs of individuals, the nature and expression of risk, and how this can be responded to. Policy in this area can be seen to be balancing so many needs and voices. Whether it succeeds in doing so is an ongoing discussion.

INTRODUCTION

On New Year's Eve 1992, Ben Silcott – a young man with schizophrenia – climbed into the lions' enclosure at London Zoo carrying two frozen chickens. Silcott believed that he had a special bond with lions and thus could relieve their suffering. He was subsequently mauled but survived. The incident was caught on camera and broadcast around the world, moving public opinion on community care for the mentally ill. The then Health Secretary, Virginia Bottomley, asked the Royal College of Psychiatrists to lead a review on the safe and secure treatment and care of mentally ill people in the community. Six months later a ten-point plan for mental health services was published detailing greater supervision of mentally ill people in the community.

This snapshot illustrates how policy making is a dynamic process subject to the influences of a range of lobbyists such as the public, professionals, the media, and interest groups. Each can exert influence in the form of personal accounts, scientific studies, or rhetoric to persuade an audience. Community care has been the dominant ideology for mental health services over the last thirty years and the treatment and care of people with psychosis have been key drivers in mental health policy making.

The 1980s saw the start of the creation of modern mental health services but also severe testing of the ideology surrounding community care. Perseverance, investment and leadership eventually produced the delivery of services with which service users were more satisfied, and the public reassured and more aware of mental health problems. In this age of austerity community care policy has persisted but shifted from prescribing specific services – often targeted at those with psychosis – to values-based practice, general wellbeing and public health initiatives. In practice, this has seen a retraction in public services for people with psychosis and for people with mental health problems as a whole.

THE ESTABLISHMENT OF MODERN COMMUNITY CARE SERVICES FOR PEOPLE WITH PSYCHOSIS

The last three decades have encompassed seven general elections split between two governing parties (Conservative 1983–1997 and Labour 1997–2010) until the Conservative-Liberal coalition government of 2010. In the early 1980s a significant proportion of people with psychosis remained in institutions despite the moral and political will to move care into the community. The 1983 Conservative government continued with the mental health policies of the previous administration, described in the policy papers *Hospital Services for the Mentally Ill* (DHSS, 1971) and *Better Services for the Mentally Ill* (DHSS, 1975). The aim of these policies was to extend the hospital closure plans of the 1960s that had been driven by the highly publicised failures of institutional care (DH and Social Services, 1969). This meant moving care from large institutions to district general hospitals, and expanding community services such as day care, residential accommodation, and greater social work support.

Investment in public health would also be required to increase work on prevention and early intervention. Reflecting a community service there would also be a new Mental Health Act giving greater rights to patients.

Community care took on the structures and working practices that we would recognise today. Community Mental Health Centres and Teams (CMHTs) began to flourish: by 1984 there were 22 of these, and by 1990 they totalled 122. These teams brought in a new practice called multidisciplinary team working, and patients who would have previously attended hospital outpatients were now cared for by a range practitioners working within these new teams. Many experienced nurses left the hospital setting to enjoy the clinical autonomy afforded to the role of community psychiatric nurse. These nurses were highly valued by GPs who now had improved access to psychiatric services. Psychiatrists were also supportive but asserted their key role in assessing and managing referrals (Royal College of Psychiatrists, 1980).

New services required additional funding but therein lay a problem – as long as the old asylums existed the money to fund these remained intact. Bridging funds would be required to overcome the gap so that new services could be created and old services run down. This type of funding was hard for mental health services to acquire for three reasons: firstly, mental health was a low priority in the budget setting when set against other departments' requirements; secondly, there was a global economic downturn and the world was in recession; and thirdly, the ideology of the Thatcher government was on reducing the size of public services and transferring services to private and third sector organisations through competitive tendering or outsourcing.

The government's expectation that mental health services should deliver community care was in no way tempered against a background of constrained funding and increasing public demand for mental health services (Pauley, 1984). Combined with a lack of understanding and guidance on how to design and administer community mental health services, the risks for service failures were increasing.

Members of the House of Commons were concerned about the state of community care and a Social Services Committee began to take evidence from professionals, voluntary groups and the public on the state of services (House of Commons, 1984). The committee heard about gaps in service provision and a lack of service user participation in shaping services. They then made key recommendations on service user involvement and the provision of a bridging fund to assist in the development of community services while closure plans were set in motion. The Conservative government responded by sending out a directive to the regional health authorities that obliged them to shut down their old asylums. The government did not centralise decision making but devolved it. At the time this was seen as a cost-saving exercise because of the limited government funding to support the programme. In spite of this the number of inpatient beds did fall from over 100,000 in 1974 to 60,000 in 1989 (Murphy, 1991).

A lack of policy development was mirrored by a lack of mental health leadership and an absence of evidence relating to service design and intervention which would have assisted service planners (Braun et al., 1981). The operational policies of CMHTs were being guided by research evidence from the USA (Stein & Test, 1980) which possessed a very different health-care system. UK research on community care was subsequently commissioned, and this included the Team for the Assessment of Psychiatric Services (TAPS) study evaluating the impact of relocating long-stay patients (Knapp et al., 1990) and the Maudsley Daily Living Programme investigating a crisis and home treatment service (Marks et al., 1988). The role of charities was important in providing support for mental health service development in the field of psychosis. Notably, the Gatsby Foundation established the National Unit for Psychiatric Research and Development (later called the Sainsbury Centre for Mental Health, and now the Centre for Mental Health).

Service users were becoming organised and establishing groups such as Survivors Speak Out and the Scottish Users Interest Group. Their activity was sobering in that it revealed the scandal of asylum life. Service users argued for people to recognise the potential within service users through the concept of recovery and efforts to reduce stigma and discrimination. They were also creating user-led innovations such as crisis cards and advanced directives. Participation in the development of services was spoken about but its realisation had to wait.

THE NEED FOR BETTER CARE CO-ORDINATION OF THOSE WITH SEVERE AND ENDURING MENTAL ILLNESS

On their discharge from hospital the treatment and care of service users would be coordinated through CMHTs. GPs were also using these services for people with common mental disorders with the overall effect of an ever-increasing demand on the new service. There were no blueprints describing how to manage crisis and home treatment, or how to work effectively with primary care. Without guidance and with a limited evidence base CMHTs began to drift away from their initial objectives, leading to open referral policies, poor multidisciplinary practice, and inadequate procedures to sustain contact with people who had severe and enduring mental health problems (Patmore & Weaver, 1991).

Anxieties about community care began to surface in the press, particularly via a series of articles in *The Times* by Marjorie Wallace, the founder of SANE (Wallace, 1985), and an Audit Commission report into community care (Audit Commission, 1984). These concerns were thrown into sharp relief in 1984 when Isabel Schwarz, a social worker, whilst at her place of work was killed by Sharon Campbell (DH and Social Services, 1998). The Stokes Inquiry that followed made a series of recommendations, one of which was the creation of a system for coordinating the care of patients in the community that later became the care programme approach (CPA).

The Conservative government accepted the recommendations of the Stokes Report but did not immediately act on these. The government's attention was on the NHS and Community Care Act 1990 which would see the creation of NHS trusts and limited competition brought into the NHS through GP fundholding (an extension of which is in place in England today under the Health and Social Care Act 2012). The act provided resources through the mental health specific grant which was available across the UK. At the same time, the government sent to NHS and social services managers in England a Department of Health circular (DH, 1990), describing the CPA. Such circulars are viewed as instructions for managers and do not represent legislation. In Scotland guidance followed in 1992 and in more detail in 1996 (Scottish Office, 1992, 1996). For Wales the CPA was initially viewed as good practice and only appeared following devolution, initially as guidance on the care-planning process and documentation in 1998 and then in its mental health strategy (Welsh Assembly Government, 2003). Northern Ireland did not adopt this process and instead emphasised existing care-planning arrangements.

The policy was to be implemented in England in 1991 but it was poorly received and followed through for some of the following reasons (North, et al., 1993; Simpson, et al., 2003):

- The circular lacked any sense of urgency or priority.
- The NHS and Community Care Act 1990 had created a system called care management which – with the CPA – created two administrative processes for mental health care, thereby bringing confusion and complexity.
- The act strengthened the role of managers and so the CPA was seen in some quarters as a bureaucratic mechanism with which to manage clinicians and clinical interventions.
- The CPA was based on a misinterpretation of intensive case management – an approach targeting people with severe and enduring mental health problems – but the CPA targeted all patients.
- The information management systems did not exist to manage such high-volume work.

The CPA and the administrative processes that it spawned burdened clinicians with a duty to evidence care co-ordination for all people with mental health disorders rather than those with just complex needs. The CPA, as a brokerage model of care management, had little UK empirical evidence to support it and was therefore openly criticised (Marshall, 1996).

The CPA did not go away: instead two highly publicised killings intensified the government's belief that it was the solution to falling confidence in community care. The first was at the end of 1991 when Ben Silcott was mauled at London Zoo, and the second came in 1992 when Jonathan Zito was killed by Christopher Clunis. Both incidents caught the public's attention for different reasons. Ben Silcott was filmed by a passer-by and the video was widely broadcast to an astonished audience: Jonathan Zito's wife Jayne initiated a vigorous and prolonged campaign for better services for the mentally ill through the Zito Trust. The role of the press was important here. *The Independent* followed the Christopher Clunis Inquiry and published related stories and their own investigation into events (Timmins, 1994). At the same time the popular print media sensationalised reports and fuelled public perception and opinion that mental illness was strongly associated with violence (Kalucy et al., 2011). The policy of community care was thus under pressure from the media, the public, and some health professionals (Coid, 1994).

The inquiries that followed found similar issues to those of the Stokes Inquiry, such as poor care coordination, poor risk assessment and risk management (in particular minimising risk), and failures in communicating early signs of deterioration (Ritchie, 1994). In response to the Silcott incident the government commissioned a review of the care and treatment of people with severe and enduring mental health problems. The committee outlined a plan for mental health (that was coined 'Bottomley's ten-point plan') which detailed steps to strengthen the implementation of the CPA and role of CMHTs in delivering mental health services for people with severe and enduring mental health problems (DH, 1995, 1996).

The remainder of the plan provided scant detail about the resources that would be made available to improve community care. Instead the focus was on increasing the control of people through the introduction of supervision registers and supervised discharge. These intentions heralded a period of legislative changes which were to make a significant impact on the rights and freedoms of people with psychosis.

LEGISLATIVE STEPS TO INCREASE CONTROL IN THE COMMUNITY

In general, people hold sympathetic and caring attitudes toward people with a mental illness and believe that we have a responsibility to care for them. Public surveys of attitudes towards mental illness and the mentally ill that were conducted by the Department of Health from 1993 to 2011 showed that the public's fear of people with mental illness significantly increased following after the introduction of the CPA and Bottomley's ten-point plan before falling and continuing to fall after 1997 (see Figure 4.1).

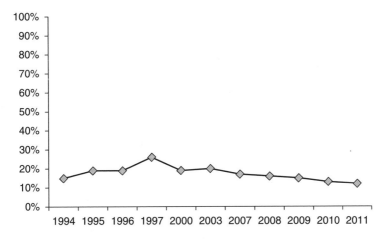

Figure 4.1 The percentage of people responding *yes* to the statement 'It is frightening to think of people with mental illness living in residential neighbourhoods'

A central part of the Bottomley plan was the Patients in the Community Act (1995) which brought in supervised discharge in England and Wales and community care orders in Scotland. Patients held under Section 3 could be placed on the order which required them to follow a treatment plan and reside in a specified place. They would then be allocated a supervisor (usually a community psychiatric nurse) who would monitor the plan, and if they refused to follow their treatment plan they could be taken and conveyed to a place where treatment could be given but not enforced. Because admission under the 1983 Act was required for compulsory treatment, supervised discharge was widely held to be 'toothless' (Pinfold et al., 1999) and thus was rarely used (i.e. one person per 100,000 of the general population). However, when it was utilised it did exert control over patients and in some cases facilitate medical treatment in the community (Pinfold et al., 2001; Atkinson et al., 2002).

Throughout the 1990s incidents of homicides and suicides were being discussed in the print media and academic press (Petch & Bradley, 1997; DH, 1999a). Whilst the statistical records showed that homicides by the mentally ill had been stable for the last forty years (Taylor & Gunn, 1999) public attention was being captured by single incidents. In 1997 the Department of Health's attitude survey revealed a significant rise in the public's fear of mentally ill people in the community. In that year there was widespread reporting of the case of Michael Stone (Francis et al., 2000) and the murder of Lin and Megan Russell.

In July 1996, Lin Russell and her two daughters were attacked, bound and beaten up whilst walking home in a country lane. Lin and Megan Russell were killed but Lucy Russell survived despite significant head injuries. Michael Stone, who had received care and treatment for a severe and dangerous personality disorder, was arrested and convicted of their murder. In the report that followed there was criticism of the mental health services and their interpretation of mental health law. At the time he was considered to be suffering from a severe and dangerous personality disorder that was not treatable and therefore was not detainable despite his repeat offending and drug use. The case added to the wider concern about public safety and increased the pressure for legislative reform.

The 1997 the new Labour government proposed a White Paper on reforming the Mental Health Act (DH, 2000). The draft bill was published in 2002 but was opposed by the Mental Health Alliance – a broad and organised group of over 30 stakeholders who feared that the bill did not adequately address the rights of patients and standards in the provision of services (Pilgrim, 2006). As a result the bill stumbled through revision after revision until it was dropped in 2006. Meanwhile legislators in Scotland had come to a workable solution and produced the Mental Health (Care and Treatment) (Scotland) Act 2003 which came into effect in October 2005. The stalled bill was revisited and for England and Wales parts of the bill were taken and used to amend the Mental Health Act 1983 and create the Mental Health Act 2007.

As regards detained patients living in England, Wales or Scotland they could now become subject to a compulsory treatment order and compelled to follow a treatment plan in the community or be recalled to hospital. Psychiatrists were initially circumspect about the value of community treatment orders but their use has exceeded expectation. From 2001 to 2012, in England there were 4,220 community treatment orders, for Wales 357, and for Scotland 744 community-based Compulsory

Treatment Orders (Health and Social Care Information Centre, 2012; Information Services Division, 2012; Welsh Government, 2012).

New powers within the Mental Health Act 2007 and the Mental Health (Care and Treatment) Scotland Act 2003 gave patients improved access to independent advocacy (a resource that has been extended in Wales through the Mental Health (Wales) Measure 2010). Qualifying patients could now benefit from an independent person representing their best interests as they navigated the mental health system. During the development of the legislation some patient groups – and notably professionals – argued that by extending the range of professionals eligible to take on statutory duties patients would benefit from improved multidisciplinary care. This opened up the way for two new roles for nurses: the Approved Mental Health Professional replacing the Approved Social Worker; and the Approved Clinician replacing the Responsible Medical Officer.

For mental health nurses working with people with severe and enduring mental health illness or intellectual impairment this provided an opportunity to locate statutory roles within advanced nursing practice and nurse consultant roles. On a wider front the modernisation of the NHS workforce nursing was also benefiting from an investment in numbers and increased responsibilities with an opportunity for better pay and increased autonomy. For people with psychosis this gave them the opportunity to have a responsible clinician with expertise in psychosocial care as well as knowledge and skills in diagnosis and prescribing medicines.

The legislative changes from 2005 to 2007 addressed a perceived failure of the Mental Health Act 1983 to provide a legal framework within the community. The use of CTOs has exceeded expectations and as with CPA is an example of reactive policy resulting in a driven rather than an evidence-based approach to service organisation and delivery. This policy has now been evaluated in Burns et al's (2013) randomised trial comparing CTOs with Section 17 leave, which showed that CTOs confer no additional benefits over the previous system but further restrict patients' freedom.

THE RISE AND FUTURE OF FUNCTIONAL TEAMS

The highly publicised tragedies of the 1990s revealed deficits in CMHTs' efforts to meet the needs of people with psychosis and schizophrenia. The resultant policy changes stressed increased care co-ordination activities and legislation to control patients. A review of care and treatment standards also showed that CMHTs were also failing to meet the physical and psychosocial care and treatment needs of this patient group (Gournay & Beadsmoore, 1995).

One response to improving standards for schizophrenia was the post-basic training of nurses and other professionals across the UK in psychological and psychosocial interventions for psychosis, in particular via the Thorn initiative (O'Carroll et al., 2004). During this time the number of CMHTs expanded and new types of teams were being developed and evaluated in the UK. These teams were known as functional teams because their efforts were focused on a specific activity – such as admission avoidance – rather than on a treatment approach or work focused on a diagnostic group. The teams included crisis, early intervention and assertive outreach teams.

The positive findings of early evaluations of functional teams (Merson et al., 1992) were being reported in new evidence summaries or briefings from the Sainsbury Centre for Mental Health (Minghell et al., 1998; Sainsbury Centre for Mental Health, 1998). These were influential because service managers and clinicians were able to quickly interpret and respond to evidence. They were also timely since they gave solutions to politicians who needed to respond to the negative events associated with community care (Francis et al., 2000).

The new Labour government of 1997 quickly set to work to improve community care, paradoxically declaring it a failure but then stating that they would stay with the policy but find a third way for mental health care (BBC, 1998). Their response was *Safe, Sound and Supportive* (DH, 1998) which described how early intervention, assertive outreach, crisis teams and modern treatments would contribute to a modern mental health service in England. Health and social care were to be devolved to the assemblies of Northern Ireland, Scotland and Wales, and the development of functional teams was described in their respective strategies.

In England the policy was supported by £300 million of investment representing a key difference from those of other nations. This new money was combined with the utilisation of clinical research to guide policy and an overarching aim of reducing inequalities in health care (described in *Our Healthier Nation,* DH, 1988). One means for reducing inequalities was the creation of national standards which would be delivered and monitored in England through the new institutions of the National Institute for Mental Health England and the Commission for Health Care Improvement.

The National Service Framework for England (DH, 1999b) made specific reference to improving mental health services for people with severe and enduring mental health problems through new service models and effective clinical interventions described by the National Institute for Clinical Evidence (NICE). Service managers and clinicians were directed – and more importantly funded – to create functional teams (DH, 2001). The detailed nature of the guidance represented micromanagement in the implementation of policy and contrasted with the preceding Conservative government's initial hands-off approach.

There was significant optimism that the new teams would provide better services for people in crisis and in significant need of help. However, not everyone anticipated that this early research would bring about better outcomes. Tom Burns, an academic psychiatrist and researcher into functional teams, drew attention to the limitations of developing services around early research findings. There was a significant risk of diverting resources away from what was confidently known to work but still poorly implemented (Burns, 2002). Much of the supporting research was from enthusiastic start-up teams within and from outside of the UK, representing different health services, team membership and control groups and with no long-term follow-up of the service.

By 2004 in England there were 168 assertive outreach teams, 263 crisis and home treatment teams, and 41 early intervention teams: by 2009 this number had risen to 250, 340 and 110 respectively (DH, 2004; Appleby, 2010). In Scotland and Wales the development of functional services or teams was described in each assembly strategy and national standards, but the money available was not ring-fenced to the same extent as England. In Wales health boards were given the freedom to decide whether a distinct team was required or whether the function could be delivered from within a CMHT.

As a result teams have been slower to develop if at all (see Table 4.1 for policy developments for the devolved governments). England's experience was a clear

Table 4.1   Key mental health policy, legislation since devolution in 1997

	England	Northern Ireland	Scotland	Wales
Policy	National Service Framework for Mental Health (1999)	Bamford Review of Mental Health and Learning Disability (Northern Ireland) (2006)	Delivering for Health (2006) Towards a Mentally Flourishing Scotland (2009)	Adult Mental Health Services for Wales: Equity, empowerment, effectiveness, efficiency (2001)
	The National Service Framework for Mental Health – Five years on (2004) New Horizons (2009) No Health Without Mental Health (2011)	Delivering the Bamford Vision: Action Plan 2009–2011 (2009)	Mental Health Strategy for Scotland: 2012–2015 (2012)	Mental Health Policy Wales Implementation Guidance: The Care Programme Approach for Mental Health Service Users (2003)
	Work, Recovery and Inclusion: Employment support for people in contact with secondary mental health services (2009)	Department for Health, Social Services and Public Safety (DHSSPS) (2009) Legislative framework for mental capacity and mental health legislation in Northern Ireland		Raising the Standard: The Revised Adult Mental Health National Service Framework and an Action Plan for Wales (2005) Together for Mental Health (2012)
Legislation	Mental Capacity Act (2005)	The Mental Health (Amendment) (Northern Ireland) Order 2004	Adults with Incapacity (Scotland) Act 2000.	Mental Capacity Act (2005)
	Mental Health Act (2007)		Mental Health (Care and Treatment) (Scotland) Act 2003	Mental Health Act (2007)
			Scottish Parliament Adult Support and Protection (Scotland) Bill (2006)	Mental Health (Wales) Measure 2010

example of how policy combined with an evidence base and financial and human resources could create real growth in the mental health infrastructure.

The specialisation of mental health teams reduced generic CMHTs to working with people with common mental health problems and people with long-term mental health problems who required specialist care or treatment or on-going supervision and support. The role of CMHTs became further diminished with the advent of Increasing Access to Psychological Therapies (IAPT) in England, and the increase in rehabilitation and recovery teams (Wolfson et al., 2009). Because of this in areas where services were highly specialised the need for a generic CMHT became less and their future uncertain.

Prior to the change of government in 2010 the dire state of public finances was being realised. The Labour government was unable to commit to further spending and in England the new mental health policy – *New Horizons* – (DH, 2009) reflected this by focusing on values rather than implementation guidance and commitments to spending.

This policy was short-lived because of the election of a new coalition government, and it was a full year before the Conservative/Social Democrat government published a health strategy for England. Entitled *No Health Without Mental Health: A Cross-Government Mental Health Outcomes Strategy for People of All Ages*, the new strategy focused on early intervention as a way to improve health, particularly in the early years (DH, 2011). The mechanism to deliver this would be through actions across departments, with the exception of continued support for IAPT, and seemed tenuously linked to mental health: for example, a method to improve mental health outcomes would be through the introduction of a 'Green

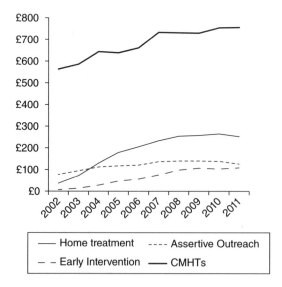

Figure 4.2 Comparison of investment in mental services from 2002 to 2011 (totals in millions) from 'Investment in mental health: working age adult and older adult reports'

deal' to support home energy improvements through the Department of Energy and Climate Change.

This strategy has resulted in the total investment in mental health services falling for the first time in ten years (DH, 2012). Assertive outreach teams started to see a reduction from 2009 and were joined by crisis and home treatment teams in 2010, whilst early intervention services saw a small rise with CMHTs still being the mainstay of the service investment in adult community services (see Figure 4.2).

The evidence base supporting functional teams has weakened. UK research into crisis, assertive and early intervention teams now questions the impact that these services make on hospital admissions and quality of life in the long term (Bird et al., 2010; Gafoor et al., 2010; Jacobs & Barrenho, 2011; Killaspy et al., 2009). Assertive outreach in particular has come under question with the discovery that CMHTs can achieve the same outcomes provided that they are organised to deliver some of the key functions of assertive outreach, such as frequent community visits and targeting the social care needs of the individual. These findings have increased the understanding of what works for whom and in what circumstances (Killaspy, 2012).

The 2010 coalition government's mental health policy is not prescriptive so service managers can freely integrate functional teams into a community mental health team and therefore reduce costs. Integrated community mental health teams are appearing in England and comprise of team members drawn from functional teams working on the specific tasks of home treatment, early intervention or assertive outreach.

The question for policy makers is whether integrated community mental health teams with small groups of practitioners can be effective when they are working within a diverse team sharing leadership, resources and wider objectives. The professionals within multidisciplinary teams are drawn together because no one individual can meet all the needs of a patient. Effective teams are known to comprise of 8 to 12 staff members who are adequately resourced and work on specific tasks with shared objectives and under good leadership. Functional teams are more likely than generic CMHTs to have these qualities (West et al., 2012).

The development of functional teams in the UK is illustrative of the dynamic relationship between evidence, policy and practice. Research and policy were combined to drive real changes to mental health services that promoted access to treatment and care for people with psychosis. Under financial constraints policy making has become less prescriptive, giving freedom to service planners to reshape teams into configurations that they believe will deliver the same benefits as stand-alone functional teams but at a lower cost.

SOCIAL INCLUSION AND RECOVERY FROM PSYCHOSIS

The term 'recovery' once described an outcome or state where the individual was free or had minimal symptoms of psychosis and was able to participate in social life. It has since moved to describing a process where resilience and fulfilment are attained in spite of symptoms. When the narrower but measurable view of recovery is taken one in seven people with schizophrenia may expect to recover (Jaaskelainen et al., 2012). This measure of clinical recovery has remained remarkably stable over time (Warner, 2004) and reminds us that the current treatments for psychosis have modest effects on symptoms and many effective treatments are difficult to access (Royal College of Psychiatrists, 2012; The Schizophrenia Commission, 2012).

Reducing symptoms and improving social functioning remain important outcomes and these have been assimilated into a revised view of recovery which includes a sense of connectedness, hope, identity, meaning and empowerment (Leamy et al., 2011). This has shifted the care focus from the biological to social and personal perspectives on positive outcomes. Recovery-based services are now concerned with empowering people with psychosis and promoting their inclusion in mainstream society (Repper & Perkins, 2003).

The 1997 Labour government wished to redress the inequalities of the Conservative years and championed social inclusion through the creation of the Social Inclusion Unit (this unit was abolished in 2010 by the coalition government, who demonstrated that the gap between rich and poor had increased under the Labour government: it was replaced by the Office for Civil Society). Labour's policy of social inclusion ran right through the government's health and social policy (Office of the Deputy Prime Minister, 2004). Its aims were to tackle the causes of exclusion such as joblessness, poverty and discrimination. In so doing it was anticipated that health inequalities would improve. This was later justified through Professor Sir Michael Marmot's (2010) review which established a clear link between social inequalities and poor health.

People with psychosis are disadvantaged economically and socially. In a European study looking into the personal impact of schizophrenia 79% were not in any work and 65% were single (Thornicroft et al., 2004). People with psychosis are also more likely to be the victims of crime (Maniglio, 2009) and experience discrimination (Thornicroft, 2006). Policy makers across the devolved nations have focused on broad initiatives that aim to tackle poor public knowledge, and prejudicial views about mental illness which could lead to discrimination and exclusion. These have included national anti-stigma campaigns such as Time to Change which have made an impact in addressing misconceptions about common and severe and enduring mental health problems (Nettle, 2013).

A specific area for policy makers was to address some of the barriers to employment. The welfare system in the UK was seen as an obstacle to people who wanted to work by paying them more to stay unemployed and not supporting people to return to work. There was also an economic argument for increasing access to effective psychological treatments because of the overall reduction in health and welfare costs (Layard et al., 2007). Investment in a new workforce for common mental health problems followed: for people with psychosis some investment found its way to NICE-recommended employment schemes such as individual place and support (IPS) (NICE, 2009). Labour's Welfare Reform Act 2007 and the coalition government's Welfare Reform Act 2012 shifted the emphasis from assessing what people could not do to what they were able do and making work pay more than being in recipt of benefits.

Whilst the current steps in welfare reform focus on reducing public costs social inclusion remains a strong aspect of mental health policy. In contrast to the 1970s, mental health service users – many of whom will have experienced psychosis – now play a key role in the commissioning of services. Numerous people have been supported back into work through IPS (Drake et al., 2012) and peer support offers a route into work for service users (a policy that positively discriminates for service users on the assertion that the lived experience of mental illness can deliver additional benefits – a claim yet to be proven, but one that tackles discrimination (Pitt et al., 2013)).

FUTURE POLICY FOR PSYCHOSIS

At the beginning of this chapter I proposed that policy development was subject to a range of individuals, groups and events that influence the decision making of politicians. This was seen in the 1980s when community care was slow to develop because of a lack of political will and therefore funding to accelerate the transition from hospital to community. Highly publicised failures in care, such as Ben Silcot and Christopher Clunis, mobilised politicians to introduce tighter controls and a new system of administering care called CPA.

These steps may have appeased the press and public who were concerned for but also fearful of the mentally ill. Such legal and bureaucratic actions have increased the administrative workload of staff and there are indications that today these systems are no better than the previous system in delivering service user-centred care (Thornicroft et al., 2013), the routine provision of effective interventions (The Schizophrenia Commission, 2012), and care for people in the least restrictive way (Burns et al., 2013).

The OCTET study (Burns et al., 2013) evaluated the impact of community treatment orders (CTOs) by randomly allocating patients to either Section 17 leave (the previous system) or CTOs and following up on the difference in outcome. This is an example of how research can test policy decisions and in this case they have tested the policy following rather than prior to implementation. The movement away from ideology and toward using research to constructing policy gathered apace under the 1997 Labour government, and continues through the Cabinet's Behavioural Insights Team and the lobbying of authors such as Ben Goldacre (Haynes et al., 2012).

Evidence coming principally from the USA and Australia was used to support the development of functional teams. The subsequent fate of assertive community treatment teams – where evidence of the clinical and financial benefits of the teams was drawn from a very different healthcare system – is illustrative of how evidence needs to be treated cautiously and critically. Promising interventions do catch the eye of policy makers but larger trials and replications are beneficial before their wider adoption.

The legacy of the Labour years has been that overall people with psychosis, particularly in England, were more likely to get help earlier, be helped to keep in contact with services, be supported back to work, and be treated at home rather than hospital during a crisis. Across the UK there is wide variation in the standards of services and still much to be concerned about (Royal College of Psychiatrists, 2012). People with psychosis continue to have problems accessing effective psychological and psychosocial interventions as opposed to pharmacological treatments (The Schizophrenia Commission, 2012). They are also likely live up to twenty years less because of the physical health problems associated with their condition, lifestyle and treatment.

The Schizophrenia Commission (2012) is an example of service users, professionals and carers attempting to influence policy makers in the way they direct funding and shape the actions of public and private service providers. Psychosis remains a disabling condition associated with an early age for onset, disability, and higher rates of mortality (Mueser & McGurk, 2004; Crump, 2013). Treating the condition remains expensive with total costs of £60,000 patient per year (Andrew et al., 2012) and with NHS costs greater than those for cancer or coronary heart disease (The Schizophrenia Commission, 2012). Mental health nurses should consider their role in influencing policy making, particularly as regards the future of policy development for psychosis. This is likely to be an argument for evidence-based teams and services that must deliver therapies – improving access to work, reducing stigma and discrimination, and gaining parity with physical health care.

Reflective Exercises

1. To what extent was policy in this area driven by political concerns regarding public safety?
2. Do you feel the emphasis on risk has given rise to a risk averse model of practice?
3. Psychosis is perhaps the most poorly understood aspect of mental health. To what extent do you think anti-stigma campaigns such as Time to Change have made a difference?
4. Co-production of care and a recovery ethos are considered fundamental to contemporary services. To what extent do you see this in current practice?

BIBLIOGRAPHY

Andrew, A., Knapp, M., McCrone, P., et al. (2012) *Effective Interventions in Schizophrenia: The Economic Case.* London: Rethink.

Appleby, L. (2010) Opening Address. Presented at Mental Health Nursing, 'On the horizon – or in clear focus?' Liverpool: Royal College of Nursing.

Atkinson, J.M. et al. (2002) The introduction and evaluation of Community Care Orders following the Mental Health (Patients in the Community) Act 1995, *Journal of Mental Health*, 11 (4): 417–429. doi:10.1080/09638230020023778.

Audit Commission (1984) *Making a Reality of Community Care*. London: HMSO.

BBC (1998, July 29) 'Third way' for mental health. Retrieved from http://news.bbc.co.uk/1/hi/health/141538.stm

Bird, V., Premkumar, P., Kendall, T., et al. (2010) Early intervention services, cognitive-behavioural therapy and family intervention in early psychosis: systematic review, *British Journal of Psychiatry*, 197 (5): 350–356. doi:10.1192/bjp.bp.109.074526.

Braun, P., Kochansky, G., Shapiro, R. et al. (1981) Overview: deinstitutionalization of psychiatric patients, a critical review of outcome studies, *American Journal of Psychiatry*, 138 (6): 736–749.

Burns, T. (2002) Mental health policy and evidence: potentials and pitfalls, *Psychiatric Bulletin*, 26 (9): 324–327. doi:10.1192/pb.26.9.324.

Burns, T., Rugkåsa, J., Molodynski, A. et al. (2013) Community treatment orders for patients with psychosis (OCTET): a randomised controlled trial, *The Lancet*. doi:10.1016/S0140-6736(13)60107-5.

Coid, J.W. (1994) The Christopher Clunis enquiry, *Psychiatric Bulletin*, 18 (8): 449–452. doi:10.1192/pb.18.8.449.

Crump, C. (2013) Comorbidities and mortality in persons with schizophrenia: a Swedish National Cohort Study, *American Journal of Psychiatry*. doi:10.1176/appi.ajp.2012.12050599.

Department of Health (1988) *Our Healthier Nation: A Contract for Health*. London: HMSO.

Department of Health (1990) *Care Programme Approach Circular HC(90)23/LASSL(90)11*. London: DH.

Department of Health (1995) *Building Bridges: A Guide to Arrangements for Interagency Working for the Care and Protection of Seriously Mentally Ill People*. London: HMSO.

Department of Health (1996) *The Spectrum of Care: Local Services for People with Mental Health Problems*. London: HMSO.

Department of Health (1998) *Modernising Mental Health Services: Safe, Sound and Supportive*. London: DH.

Department of Health (1999a) *Safer Services: Report of the National Confidential Inquiry into Suicide and Homicide by People with Mental Illness*. London: DH.

Department of Health (1999b) *National Service Framework for Mental Health: Modern Standards and Service Models*. London: DH.

Department of Health (2000) *Reforming the Mental Health Act*. London: HMSO.

Department of Health (2001) *The Mental Health Policy Implementation Guide*. London: DH.

Department of Health (2004) *The National Service Framework for Mental Health: Five Years On*. London: DH.

Department of Health (2009) *New Horizons: A Shared Vision for Mental Health*. London: DH.

Department of Health (2011) *No Health Without Mental Health: A Cross-Government Mental Health Outcomes Strategy for People of All Ages*. London: DH.

Department of Health (2012) *Investment in Mental Health: Working Age Adult and Older Adult Reports*. London: DH.

Department of Health and Social Services (1969) *Report of the Committee of Inquiry into Allegations of Ill-treatment of Patients and other Irregularities at the Ely Hospital, Cardiff*. London: HMSO.

Department of Health and Social Services (1998) *Report of the Committee of Inquiry into the Care and After-care of Miss Sharon Campbell* (Vol. Cm 440). London: HMSO.

DHSS (1971) *Hospital Services for the Mentally Ill*. London: HMSO.

DHSS (1975) *Better Service for the Mentally Ill*. London: HMSO.

Drake, R.E., Bond, G.R. & Becker, D.R. (2012) *Individual Placement and Support: An Evidence-Based Approach to Supported Employment*. Oxford: Oxford University Press.

Francis, R., Higgins, J. & Cassam, E. (2000) *Report of the Independent Inquiry into the Care and Treatment of Michael Stone*. South East Coast Strategic Health Authority. Retrieved from www.mentalhealthalliance.org.uk%2Fpolicy%2Fdocuments%2FMichael_Stone_briefing.pdf&ei=-OZIUPu3AsKg0QWP34GoBA&usg=AFQjCNFKQQOCX_p3pIp3iXlaS6zK_gGNvA

Gafoor, R., Nitsch, D., McCrone, P., et al. (2010) Effect of early intervention on 5-year outcome in non-affective psychosis, *British Journal of Psychiatry*, 196 (5): 372–376. doi:10.1192/bjp.bp.109.066050.

Gournay, K. & Beadsmoore, A. (1995) The report of the clinical standards advisory group: standards of care for people with schizophrenia in the UK and implications for mental health nursing, *Journal of Psychiatric and Mental Health Nursing*, 2 (6), 359–364. doi:10.1111/j.1365-2850.1995.tb00106.x

Haynes, L., Service, O., Goldacre, B. & Allen, D. (2012) *Test, Learn, Adapt: Developing Public Policy with Randomised Controlled Trials*. London: The Cabinet Office.

Health and Social Care Information Centre (2012) *Inpatients Formally Detained in Hospitals under the Mental Health Act 1983, and Patients Subject to Supervised Community Treatment, Annual Figures, England, 2011/12*. London: Government Statistical Service.

House of Commons (1984) *Report of the House of Commons Social Services Committee Inquiry Into Community Care for Adult Mentally Ill and Mentally Handicapped People*. London: HMSO.

Information Services Division (2012) *Adult Mental Health Benchmarking Toolkit*. Edinburgh: Information Services Division.

Jaaskelainen, E., Juola, P., Hirvonen, N., et al. (2012) A systematic review and meta-analysis of recovery in schizophrenia, *Schizophrenia Bulletin*. doi:10.1093/schbul/sbs130

Jacobs, R. & Barrenho, E. (2011) Impact of crisis resolution and home treatment teams on psychiatric admissions in England, *British Journal of Psychiatry*, 199 (1): 71–76. doi:10.1192/bjp.bp.110.079830

Kalucy, M., Rodway, C., Finn, J., et al. (2011) Comparison of British national newspaper coverage of homicide committed by perpetrators with and without mental illness, *Australian and New Zealand Journal of Psychiatry*, 45 (7): 539–548. doi:10.3109/00048674.2011.585605

Killaspy, H. (2012) Importance of specialisation in psychiatric services: Commentary on... How did we let it come to this?, *The Psychiatrist*, 36 (10): 364–365. doi:10.1192/pb.bp.112.039537.

Killaspy, H., Kingett, S., Bebbington, P., et al. (2009) Randomised evaluation of assertive community treatment: 3-year outcomes, *British Journal of Psychiatry*, 195 (1): 81–82.

Knapp, M., Beecham, J., Anderson, J., et al. (1990) The TAPS project. 3: Predicting the community costs of closing psychiatric hospitals, *British Journal of Psychiatry*, 157 (5): 661–670. doi:10.1192/bjp.157.5.661.

Layard, R., Clarke, D., Knapp, M. & Mayraz, G. (2007) *Cost-benefit Analysis of Psychological Therapy*. London: London School of Economics and Political Science.

Leamy, M., Bird, V., Le Boutillier, C., et al. (2011) Conceptual framework for personal recovery in mental health: systematic review and narrative synthesis, *British Journal of Psychiatry*, 199 (6): 445–452. doi:10.1192/bjp.bp.110.083733.

Maniglio, R. (2009) Severe mental illness and criminal victimization: a systematic review, *Acta Psychiatrica Scandinavica*, 119 (3): 180–191. doi:10.1111/j.1600-0447.2008.01300.x

Marks, I., Connolly, J. & Muijen, M. (1988) The Maudsley Daily Living Programme: a controlled cost-effectiveness study of community-based versus standard in-patient care of serious mental illness, *Psychiatric Bulletin*, 12 (1): 22–24. doi:10.1192/pb.12.1.22.

Marmot, M. (2010) *Marmot Review: Fair Society, Healthy Lives – Strategic Review of Health Inequalities in England Post 2010*. London: Marmot Review.

Marshall, M. (1996) Case management: a dubious practice, *BMJ*, 312 (7030): 523–524. doi:10.1136/bmj.312.7030.523.

Merson, S., Tyrer, P., Lack, S., et al. (1992) Early intervention in psychiatric emergencies: a controlled clinical trial, *The Lancet*, 339 (8805): 1311–1314. doi:10.1016/0140-6736(92)91959-C

Minghell, E., Ford, R., Freeman, T., et al. (1998) *Open All Hours: 24-hour Response for People with Mental Health Emergencies*. London: Sainsbury Centre for Mental Health.

Mueser, K.T. & McGurk, S.R. (2004) Schizophrenia, *The Lancet*, 363 (9426): 2063–2072. doi:10.1016/S0140-6736(04)16458-1.

Murphy, E. (1991) *After the Asylums: Community Care for People with Mental Illness*. London: Faber and Faber.

Nettle, M. (2013) Time to Change campaign through the eyes of a service user. Invited commentary on … Evaluation of England's Time to Change programme, *British Journal of Psychiatry*, 202 (s55): s102–s103. doi:10.1192/bjp.bp.113.127423

NICE (2009) *Schizophrenia (CG82): Core Interventions in the Treatment and Management of Schizophrenia in Primary and Secondary Care (update)*. London: NICE.

North, C., Ritchie, J. & Ward, K. (1993) *Factors Influencing the Implementation of The Care Programme Approach*. London: HMSO.

O'Carroll, M., Rayner, L. & Young, N. (2004) Education and training in psychosocial interventions: a survey of Thorn Initiative course leaders, *Journal of Psychiatric and Mental Health Nursing*, 11 (5): 602–607. doi:10.1111/j.1365-2850.2004.768.x

Office of the Deputy Prime Minister (2004) *Mental Health and Social Exclusion*. London: HMSO.

Patmore, C. & Weaver, T. (1991) *Community Mental Health Teams: Lessons for Planners and Managers*. London: Good Practices in Mental Health.

Pauley, R. (1984, November 13) The Economic Statement: NHS faces squeeze, *The Financial Times*, p. 13.

Petch, E. & Bradley, C. (1997) Learning the lessons from homicide inquiries: adding insult to injury?, *Journal of Forensic Psychiatry*, 8 (1): 161–184. doi:10.1080/09585189708412002

Pilgrim, D. (2006) New 'mental health' legislation for England and Wales: some aspects of consensus and conflict, *Journal of Social Policy*, 36 (01): 79–95. doi:10.1017/S0047279406000389

Pinfold, V., Bindman, J., Friedli, K., et al. (1999) Supervised discharge orders in England: compulsory care in the community, *Psychiatric Bulletin*, 23 (4): 199–203. doi:10.1192/pb.23.4.199.

Pinfold, V., Bindman, J., Thornicroft, G., et al. (2001) Persuading the persuadable: evaluating compulsory treatment in England using Supervised Discharge Orders, *Social Psychiatry and Psychiatric Epidemiology*, 36 (5): 260–266. doi:10.1007/s001270170058.

Pitt, V., Lowe, D., Hill, S., et al. (2013) 'Consumer-providers of care for adult clients of statutory mental health services'. In The Cochrane Collaboration and D. Lowe (eds), *Cochrane Database of Systematic Reviews*. Chichester: Wiley. Retrieved from http://doi.wiley.com/10.1002/14651858.CD004807.pub2

Repper, J. and Perkins, R. (2003) *Social Inclusion and Recovery: A Model for Mental Health Practice*. Edinburgh: Baillière Tindall.

Ritchie, J.H. (1994) *The Report of the Inquiry into the Care and Treatment of Christopher Clunis*. London: HMSO.

Royal College of Psychiatrists (1980) A discussion document by a working party of the Social and Community Psychiatry Section, *Psychiatric Bulletin*, 4 (8): 114–118. doi:10.1192/pb.4.8.114.

Royal College of Psychiatrists (2012) *National Audit of Schizophrenia*. London: Royal College of Psychiatrists.

Sainsbury Centre for Mental Health (1998) *Keys to Engagement: Review of Care for People with Severe Mental Illness Who Are Hard to Engage with Services*. London: Sainsbury Centre For Mental Health.

Scottish Office (1992) *Community Care: Guidance on Care Programmes for People with a Mental Illness Including Dementia, Circular SWSG 1/92*.

Scottish Office (1996) *Community Care: Care Programme Approach for People with Severe and Enduring Mental Illness Including Dementia, Circular SWSG16/96*. Retrieved from http://mars.northlan.gov.uk/xpedio/groups/public/documents/report/053729.pdf

Simpson, A., Miller, C. & Bowers, L. (2003) The history of the care programme approach in England: Where did it go wrong?, *Journal of Mental Health*, 12 (5): 489–504.

Stein, L.I. & Test, M.A. (1980) Alternative to mental hospital treatment. I. Conceptual model, treatment program, and clinical evaluation, *Arch Gen Psychiatry*, 37: 392–397.

Taylor, P.J. & Gunn, J. (1999) Homicides by people with mental illness: myth and reality, *British Journal of Psychiatry*, 174 (1): 9–14. doi:10.1192/bjp.174.1.9

The Schizophrenia Commission (2012) *The Abandoned Illness*. London: Rethink.

Thornicroft, G. (2006) *Shunned: Discrimination against People with Mental Illness*. Oxford: Oxford University Press.

Thornicroft, G., Farrelly, S., Szmukler, G., et al. (2013) Clinical outcomes of Joint Crisis Plans to reduce compulsory treatment for people with psychosis: a randomised controlled trial, *The Lancet*. doi:10.1016/S0140-6736(13)60105-1

Thornicroft, G., Tansella, M., Becker, T., et al. (2004) The personal impact of schizophrenia in Europe, *Schizophrenia Research*, 69 (2–3): 125–132.

Timmins, N. (1994, February 25) Christopher Clunis Report: Schizophrenic made 'series of violent attacks', *The Independent*.

Wallace, M. (1985, December 17) Spectrum: Through an open door to despair, *The Times*.

Warner, R. (2004) *Recovery from Schizophrenia: Psychiatry and Political Economy*. Hove: Brunner-Routledge.

Welsh Assembly Government (2003) *Mental Health Policy Wales: Implementation Guidance: The Care Programme Approach for Mental Health Service Users*. Cardiff: Welsh Assembly Government.

Welsh Government (2012) *Admission of Patients to Mental Health Facilities in Wales, 2011–12 (including patients detained under the Mental Health Act 1983) and Patients Subject to Supervised Community Treatment*. Cardiff: Welsh Government.

West, M., Alimo-Metcalfe, B., Dawson, J., et al. (2012) *Effectiveness of Multi-Professional Team Working (MPTW) in Mental Health Care*. London: National Institute for Health Research.

Wolfson, P., Holloway, F. & Killaspy, H. (2009) *Enabling Recovery for People with Complex Mental Health Needs*. London: Royal College of Psychiatrists.

5 OLDER PEOPLE

Elizabeth Collier and Catherine McQuarrie

Chapter Overview

Ageing remains inevitable and not (currently) subject to choice, yet in this chapter the authors will argue that how we as a society respond to the needs of those who age and indeed require mental health care is a matter of choice. It has been speculated that the general level of hostility expressed towards those who age (all of us surely) is really an expression of the fear of the ageing process and the losses people may experience.

Yet the provision of services to older clients has never been more necessary as the demographics of the society we live in are transformed by the growing number of older people. People are living longer and thus accordingly requiring services for a longer period of time. Individuals with substance use issues may realistically be expected to live to an age where they will receive service for older people as will those who are HIV positive. This changing client profile will require a rethink amongst service providers. As a consequence of the economic situation in Britain at the time of writing there are proposed changes to when individuals can retire and receive their pension. The current arbitrary age of 65 as the threshold for old age would seem to be about to be redefined.

Our understanding of what actually constitutes old age or being elderly may be about to be transformed. You can usefully consider these issues when you have read the chapter by considering the questions at the end of the chapter.

INTRODUCTION

Reference to delineated age groups is a fairly universal way of organising health services, and the UK is no exception. In England and Wales mental health policy has historically remained focused on adults of working age, that is 18 to 64, although

Scotland has maintained an inclusive policy for all ages. Northern Ireland has organised mental health policy around psychiatric diagnosis rather than age, however older people are categorised as having specific needs. An age-inclusive approach has recently been adopted in England with the publication of *No Health Without Mental Health* (DH, 2011). Implementing policy focused around mental health/ill health for the benefit of people who are older is recognised as a challenge because of age discrimination (Bytheway et al., 2007; Collier, 2007; DH, 2008; Scottish Government, 2011). Age discrimination has been commonplace in health and social care (Welsh Assembly Government, 2006; Age Concern, 2008; Beecham et al., 2008; DH, 2009a; Mental Health Foundation, 2009; RCP, 2009b; CPA, 2009) and at its worst in mental health care (Anderson, 2011). For this reason challenging age discrimination has been common to policies focused on older people internationally, as have mental health promotion, healthy living, independence, and aims for integrated services (Adams & Collier, 2009).

Public health policy focuses on prevention and staying healthy, but for the people we meet in specialist mental health services their goals will usually relate to recovering in the context of existing mental health problems. This may complicate the implementation of public health policy when people with mental health problems may be denied access to public health initiatives, which is potentially more likely when they are older (Scottish Government, 2012).

This chapter aims to provide a context by which to understand older people's mental health policy, and will discuss several issues that are implicated in how policy guides practice in relation to mental health care for people who are older. It will also explore how an older person is defined together with the historical influence regarding older people and mental illness and how this has influenced policy, before going on to focus on mental health policy in the context of social inclusion for older people.

HOW AN OLDER PERSON IS DEFINED

The age of 65 has traditionally delineated between adulthood and old age and this has largely informed health and social care organisation since the mid-twentieth century. This may be a useful framework for the organisation of services but it is an arbitrary figure: 50 years of age is recognised as a defining feature and common reference point for older age (DH, 2001a; DWP, 2005; Welsh Assembly Government, 2006; Scottish Government, 2012). Average life expectancy in the UK is now 82.1 for women and 78.1 for men (ONS, 2008–2010) and perceptions of middle age have been reported as 63 (Panayotes et al., 2007). This raises many questions about public and private definitions of old age and so it remains a relative concept. However one consistent challenge for people perceived as older is discrimination and negative attitudes.

Most research studies on the experience of long-term mental illness do not include people over the age of 65, and in studies where age groups are indicated these will often appear by decade up to the age of 65 and then with an over-65 category (Collier, 2012). This reflects an attitude that is pervasive across mental

Table 5.1 Estimated population figures for over 50s in the UK 2010

Age	Number of people
50–59	7,558,000
60–69	6,692,000
70–79	4,471,000
80–89	2,787,000
90–99	465,000
100+	12,000

(ONS, 2011)

health research, policy and practice (i.e. older people seen as an homogeneous group). It can be seen from Table 5.1 that there are four more categories of age by decade after age 65, and it is recognised that many of these people may be carers for their own parents (DH, 2010).

Approximately 8% of over 60s in England and Wales are from Black and minority ethnic (BME) groups (Falkingham et al., 2010).

OLDER PEOPLE AND MENTAL ILLNESS

In order to understand the mental health policy of the present day it is important to consider first where this has come from from a historical point of view, and how the conceptualisation of mental ill health in later life has changed and developed. Dementia has traditionally been perceived as a normal part of the ageing process, and this has contributed to nihilistic attitudes to older age resulting in beliefs that older people cannot be treated (Hilton, 2005). Evidence to the contrary slowly emerged throughout the twentieth century, and prevalence figures for dementia in the over 65s are now reported, for example, as 1.3% for 60 to 69 year olds and 20.3% for 85 to 89 year olds (Alzheimer's Society, 2007). However, there is a disproportionate focus on dementia and mental capacity in academic literature (Cohen et al., 2000; Collier, 2006). It is the mental health of older people (and indeed young people) that is most negated (MIND, 2005), and there is evidence that old age is still equated with inevitable cognitive decline by some professional staff who may also believe that nothing can be done for older people with depression (DH, 2008).

It is unclear whether psychiatric classifications have influenced ageist beliefs, or that society's ageist beliefs have influenced psychiatric classifications (Collier, 2008). Nevertheless psychiatric classification has been criticised for being developed with younger samples and thus older people are outside the threshold for diagnosis (Beekman et al., 1999). In addition, cultural differences are poorly understood (DH, 2001a; Audit Commission, 2002). The ageist idea of old age being synonymous with ill health and disability is demonstrated by use of the term 'old old' which has come to refer not only to the over 85s but to people over 65 who are chronically ill and/or disabled regardless of their chronological age (Komp et al., 2009). This contributes to two main tensions in health and social care policy for older people: the promotion of active, healthy, person-centred and individualistic approaches which contrast with those suggestive of passivity, decline, loss and categorisation (DH, 2008). The latter contributes to a view of long-term care needs as associated with disability, frailty and continuing chronic conditions such as stroke and dementia (DH, 2005d; 2008).

The discrimination associated with having mental illness is well established, and older people with mental health problems may experience the double jeopardy of discrimination on the basis of being both old and mentally unwell (Jenkins & Laditka, 1998). This idea of double jeopardy has also been applied to older people from BME populations because of being older and from an ethnic minority who are further marginalised from having their needs met (DH, 2009b), so if mental illness is added here older people with mental health problems from black and minority ethnic origins potentially face multiple barriers to equality. Ethnic origin however was not indicated as a risk for social exclusion by the Institute of Fiscal Studies (2006), who reported that the risk factors for social exclusion comprised of:

- being 80 and over;
- living alone;
- having no living children;
- having poor mental or physical health;
- having no access to a private car and never uses public transport;
- living in rented accommodation;
- having a low income with benefits as the main source of income;
- living without access to a telephone.

OLDER PEOPLE AND MENTAL HEALTH POLICY

Public health policy across the UK tends to be categorised with reference to age and stage of life, such as starting well in children and young people, developing well, living well, employment and working life, and ageing well in later life (Scottish Executive 2003; www.dh.gov.uk/health/category/ageing/), with 'ageing well' referring to people aged 45 or older. Service frameworks focused on the needs of older people have many similarities, such as rooting out age discrimination, promoting health, preventing falls and stroke, and intermediate care and mental health (DH, 2001a; Welsh Assembly Government, 2006; DHSSPS, 2009), though Northern Ireland also includes dental and sexual health. Scotland's plan for an ageing population focuses on issues such as the links between generations, quality of life, housing, transport and infrastructure, and learning opportunities, as well as removing barriers to these for older people (Scottish Executive, 2007).

Policies for older people are often dominated by a biomedical model of ageing (DH, 2008), and have been inadvertently ageist themselves (Baldwin, 2003; Benbow, 2005; Collier, 2005) in terms of access to comprehensive mental health policy developments aimed at 18 to 64 year olds (DH, 1999, 2001b; Welsh Assembly Government, 2005), a risk that is recognised even within the existing age-inclusive mental health policy for Scotland (Scottish Government, 2011). In addition, it has been recognised that assessments of mental health in older people may be culturally biased (DH, 2001b; Audit Commission, 2002), with assumptions being made regarding, for example, family willingness to act as primary carers for older relatives (Shah, 2009). Paradoxically, Asian older people have been reported as interpreting offers of help as questioning the presence and willingness of family support (DH, 2008).

The Equality Act (2010) has formalised the need to ensure older people are not excluded from services as it has long been recognised that health services should be accessible on the basis of clinical need rather than age (MIND, 2005; DH, 2005a, 2005c, 2006, 2008). However, people who enter 'old age' with pre-existing mental health problems (formerly referred to as graduates; Campbell & Ananth, 2002) were traditionally transferred from adult to old age services at age 65. This practice was recognised as problematic as many people became lost to services at this transition point, some as a result of death by natural causes, suicide or homelessness (Abdul-Hamid et al., 1998; Campbell & Ananth, 2002). One of the few studies examining this issue found that being transferred between services resulted in reconfigured relationships, resigned acceptance, and a catalyst for re-examining what it meant to get old with access to certain types of care becoming limited or impossible (Dadswell, 2005). To try to resolve such problems, transition policies were encouraged for people being transferred from adult to old age services (RCP, 2002; DHSSPS, 2010) in order to meet age equality requirements (National Mental Health Development Unit, 2011a, 2011b). The Royal College of Psychiatrists (2002) also recommended that GPs find out how many graduates there were registered in primary care but this was ignored (Bawn et al., 2007), with the result that no figures exist for this group.

Debate continues between rehabilitation, adult and old age psychiatry about who should be providing a service for older people with long-term mental health problems (Abdul-Hamid et al., 2011). However, the practice of transition from adult to old age services at age 65 appears to be gradually changing so that this only happens for people who also develop complex physical health needs or dementia (RCP, 2009a; Healthcare Commission, 2009). The distinction between the needs of people who present for the first time in later life and those who enter old age with pre-existing mental health problems is important because of the potential for differing needs, for example the long-term effect of social and economic disadvantage and disruptions in relationships from earlier adulthood for the latter (Cummings & Kropf, 2011; Collier, 2012). The potentially complex needs of older people who have pre-existing mental health problems are not well understood (Collier, 2012) and this makes them invisible to policy makers (Abdul-Hamid et al., 1998; Cohen et al., 2000; Wrigley et al., 2006). There is a risk that they will be ignored by both general psychiatry (adult services) and old age psychiatry (Campbell & Ananth, 2002).

Current mental health policy aims to reduce stigma and discrimination in relation to mental illness (Welsh Assembly Government, 2005; DHSSPS, 2010; DH, 2011; Scottish Government, 2011) but does not maintain previous policy initiatives to root out age discrimination. This is unfortunate, particularly as in England for example older people were included in mental health policy directly for the first time in 2011. However, indirect discrimination (that is, discrimination communicated in assumptions and attitudes) remains a risk (CPA, 2009), and this may compromise meeting the needs of people who are older (Scottish Government, 2011). The experience of age discrimination itself can have an impact on a person's mental health (www.wellscotland.info).

Recovery approaches have developed to form the cornerstone of much mental health policy (DH, 2005b; Smith-Merry et al., 2010) which aims to provide a framework of positive expectations in relation to people who use mental health services. If older people are going to benefit from their inclusion in a mental health policy for all adults then there are many challenges, not least as to how the principles of recovery can be adopted with people who may have negative assumptions made about them. Other perceptions of the needs of older people may not match those of the people themselves (Heikkinen, 2000; Dadswell, 2005; Strauss, 2008). Heikkinen (2000) found that no sense of being old emerged until after the age of 85 when the physical body became an explicit concern and physical props such as walking aids affected how others perceived them. The mental health needs of people who are older and physically frail therefore have to be addressed within the particular life context and not assumed, and perhaps disbelief has to be suspended (Perkins & Tice, 1995). It is here where the tensions become apparent, as there will be people who continue to have high support needs (as do people of all ages) and many of these needs may concern a lack of access to information, money, technology, equipment and transport (Blood, 2010). For this reason the remainder of the chapter will focus on mental health promotion in the context of social inclusion, with a view to exploring how positive expectations and attitudes might be nurtured in the context of people who are older.

Promoting mental health is common across UK mental health policy and this includes paying particular attention to social inclusion. However, people who are older have not necessarily benefitted from these initiatives, possibly because of the persistent care narratives evident in discourse about older people rather than a recognition of older people as citizens with aspirations (Bowers et al., 2005). One example of this attitude is demonstrated in the national minimum standards for care homes documents published by the Department of Health (England) (2003a, 2003b) where reference to aspirations appears only in the document relating to 'adults (18–64)' but is missing from that which refers to older people (Collier & Yates-Bolton, 2011). There is a danger that health and social services become preoccupied with health and social care needs, and thus risk missing quality of life issues that are important protective factors in mental health and wellbeing, in particular for older adults (Katz et al., 2011).

For people with mental health problems who are older, the challenge in adopting recovery values and positive expectations of their abilities is a work in progress. Despite the vast literature on recovery, there appears to be only one research study that specifically asked older people about their experiences. The paper by Daley et al. (2012) found three distinct components of recovery for older people which differed from those found with younger people. These were: the significance of an established and enduring sense of identity, coping strategies which provide continuity and reinforce identity, and the associated impact of physical illness. One principle of contemporary recovery is the need to have positive expectations of people with mental illness, as psychiatric patients are citizens capable of contributing and being included in society (Sayce, 2000; Repper &

Perkins, 2003). This sense of citizenship is also of paramount importance to people who are older (Craig, 2004; DWP, 2005). The values of contemporary recovery are mirrored to a certain extent in some older people policy where there is an emphasis on remaining active and healthy, on active agency in ageing, and on the promotion of wellbeing and choice (DH, 2008), all of which will have implications for mental health. In 2005 the Department of Work and Pensions stated:

> During the 20th century the state gradually assumed an increasing share of responsibility for people past State Pension Age, on the patronising assumption that age equalled dependence. It is clear that in the 21st century we need a new and more sophisticated model, which recognises the potential of older people and the need to reflect that in a changed role in society. We must support independence rather than enforcing dependence, and develop policies and services that respond to need rather than simply to chronological age. (DWP, 2005: viii/ix).

The Scottish Government has recognised the need for social justice and independence which views the skills of older people as an asset and strives to remove the barriers to occupational activity, such as paid and volunteering work, learning opportunities, leisure culture and sport (Scottish Executive, 2007).

OLDER ADULTS, MENTAL HEALTH PROMOTION AND SOCIAL INCLUSION

Social exclusion has been defined as 'a shorthand term for what can happen when people or areas suffer from a combination of linked problems such as unemployment, poor skills, low incomes, poor housing, high crime, bad health and family breakdown' (SEU, 2005: 3). It has also been described as society's inability to keep all groups and individuals within reach of what we would expect as a society (Levitas, 1998). The impact this can have on people's mental health and wellbeing has many dimensions. This can take the form of a combination of isolation and alienation from economic, social, political and cultural life (Oppenheim, 1998).

A Life Course Approach to health inequalities has particular relevance to the issue of social inclusion. This approach exposes the hazards that people are exposed to in life, and the impact these hazards can have if they accumulate over time to impact on health and inequalities (Bartley, 2004). In relation to mental health and social inclusion a life-course perspective indicates that poor educational attainment, coming from poorer households and disadvantage in life can all contribute to someone's mental health status in later life (CAB, 2003). However, people of working age with long term-mental ill health and without access to specialist support have been recognised as a neglected majority (Rethink, 2004; SCMH, 2005). It may be that older people with long-term mental health problems can be considered the neglected minority of the neglected majority, as they remain invisible (McKay, 2010) despite having special needs (Jolley et al., 2004).

Feelings of stigma and discrimination around mental health problems can have a considerable impact on whether someone finds support, as these can even prevent discussing illness with friends and family (CAB, 2003). Black older people have been found to believe that mental health services have no relevance for them (Marwaha & Livingstone, 2002). Stigma and discrimination are still, despite various campaigns to tackle these issues, prevalent for people with mental health problems (Social Exclusion Unit, 2004). Joint working with employment, education, housing, voluntary sector and leisure providers, so that people can make a seamless transition from using mental health services to engaging in these other roles in the community, needs to be considered in promoting inclusion (SCMC, 2002).

The Social Care Institute for Excellence (SCIE, 2010) detailed six areas that were conducive to the development of social inclusion in practice:

- Access to social networks should be promoted and supported.
- Transport issues should be resolved so that people can be involved in activities in the wider community.
- Strong links should be built with community centres and schools to increase the levels of social contact between different age groups.
- People's skills should be identified, respected and used, thereby giving people ordinary opportunities to participate in the wider community through the use of developed person-centred planning.
- People should be involved in service planning, taking into account their ideas and suggestions.

Mental health problems can result from a range of adverse factors associated with social exclusion, for example in relation to employment and poverty. Unemployed people are twice as likely to have depression as people in work, and children in the poorest households are three times more likely to have mental health problems than children in well-off households (DH, 1999). There has been evidence to suggest that there is a positive association between mental health and employment, with people in work enjoying better mental health than those who are unemployed, and that the longer someone is out of work the greater the impact this will have on someone's mental health and wellbeing (Scottish Association of Mental Health, 2011). Indeed it is people who use mental health services that are likely to be poor, unemployed, living in substandard housing and socially isolated (SCMH, 2002). People with mental health problems face severe issues in the employment market: losing a job because of ill health and failing to regain employment following a period of illness contribute to users of mental health services being the most severely hit of all disabled groups, with the lowest rate of employment (CAB, 2004). In their 2006 report, 'Paying the Price: The real costs of illness and disability for CAB clients', Citizens Advice Scotland found that only as few as 13% of their clients who had mental health problems were in employment (CAS, 2007).

Employment is seen as one of the most conducive factors in maintaining mental health and wellbeing and promoting inclusion. Unemployed people are at a significant risk of becoming socially excluded and experiencing mental health problems, with suicide being a high risk within this group. The change of role experienced on retirement and the loss of social connection that the function of work gives can often lead to feelings of isolation and loneliness. Involvement in the workforce can decrease stigma and remains important throughout life (McKay, 2010) and this includes the wider concept of occupation, for example volunteering.

In England 65 to 74 year olds have the highest rate of formal volunteering for adults over the age of 16 (Communities and Local Government, 2007/8). However, the European Foundation for the Improvement of Living and Working Conditions has stated:

> The population beyond retirement age is, of course, large – and growing – but also diverse, with different economic, health and social resources. These different conditions and experiences influence opportunities and preferences for participation in voluntary activities. One of the main reasons for lower rates of volunteering is the poor living conditions of some groups of people, who often have to cope not only with low income but also with physical disabilities. It is important, therefore, to strengthen broader policy strategies such as national health and income policies that target the general improvement of living conditions of older people. Programmes tailored specifically to the involvement of older people as volunteers are rare. (Ehlers et al., 2011: 8)

ACTIVITY 1

Read Vignette 1 below. How would you respond to Roy's question and help facilitate his goal?

Vignette 1

Jane is a student nurse who meets Roy on an assessment ward for older people. Roy is 66 years old and has been experiencing depression for some time. In a conversation with Roy, Jane learns that he really misses going out for long walks with his dog. Roy's dog Sandy died a year ago and he remains distressed about this loss as Sandy was his long-term companion and he had shared his life with him for twenty years. Jane is aware of a local animal sanctuary that uses volunteer dog walkers and asks Roy if he would like to visit. Roy enjoys the experience and asks how he would go about becoming a regular volunteer.

The statutory retirement age is increasing and the state pension age will increase to 65 for all by November 2018, 66 by 2020, and 68 between 2044 and 2046 (House of Commons, 2012): older people may then be seen to remain longer or wish to re-enter the workplace. One of the key policy considerations from some governments is that of identifying how labour market participation can be increased for older age groups (Scottish Government, 2010). However, an examination of training participation by age amongst unemployed and inactive people identified that for older adults (50+)

some of the major barriers to their gaining employment from a personal perspective was a lack of confidence and qualifications, and from an employer perspective, negative attitudes to training older people and the length of time they may have been unemployed (Newton et al., 2005). These problems may be compounded by long-term mental ill health as this has been found to result in early retirement from the workforce (Rice et al., 2011; Collier, 2012). Newton et al. (2005) also found that people felt tarnished by the stigma of redundancy, as well as being seen as unable to deal with change, slow to learn and forgetful. Discrimination in employment on the basis of age has also been found for people over the age of 40 (Joseph Rowntree Foundation, 2002).

In 2006, The Sure Start to Later Life (Office of Deputy Prime Minister, 2006) report stated that:

- 9 out of 10 older people believed that employers discriminate against them;
- a quarter spoke from experience;
- 10% of companies did not employ persons aged over 50;
- One million people over the state pension age were in paid employment;
- the majority of people said they would consider working after formal retirement, but would do so on a part-time or flexible basis;
- feeling valued, in control and having job flexibility were important factors in staying in work up to and beyond state retirement age.

The report also stated:

> Older people have told us that they see employment past retirement age as an opportunity. For some it can provide a much needed supplement to pension income. For others the main motivation is a sense of worth and of contributing and of identity ... It is estimated that the relatively lower level of employment among older workers costs the economy £19–£31 billion a year in lost output and taxes and increased welfare payments. (2006: 100)

The Foresight Mental Capital and Wellbeing Project (2008) reported in relation to older people that there was a need to 'reverse the continued negative stereotyping and massive under-utilisation of their mental capital', thus bring positive improvements for older adults and society as a whole. They also advocated that the government adopted a life-course approach and the appointment of a 'high level lead within government to ensure sustainable long term action' (2008: 32). Although the Department of Health in England has since responded with a life-course policy in No Health Without Mental Health (DH, 2011), there is still a risk of people being categorised into delineated age categories.

ACTIVITY 2

Read Vignette 2 below. How will you assist Eleanor with her aspiration and what agencies could you utilise in supporting her? (Some potential resources are shown at the end of the chapter.)

Vignette 2

Eleanor is a 69 year old woman who attends the CMHT drop-in cafe and has mentioned to you that she misses work. She feels that she would like to re-enter the work force in some capacity as she believes it will give her a purpose and structure to her life as well as social contact, something she has been missing following the death of her husband eighteen months previously.

CONCLUSION

In relation to older adults there is some suggestion that this group are particularly vulnerable to becoming socially excluded from society (SEU, 2005). Social isolation is an important risk factor in relation to mental health and wellbeing, and a combination of factors in later life can impact on someone's ability to maintain their role as an active citizen. Mental wellbeing is crucial to fulfilling life roles and enabling people to realise their personal potential. At a societal level, mental wellbeing is a resource for social cohesion and better social and economic welfare (Keyes, 2002).

There is a need to harness the experience and wealth of knowledge that exists within the older adult population and challenge our assumptions about the abilities or needs that older people with mental health problems have. Utilising mental wealth (such as cognitive and emotional resources, emotional intelligence, social skills and resilience) will create an environment where people will feel able to contribute to their community (Beddington et al., 2008).

This chapter has highlighted the particular challenges in relation to mental health policy in the context of people who are older. It remains to be seen how practitioners involved in implementing mental health policy in practice can contribute to shifting attitudes towards older people, and ensure equal access to initiatives aimed at occupation and employment despite their on-going mental health difficulties and their age.

Reflective Exercise

1. How would you define an older person?
2. How do you think everyday jokes, for example about having 'senior moments', may contribute to perpetuating negative attitudes towards being older?
3. Do you think that policy for older people with mental illness should focus on needs relating to mental illness, or those relating to being older?
4. Do you think a lifespan policy (age blind) will change attitudes towards older people?
5. How do you think recovery principles apply to people in later life?

DISCUSSION ON THE ACTIVITIES

Activity 1

This vignette was based on the real experiences of a student nurse who put this into practice on a placement and reported it in a mental health promotion assignment. Although Roy (a pseudonym) did not feel he could own another dog himself, he became a regular dog-walking volunteer, and also happened to meet an old friend at the sanctuary with whom he rekindled his friendship. His depression became very much improved and he was discharged from inpatient care soon after. His wife thanked the student nurse for giving her back her husband.

Activity 2

The following are useful resources:

Department for Work and Pensions: Age Positive publications
www.dwp.gov.uk/age-positive/

Access to work
Mental Health Support service
www.direct.gov.uk/en/DisabledPeople/DG_201750

50+ Works
www.50plusworks.com
Working past state pension age: your options
www.direct.gov.uk/en/Pensionsandretirementplanning/PlanningForRetirement/DG_183723

BIBLIOGRAPHY

Abdul-Hamid, W., Holloway, F. & Silverman, M. (1998) Psychiatric care needs of elderly graduates: unanswered questions, *Aging and Mental Health*, 2 (3): 167–170.

Abdul-Hamid, W., Holloway, F. & Silverman, A.M. (2011) Care of elderly patients with functional disorders: a UK debate, *Psychiatric Services*, 62 (1): 104–105.

Adams, T. & Collier, E. (2009) 'Services for older people with mental health conditions'. In *Psychiatric and Mental Health Nursing: The Craft of Caring* (2nd edition). London: Hodder Arnold. pp. 486–492.

Age Concern (2008) *Primary Concerns: Older People's Access to Primary Care*. London: Age Concern. Available at http://www.ageuk.org.uk/documents/en-gb/for-professionals/research/primary%20concerns%20(2008)_pro.pdf?dtrk=true accessed (last accessed 7 November 2013).

Alzheimer's Society (2007) *Dementia UK: Summary of Key Findings*. London: LSE/ King's College/ Alzheimer's Society. Available at http://www.alzheimers.org.uk/site/scripts/download_info.php?fileID=1 (last accessed 7 November 2013).

Anderson, D. (2011) Age discrimination in mental health services needs to be understood, *The Psychiatrist*, 25 (1) January: 1–4.

Audit Commission (2002) *Directions in Diversity: Current Opinions and Good Practice.* London: Audit Commission.

Baldwin, R.C. (2003) National Service Framework for older people, Editorial, *Psychiatric Bulletin*, 27: 121–122.

Bartley, M. (2004) *Health Inequality: An Introduction to Theories, Concepts and Models.* Cambridge: Polity.

Bawn, S., Benbow, S., Jolley, D. et al. (2007) Transitions graduating between general and old age psychiatry services in England and Wales, *Mental Health Review*, 12 (1): 21–26.

Beddington, J., Cooper, C., Field, J. et al. (2008) The mental wealth of nations, *Nature*, vol 455/23: 1057–1060.

Beecham, J., Knapp, M., Fernandez, J. et al. (2008) *Age Discrimination in Mental Health Services.* PSSRU discussion paper 2536. Available at www.pssru.ac.uk

Beekman, A.T., Copeland, J.R. & Prince, M.J. (1999) Review of community prevalence of depression in later life, *British Journal of Psychiatry*, 174: 307–311.

Benbow, S. (2005) *'One 'ism too Many': Ageism and Dementia.* Royal College of Psychiatrists, Summer newsletter no. 38. Available at www.rcpsych.org.uk

Blood, I. (2010) *Older People with High Support Needs: How Can We Empower Them to Enjoy a Better Life?* Better life programme. London: Joseph Rowntree Foundation.

Bowers, H., Eastman, M., Harris, J. & Macadam, A. (2005) *Moving Out of the Shadows: A Report on Mental Health and Wellbeing in Later Life.* London: Help and Care Development Ltd.

Bytheway, B., Ward, R., Holland, C. & Peace, S. (2007) *Too Old: Older People's Accounts of Discrimination, Exclusion and Rejection.* A report from the Research on Age Discrimination Project (RoAD) to Help the Aged. London: Help the Aged.

Campbell, P. & Ananth, H. (2002) Graduates. In R. Jacoby and C. Oppenheimer (eds), *Psychiatry and the Elderly*, 3rd edition. Oxford: Oxford University Press. pp.762–798.

Centre for Policy on Ageing (2009) *Age and Age Discrimination in Secondary Health Care in the United Kingdom: A Review from the Literature.* London: CPA.

Citizens Advice Bureau (2003) *Mental Health and Social Exclusion.* London: CAB.

Citizens Advice Bureau (2004) *Out of the Picture: CAB Evidence on Mental Health and Social Exclusion.* London: CAB.

Citizens Advice Scotland (2007) 'Illness and disability in detail: CAB clients with mental health issues'. Briefing Paper 23a. Edinburgh: CAS.

Cohen, C.I., Cohen, G.D., Blank, K. et al. (2000) Schizophrenia and old adults: an overview: directions for research and policy, *American Journal of Geriatric Psychiatry*, 8 (1): 19–28.

Collier, E. (2005) Latent age discrimination in mental health care, *Mental Health Practice*: 42–49.

Collier, E. (2006) Mental health and functional mental disorder in older adults, *Nursing Older People*, 18 (9): 25–32.

Collier, E. (2007) 'Approaches to help support and care'. In R. Neno, B. Aveyard and H. Heath (eds), *Older People and Mental Health Nursing: A Handbook of Care.* Oxford: Blackwell. pp. 53–66.

Collier, E. (2008) Historical development of psychiatric classification, *British Journal of Nursing*, 17 (14): 890–894.

Collier, E. (2012) A biographical narrative study exploring mental ill health through the life course. Unpublished PhD thesis, University of Salford, UK.

Collier, E. & Yates-Bolton, N. (2011) 'Older people in mental health care'. In P. Barker (ed.), *Mental Health Ethics: The Human Context.* London: Routledge. pp. 239–249.

Communities and Local Government (2007/8) *2007/8 Citizenship Survey:Volunteering and Charitable Giving Topic Report, Communities and Local Government*. Available at http://data.gov.uk/dataset/citizenship_survey-volunteering_and_charitable_giving_topic_report (last accessed 7 November 2013).

Craig, G. (2004) Citizenship, exclusion and older people' *Journal of Social Policy,* 33 (1): 95–114.

Cummings, S.M. & Kropf, N.P. (2011) Aging with a severe mental illness: challenges and treatments, *Journal of Gerontological Social Work,* 54: 175–188.

Dadswell, R.A. (2005) What does it feel like to be transferred from adult mental health services, to services for older people on reaching the age of 65 years? The lived experience is explored using a phenomenological approach. Unpublished MSc thesis, Advanced Practice (Mental Health), University of Surrey.

Daley, S., Newton, D., Slade, M., Murray, J. & Banerjee, S. (2012) Development of a framework for recovery in older people with mental disorder, *International Journal of Geriatric Psychiatry,* 28: 522–529.

Department of Health (1999) *The National Service Framework for Mental Health.* London: DH.

Department of Health (2001a) *The National Service Framework for Older People.* London: DH.

Department of Health (2001b) The *Mental Health Policy Implementation Guide.* London: DH.

Department of Health (2003a) *Care Homes for Older People: National Minimum Standards.* London: HMSO.

Department of Health (2003b) *Care Homes for Adults (18–65): National Minimum Standards.* London: HMSO.

Department of Health (2005a) *Securing Better Mental Health for Older Adults.* London: DH.

Department of Health (2005b) NIMHE *Guiding Statement on Recovery.* London: DH. Available at www.psychminded.co.uk/news/news2005/feb05/nimherecovstatement.pdf (last accessed 11 December 2008).

Department of Health (2005c) *Everybody's Business: Integrating Mental Health Services For Older Adults.* London: Care Services Improvement Partnership (CSIP).

Department of Health (2005d) *The National Service Framework for Long Term Conditions.* London: DH.

Department of Health (2006) *A New Ambition for Old Age: Next Steps in Implementing the National Service Framework for Older People.* London: DH.

Department of Health (2008) *Health and Care Services for Older People: Overview of a Report on Research to Support the NSFOP.* London: DH.

Department of Health (2009a) *Ageism and Age Discrimination in Mental Health Care in the United Kingdom: Review from the Literature* (Centre for Policy on Ageing). London: DH.

Department of Health (2009b) *Delivering Race Equality in Mental Health: A Review.* London: DH.

Department of Health (2010) *Healthy Lives, Healthy People: Our Strategy for Public Health in England.* London: DH.

Department of Health (2011) *No Health Without Mental Health.* London: DH.

Department of Health Social Services and Public Safety (2009) *Service Framework for Health and Wellbeing of Older People.* Belfast: Northern Ireland DHSSPS.

Department of Health, Social Services and Public Safety (2010) *Service Framework for Mental Health and Wellbeing Consultation.* Belfast: Northern Ireland DHSSPS.

Department of Work and Pensions (2005) *Opportunity Age: Opportunity and Security Throughout Life.* London: DWP.

Ehlers, A., Naegele, G. & Reichert, M. (2011) *Volunteering by Older People in the EU: European Foundation for the Improvement of Living and Working Conditions.* Luxembourg: Publications Office of the European Union.

Falkingham, J., Evandrou, M., McGowan, T. et al. (2010) 'Demographic issues, projections and trends: Older people with high support needs in the UK'. JRF programme paper: *Better Life*. London: ESRC Centre for Population Change.

Foresight Mental Capital and Wellbeing Project (2008) *Final Project Report – Executive Summary*. London: The Government Office for Science.

Healthcare Commission (2009) *Equality in Later Life: A National Study of Older People's Mental Health Services*. London: Commission for Healthcare Audit and Inspection.

Heikkinen, R. (2000) Ageing in an autobiographical context, *Ageing and Society* 20 (4): 467–483.

Hilton, C. (2005) The clinical psychiatry of late life in Britain from 1950 to 1970: an overview, *International Journal of Geriatric Psychiatry*, 20: 423–428.

House of Commons (2012) *State Pension Age*. Standard note SN 02234. London: House of Commons.

Institute of Fiscal Studies (2006) *The Social Exclusion of Older People: Evidence from the First Wave of the English Longitudinal Study of Ageing* (ELSA). London: Social Exclusion Unit. Available at www.communities.gov.uk/documents/corporate/pdf/143564.pdf

Jenkins, C.L. & Laditka, S.B. (1998) Double jeopardy: the challenge of providing mental health services to older people, *Administration and Policy in Mental Health* 26 (1): 65–74.

Jolley, D., Kosky, N. & Holloway, F. (2004) Older people with long-standing mental illness: the graduates, *Advances in Psychiatric Treatment*, 10: 27–36.

Joseph Rowntree Foundation (2002) *Past it at 40? A Grassroots View of Ageism and Discrimination in Employment*. Bristol: The Policy Press.

Katz, J., Holland, C., Peace, S. & Taylor, E. (2011) *A Better Life: What Older People with High Support Needs Value*. London: Joseph Rowntree Foundation.

Keyes, C.L.M. (2002) The mental health continuum: from languishing to flourishing in life, *Journal of Health and Social Research*, 43: 207–222.

Komp, K., Van Tilburg, T. & Van Groenou, M.B. (2009) The influence of the welfare state on the number of young old persons, *Ageing and Society*, 29: 609–624.

Levitas, R. (1998) *The Inclusive Society? Social Exclusion and New Labour*. London: Macmillan.

Marwaha, S. & Livingstone, G. (2002) Stigma, racism or choice: Why do depressed ethnic elders avoid psychiatrists?, *Journal of Affective Disorders*, 72: 257–265.

McKay, E.A. (2010) 'Rip that book up, I've changed': unveiling the experiences of women living with and surviving enduring mental illness, *British Journal of Occupational Therapy*, 73 (3): 96–105.

Mental Health Foundation (2009) *All Things Being Equal: Age Equality in Mental Health Care for Older People in England*. London: MHF.

MIND (2005) *Access All Ages: Survey of Older People with Mental Health Problems Over 50*. London: MIND.

National Mental Health Development Unit (2011a) *A Long Time Coming: Strategies for Achieving Age Equality in Mental Health Services*, Part 1. Bath: NDTi.

National Mental Health Development Unit (2011b) *A Long Time Coming: Achieving Age Equality in Local Mental Health Services*, Part 2. Bath: NDTi.

Newton, B., Hurstfield, J., Miller, L. et al. (2005) *Training Participation by Age amongst Unemployed and Inactive People*. Leeds: Department for Work and Pensions.

Office for National Statistics (2008–2010) *Interim Life Tables* (released 29 September 2011). Available at www.ons.gov.uk/ons/rel/lifetables/interim-life-tables/2008-2010/index.html (last accessed 3 July 2012).

Office for National Statistics (2011) *'Ageing in the UK' Datasets, 2010 Mid-Year Estimates Update*. Available at www.ons.gov.uk/ons/publications/re-reference-tables. html?edition=tcm%3A77-248402

Office for the Deputy Prime Minister (2006) *A Sure Start to Later Life: Ending Inequalities for Older People: A social exclusion unit final report*. London: DWP, DH, SEU.

Oppenheim, C. (ed.) (1998) *An Inclusive Society: Strategies for Tackling Poverty*. London: IPPR.

Panayotes, D., Edlira, G. & James, N. (2007) *Age Identity, Age Perceptions, and Health. Evidence from the English Longitudinal Study of Ageing Annals of the New York Academy of Sciences*, Vol.1114, *Healthy Aging and Longevity*. DOI: 10.1196/annals.1396.021

Perkins, K. & Tice, C. (1995) A strengths perspective in practice: older people and mental health challenges, *Journal of Gerontological Social Work*, 23 (3/4): 83–97.

Repper, J. & Perkins, R. (2003) *Social Inclusion and Recovery: A Model for Mental Health Practice*. Edinburgh: Ballière Tindall.

Rethink (2004) *Lost and Found: Voices from the Forgotten Generation*. London: Rethink.

Rice, N.E., Lang, I.A., Henley, W. & Melzer, D. (2011) Common health predictors of early retirement: findings from the English Longitudinal Study of Ageing, *Age and Ageing*, 40: 54–61.

Royal College of Psychiatrists (2002)'Caring for people who enter old age with enduring or relapsing mental illness ('graduates')'.Council report CR110. London: RCP.

Royal College of Psychiatrists (2009a) 'Age discrimination in mental health services: making equality a reality'. Position statement PS2/2009/. London: Royal College of Psychiatrists.

Royal College of Psychiatrists (2009b) 'Links not boundaries: service transitions for people growing older with enduring or relapsing mental illness'. CR153. London: Royal College of Psychiatrists.

Sainsbury Centre for Mental Health (2002) *An Executive Briefing on 'Working for Inclusion'*. London: The Sainsbury Centre for Mental Health.

Sainsbury Centre for Mental Health (2005) *The Neglected Majority: Developing Intermediate Mental Health Care in Primary Care*. London: Sainsbury Centre.

Sayce, L. (2000) *From Psychiatric Patient to Citizen Overcoming Discrimination and Social Exclusion*. London: Macmillan.

Scottish Association of Mental Health (2011) 'What's it worth now? The social and economic costs of mental health problems in Scotland'. *Full Report*. Glasgow: SAMH.

Scottish Executive (2003) *National Programme for Improving Mental Health and Wellbeing Action Plan 2003–2006*. Edinburgh: The Scottish Executive.

Scottish Executive (2007) *All Our Futures: Planning for a Scotland with an Ageing Population*. Edinburgh: Scottish Executive.

Scottish Government (2010) *Demographic Change in Scotland*. Available at www.scotland. gov.uk/publications/2010/11/24111237/4

Scottish Government (2011) *Mental Health Strategy for Scotland 2011–2015: A consultation*. Edinburgh: The Scottish Government.

Scottish Government (2012) *Mental Health Strategy for Scotland: 2012–2015*. Edinburgh: The Scottish Government.

Shah, A. (2009) Psychiatry of old age and ethnic minority older people in the United Kingdom, *Reviews in Clinical Gerontology*, 19: 119–134.

Smith-Merry, J., Sturdy, S. & Freeman, R. (2010) Recovering mental health in Scotland: 'recovery' from social movement to policy goal, Knowledge and Policy in Education and Health Sectors. Available at www.knowandpol.eu

Social Care Institute for Excellence (2010) *Dignity in Care Factsheet*. London: Social Care Institute for Excellence.

Social Exclusion Unit (2004) *Mental Health and Social Exclusion.* London: Office of the Deputy Prime Minister.

Social Exclusion Unit (2005) *Excluded Older People: Social Exclusion Unit Interim Report.* London: Office of the Deputy Prime Minister.

Strauss, J. (2008) Prognosis in schizophrenia and the role of subjectivity, *Schizophrenia Bulletin,* 34 (2): 201–203.

Welsh Assembly Government (2005) *Adult Mental Health Services: Raising the Standard – The revised adult mental health National Service Framework and an action for Wales.* Cardiff: Welsh Assembly Government.

Welsh Assembly Government (2006) *National Service Framework for Older People in Wales.* Cardiff: Welsh Assembly Government.

Wrigley, M., Murphy, B., Farrell, M. et al. (2006) Older people with enduring or recurrent severe mental illness in the eastern region of Ireland, *Irish Journal of Psychological Medicine,* 23 (4): 145–150.

6 DEMENTIA

Trevor Adams

Chapter Overview

Care of those with dementia has had a very chequered history in mental health services. In the era of institutional care it could be characterised as the worst excesses of warehousing: large numbers of individuals cared for in crowded 'psycho-geriatric' wards and exposed to a grinding routine of tasks carried out by a workforce that were neither valued nor indeed cared for themselves.

This chapter will illuminate the transformation that has occurred and how policy and legislation have brought real change to the services provided. The changing nature of services for people with dementia has come about by changes in the values underpinning practice just as much as the policy informing it. There has been a growing and assertive service user movement that has insisted upon dementia as being something one 'has' rather than something one 'is'. That change – coupled and informed by changes such as advanced directives – have facilitated a growing engagement with a different ethos of care.

The emergence of choice and a greater sense of control over events have required those who provide services to offer a more person-centred service. A growing sense of optimism evidenced by therapeutic advances and services that are offered far earlier has changed the landscape of services for those with dementia. As will be seen in the chapter policy today is now moving away from care and treatment initiatives on their own but also considering the structure and design of the communities we live in. The aspiration of a 'dementia friendly community' may be realised sooner than we think.

INTRODUCTION

This chapter reviews developments in health and social policy in the United Kingdom that affect the mental health nursing of people with dementia, and argues that the speciality has a lot to offer the future provision of support to people with dementia. There are two reasons for this optimism. The first is that mental health nurses base their practice on a set of ideas that draws equally from bio-medical *and* psycho-social approaches. This means that mental health nurses are able to offer a 'one stop' service that is more comprehensive and holistic than many other health and social care professions, such as Medicine or Clinical Psychology who only draw on one theoretical approach. For this reason mental health nursing is very practical and concerned with supporting people who have dementia and helping their families address everyday situations. One area of expertise that mental health nurses often display is their use of everyday language to help people with dementia and their family carers understand the implications of dementia on their life. This is greatly valued by families and often places mental health nurses in a significant and influential position within community mental health teams. While mental health nurses are often valued by people with dementia and their family members, they regularly find themselves sidelined and marginalised within mental health nursing itself.

While mental health nursing has a lot to offer, the speciality is presently facing a crisis that has arisen for three reasons. Firstly, there is currently an absence of leadership in mental health nursing, although sometimes it is the case that the views of existing leaders in the speciality are actually not sought – as I believe was the case in the development of a recent directive from the Department of Health, *Making a Difference in Dementia: Nursing Vision and Strategy* (DH, 2013). Secondly, mental health nursing has not kept up-to-date with recent thinking on how people with dementia should best be supported, including the recent ideas set out in 'Caring for Our Future: Reforming Care and Support' (DH, 2012a). Thirdly, mental health nurses have not entered into the discussion about where nursing expertise lies within dementia nursing. I believe that mental health nurses specialising in people with dementia and their families are the point at which professional expertise and specialism lie, though other groups – such as Admiral Nursing – are likely to have an overlapping expertise with family carers who are their particular focus.

This chapter argues that mental health nurses specialising in people with dementia and their family carers are the natural source of specialism within dementia nursing. However, recent ideas regarding giving support to people with dementia have now moved on and there is an urgent need for mental health nurses to catch up and align themselves with recent shifts in health and social policy. Mental health nurses have developed a person- and relationship-centred approach that highlights the person with dementia within the context of mutual and reciprocal relationships between themselves and family carers and health-care professionals. Other nursing groups such as the Admiral Nurses adopt a different approach which focuses on supporting family carers. This chapter supports approaches by mental health nurses in which the person with dementia and their family carers are together the focus of support, but also argues that this approach should be extended so that the ability of people with dementia and their family carers to make optimal choices is extended. This is not an over-dramatic viewpoint, but I do believe that if mental health nurses do not extend their basis of practice, they may well find their work taken over by others – and this would be a great shame.

HEALTH CARE POLICY AND ITS IMPLICATIONS FOR THE MENTAL HEALTH NURSING OF PEOPLE WITH DEMENTIA

One of the difficulties in looking at the policy for the mental health nursing of people with dementia is that very little policy actually exists. One main reason for this absence is the widespread ageism that exists both in society and in mental health nursing itself. To a large extent people with dementia were uncategorised before the beginning of the twentieth century and as a result were undifferentiated from other people with mental health conditions. They were a hidden group within the provision of institutional care and as such 'swept under the carpet' of the asylum system. People with dementia found themselves marginalised and without a voice in institutions and the rest of society. In the absence of policy specifically relating to people with dementia, health and social policy generic documents relating to community care, informal care, mental health and mental health nursing were often applied to people with dementia even though they never quite fitted. People with dementia themselves were hardly ever considered and they remained as hidden and silent as ever, with their voices never really heard.

The marginalisation and silencing of people with dementia emerged within asylum-based mental health nursing (or as it was then called, 'mental nursing') and were underpinned by a medical understanding of people with dementia that remained unchallenged until the 1960s. This approach saw people with dementia as having a disease of the brain that severely and progressively affected their cognitive ability. The philosophical basis of this 'defectological' approach in which people with cognitive difficulties were seen as having a 'defect' was defined by the medical profession and emerged through ideas developed in the Enlightenment of the eighteenth century. This approach saw people's ability to think as the distinctive feature of what it means to be human. As Descartes asserted, 'I think therefore I am'. In this way, people with dementia were regarded as less human than other people and also defective. This approach gave rise to people with dementia being taken out of mainstream society and finding themselves placed in asylums and long-stay hospitals.

While long-stay asylums no longer exist, many people with dementia are still institutionalised and nursed in long-stay wards and residential care homes. These places often still see people with dementia as having little ability to make their views and opinions known: indeed in some, they are given poor care and treated with emotional and physical abuse. Moreover, the views of people with dementia and their family carers who are living at home are hardly ever considered and little attempt is made to ask them what sort of care they want. While asylums and institutions no longer exist, the views and attitudes of some nurses are reminiscent of those that held sway in the asylum system.

This way of seeing people with dementia was taught to student nurses up until the late 1960s and perhaps even later. Houliston (1961: 65) for example – in her standard textbook on mental nursing – states that dementia is 'a state of permanent mental enfeeblement due to disease or decay of the brain. Unlike the mental defective who never was normal, the dement was normal once'. Later still in 1969, Altschul and Simpson suggested that people with dementia displayed 'degraded behaviour', and commended 'ward routine' as a stabilising factor concerned with vigilance, perseverance and scrupulous punctuality. The end result of seeing people with dementia in this way is clearly visible in the disturbing and alarming description of long-stay dementia 'care' given by Tony Whitehead, a leading consultant in the psychiatry of old age:

> Patients were herded together in old, bleak, neglected buildings with large dark wards, closely placed rows of beds, little furniture and frightening inactivity. Multiple regulations curtail the patient's freedoms and reduce their contact with the outside world. They may be confined to the ward and allowed out only in large supervised groups. Privacy, usually valued by the elderly, is often nonexistent. Bathing is supervised and may take place in a communal bathroom. Visiting is restricted to a few hours a week and children are often prohibited. To visit some wards for the elderly is to visit the annex to the mortuary. Rows of old people lie in bed with legs bent and muscles wasted by lack of use, eyes dull and vacant, waiting to die. (Whitehead, 1970)

As Tony Whitehead was writing this, others such as Barbara Robb (in her book *Sans Everything* (1970)) were bringing to light further evidence of dehumanising practices on people with dementia in long-stay hospitals. But in spite of this growing and worrying concern, the Department of Health at the time did little to offer new policies and practices that specifically related to the growing number of people with dementia. Interestingly, however, change did occur through the influential and significant work of innovative psychiatrists such as Tony Whitehead together with clinical psychologists like Bob Woods. Through their work, the new and progressive speciality of 'Psychiatry of Old Age' emerged and helped dismantle the old hospital-based mental health services for older people to offer instead a new community-based and multi-disciplinary approach to people with dementia. I would say that it was their work that kick-started the developments associated with supporting people with dementia, and which flourished latterly.

More fundamental changes regarding service only came about in the early 1980s following the publication of the Health Advisory Service document, *The Rising Tide* (HAS, 1982). This small document laid down significant guidelines relating to the provision of support to older people with dementia, and stimulated the government investment into developing new 'demonstration services' that offered examples of good practice to people with dementia. These innovations occurred at the same time as the development of 'community care' as outlined in *Making a Reality of*

Community Care, (Audit Commission, 1986) and *Caring for People: Community Care in the Next Decade and Beyond* (DH, 1989). Often ascribed to the Thatcher administration, community care had been around since the late 1950s, and many of the mental hospitals had by the 1980s lost over half of their patients. Yet what was new here was not community care itself, rather that the main source of support was not 'the state' but 'the community' and what was once called 'care in the community' had become 'care by the community'.

The main thrust within the community care programme was concentrated on people living in mental hospitals, many of whom had schizophrenia and other functional mental illnesses. These people had found themselves living in mental hospitals for many years and had thus become institutionalised. This client-group differed from many people with dementia who lived at home, and for them community care was more concerned with enabling them to remain in their own home and preventing their admission into long-stay care. This required mental health nurses to underpin their work with a different set of ideas and skills from those they had developed within mental hospitals.

POLITICS, IDEOLOGY AND DEMENTIA CARE

During the 1980s political and ideological changes substantially affected the organisation of health and social policy, and affected the scope and direction of mental health nursing for people with dementia. However, these ideas have not gone away and present-day policy has built on, extended, and further developed these.

In the 1980s the economic and social difficulties of the 1970s were beginning to be tackled, not least the high rate of inflation and its severe economic implications. The dominant remedy put forward at the time was associated with the political and economic views of the 'New Right' that were concerned with reducing the level of inflation by cutting public expenditure.

In 1977, the Labour Prime Minister James Callaghan applied to the International Monetary Fund for a loan to address the substantial economic difficulties at the time. This loan was granted, but came with various conditions attached that corresponded to the views of the New Right. While this policy was initiated by the Labour administration of James Callaghan, it was soon continued by the new prime minister Margaret Thatcher, who gained power in 1979 and remained so throughout the 1980s. This policy gave rise to strenuous and far-reaching moves to reduce government spending, not least in the increasingly expensive area of health and social care.

One way by which the Thatcher administration sought to reduce government spending was to transfer responsibility for the provision of services from the state to other agencies such as the private sector and indigenous sources of support within the community such as family, friends and neighbours. This approach was outlined in an early document from the Thatcher administration, *Growing Older* (DHSS,

1981). In addition, to gain financial control and limit public spending tighter management processes were put into place. For example, Sir Roy Griffith who was Managing Director of Sainsbury's at the time, was asked to chair a small group that produced *The Management Inquiry, National Health Service* (DH, 1983) which advocated new and better structures of management for the National Health Service. This document was indicative of the managerialism that had begun to emerge in the health and social sector and would lead to a considerable amount of reorganisation, such as that displayed in the 1989 White Paper *Working for Patients*.

It is noteworthy that underpinning the Thatcher administration's ideology was the idea that people should have the freedom to make choices based on their personal desires and wishes (i.e. without government interference). Moreover, each person was seen as having a position in the marketplace that enabled them to make choices about the sort of health and social care they wanted, whether statutory, private or voluntary. The idea here was that the consumer was king and people were seen as having the right to purchase what they wanted from the market. While it must be argued whether people have sufficient money to buy the services they desire, in the case of people with dementia we must also ask whether they have the cognitive ability to make worthwhile choices.

It is within this context that the state increasingly removed itself from the role of main provider of services to one in which it increasingly took on the role of regulating services. The Care Quality Commission is a present-day example of a government-initiated regulatory body set up to ensure good health and social care practice. But the point that must be made in the context of this chapter is that the Thatcher administration helped create a social context which encouraged the idea that people had the right to make choices about the sort of health and social care they wished to have. As we shall see, this idea is now one of the main ideas within health and social care policy to all people, including people with dementia.

As a result of the Thatcher administration, health and social care for people with dementia took on a completely different landscape that was underpinned by an entirely new ideology. For mental health nurses working alongside people with dementia, this new landscape meant that if they were to offer the sort of support that was now expected they had to integrate this new ideology within their practice. Two of the most significant areas of ideology related to the 'the family carer' and 'the person with dementia'.

Families have always supported their sick or disabled relatives, at least until they entered long-stay care. One of the things the new ideological understanding brought to community care was a reliance on 'family carers' and the expectation that someone in the family would identify themselves – or find themselves identified – as the 'primary carer' and the main source of support for the relative with dementia. This ideological commitment to 'the carer' underpinned much government thinking at the time and can be seen in *Caring About Carers: A National Strategy for Carers* (DH, 1989): it has continued up until the present. This ideology not only highlights the contribution of family carers but also constructs and identifies 'family carers' as a legitimate power group within dementia care and allows them to be regarded by themselves and others as having legitimate needs and rights.

The increased recognition and reliance on the family as an important source of support within community care came under substantial critique. The main area for this was that health and social policy was thought to be reverting back to a traditional and outdated model of the family in which women were the main source of support for dependent members, one which failed to take into account the fact that many woman today are in paid employment. This critique was supported by anecdotal and empirical evidence which showed that many family carers found looking after a relative with dementia physically and emotionally demanding, and this could give rise to them experiencing mental health problems.

The rise of 'the carer' as the primary source of support for people with dementia led to the development of a range of practical approaches and interventions to family carers. One such approach was the Stress-Management Model developed by Zarit et al. (1986) which sought to address the stress families experience as they support relatives with dementia. Moreover, a new breed of nurse emerged called 'the Admiral Nurse', who worked alongside traditional mental health nurses and whose primary focus was the primary family carer. Admiral Nurses:

- offer a skilled assessment of the needs of family carers and people with dementia;
- provide information and practical advice for family carers on different aspects of caring for a relative/friend with dementia;
- work with families at the point of diagnosis and throughout the caring journey, providing emotional and psychological support and guidance about accessing services;
- help family carers and people with dementia to develop and improve skills to assist with care giving and promote positive approaches to living with dementia;
- work collaboratively with other professionals and organisations to facilitate co-ordinated care provision;
- work with family carers to enable them to express their wishes and views about the services they receive;
- (See www.dementiauk.org/what-we-do/admiral-nurses/what-admiral-nurses-do/ (last accessed 29 March 2013).)

New Admiral Nursing services are set up through funds from outside the NHS by its parent body 'For Dementia' which has charity status. Over time, Admiral Nurses have become a valued source of support for relatives of people with dementia. Admiral Nursing however is not without critics. For example, Admiral Nurses claim that their distinctiveness is that they work with carers, but this raises the question about whether they are marginalising the person with dementia and thus are only listening to and addressing the needs of family carers. In addition, there is the question of whether Admiral Nurses merely duplicate the work of community mental health nurses, and if this is so whether it is needless, costly and contributes to bad communication. To a large extent Admiral Nurses have pushed the claim that their value lies in the fact that they are dementia specialists. A recent document *Making a Difference in Dementia: Nursing Vision and Strategy* (DH, 2013) identifies Admiral Nurses as a source of specialism in Dementia Nursing, yet this is questionable as their focus is not on people with dementia but their carers, and perhaps reflects limitations in how the document was written.

Another identity developed in the 1980s, though this time not as a result of the Thatcher administration: instead it appeared via the emergence of 'dementia studies' as a discipline with the idea of 'the person with dementia'. As we have already seen, the medical profession gave rise to people with dementia being seen as having a disease of the brain and this caused them to be objectified by depersonalising professional practices. In the late 1980s and early 1990s a new way of thinking about people with dementia developed through the pioneering work of Tom Kitwood, which he described as 'person-centred care'. Its main concern was that 'the person comes first' and it argued that personhood in people with dementia arose out of the relationship other people have with them. This approach challenged traditional practices and interaction within service delivery to people with dementia that gave rise to their depersonalisation in long-stay care homes and hospitals.

These developments – together with increased recognition of the increasing numbers of people with dementia – led to the establishment of dementia nursing as a specialism within mental health nursing (Adams, 1996). It is important to note that these developments largely occurred outside and without reference to other areas of mental health nursing. As a result, a dichotomy arose in mental health nursing between people of working age and those with dementia, with each side having their own ideas, vocabulary, skills and practice. While mental health nurses working alongside people with dementia had gained some visibility within the profession, not least by their sheer number, the dominant group within the profession was still aligned to people of working age.

DEVELOPMENTS IN MENTAL HEALTH NURSING IN THE 1980s AND 1990s

Various developments occurred in mental health nursing in the 1980s and 1990s that arose from the significant unrest that existed within the profession at that time. These developments were precipitated, in part, by the introduction of Project 2000 which sought to bring nursing into the university system of higher education. While the implementation of Project 2000 was problematic for a number of reasons, the issue that alarmed many mental health nurses was the identity and position it offered mental health nursing. Within Project 2000, mental health nursing was merely given the status of a branch that followed an initial core common foundation programme that was largely orientated towards general nursing. This unrest had its roots in the early part of the twentieth century when mental health nursing ceased to be controlled by the medical profession and came under the regulation of the General Nursing Council with its historic and ideological commitment to general nursing. In the 1990s these concerns led to a re-examination of what constituted the focus for mental health nursing, and for some the belief that it should leave 'nursing' and become a generic mental health profession. Concerns about Project 2000 were supported by strong leadership offered by professional organisations within mental health nursing, and also by a number of vocal, articulate, university-based and popular representatives of the profession such as Tony Butterworth and Charlie Brooker. This discussion was continued in a DH review of mental health nursing, *Working in Partnership,* under the chairmanship of Tony Butterworth. The report was the first major review of the profession since the publication of *Psychiatric Nursing Today and Yesterday* in 1968, and explored the social changes that had occurred since that time and their implications on practice, education, research and management within mental health nursing.

A key recommendation within *Working in Partnership* was that mental health nursing should focus on people with serious and enduring mental illness and that this should include older people, although the report gave few references and examples of how this might be done. Nevertheless, this reference to older people in the report was a timely recognition of the growing number of mental health nurses who were working with people with dementia, and that the speciality was a legitimate, important and valued part of the profession. This had not previously been the case in mental health nursing, though it has to be said that many leading writers on mental health nursing still understood 'long-term conditions' in relation to people of working age rather than older people with dementia. This perpetuated the longstanding ageism within mental health nursing.

Just over ten years later, two further reports were published – *The Chief Nursing Officer's Review of Mental Health Nursing in England* and *Rights, Relationships and Recovery* (Scottish Executive, 2006) – which concerned the development of mental health nursing in Scotland. Each report placed recovery at the core of its recommendations, and despite some differences in health and social care policy and health outcomes in both countries, the reviews covered similar ground in their focus on recovery, developing capabilities for the mental health nursing workforce, preparing students with the best education for practice, and highlighting the importance of leadership and support. With regard to the mental health nursing of people with dementia they are regularly cited in the two reports, and at times the use of the recovery approach with people with dementia is at least mentioned.

RECOVERY

As we have seen recovery became an important therapeutic approach within mental health nursing and remains so. The importance of recovery as an underpinning idea within the mental health nursing of people with dementia is recognised by Keady et al. who suggest that '[R]ecovery has a place within dementia care nursing' and also that 'one of the most pressing challenges ahead is to use, adapt and (potentially) modify this approach for the dementia care field' (2009: 570).

At first sight the idea of recovery does not look as though it has much to offer people with dementia, as they are widely understood as having no expectation of a cure. Some would say that even talking about recovery might give some family carers the false idea that their relative may eventually be cured. It should be noted that this way of thinking is based on a medical understanding of dementia – one that was challenged by Kitwood who argued that people with dementia have the capacity of gaining an enhanced sense of personhood and may experience 'rementia'. I would add that recovery has something positive to offer people with dementia, and perhaps also holds out the possibility of bringing together the mental health nursing of people of working age with the mental health nursing of older people through shared use of the same concept (Adams, 2010b).

Anthony defines 'recovery' as a 'unique process of changing one's attitudes, values, feelings, goals, skills, and/or roles. It is a way of living a satisfying, hopeful, and contributing life even with limitations caused by illness. Recovery involves the development of new meaning and purpose in one's life as one grows beyond the catastrophic effects of mental illness' (1993:15). This definition highlights that recovery is a process by using a journey metaphor.

Thinking about recovery as a means of promoting wellbeing offers the mental health nursing of people with dementia a new approach that extends Kitwood's understanding of 'person-centred care'. The distinctive nature of this new recovery-based approach is that people with dementia are seen as having increased agency and the ability to make choices and have control. While not directly offering people with dementia the ability to make choices and have control, the idea of recovery offers them much more self-direction than institutional approaches and also person-centred care. The idea of recovery has been applied to the mental health nursing of people with dementia, and various interventions have been identified based on the recovery approach (Adams, 2010b).

PEOPLE WITH DEMENTIA AND SOCIAL POLICY SINCE THE NEW MILLENNIUM

Over the last few years, older people with dementia have increasingly been included in government health and social policy reports and objectives. The most important example here has been the National Strategy for Dementia, *Living Well with Dementia* (DH, 2009), which outlines 17 objectives regarding the development of services for people with dementia. These comprise:

- an improved public and professional awareness and understanding of dementia;
- good quality early diagnosis and intervention for all;
- good quality information for those diagnosed with dementia and their carers;
- easy access to care, support and advice following a diagnosis, facilitated by a dementia advisor;
- structured peer support and learning networks;
- community personal support services;
- services within the Carers' Strategy;

- good quality care in general hospitals;
- intermediate care for people with dementia;
- good housing, housing-related and telecare support;
- high quality services within care homes
- good end-of-life care;
- an informed and effective workforce across all services;
- a joint commissioning strategy;
- better regulation and assessment;
- a review of the research;
- national and regional implementation support.

These objectives were later combined with concerns about the over-prescription of antipsychotic medication to people with dementia and this led to the identification of four priority objectives. These objectives are:

- good-quality early diagnosis and intervention for all;
- improved quality of care in general hospitals;
- living well with dementia in care homes;
- reduced use of antipsychotic medication.

A further document, *No Health Without Mental Health: A Cross-Government Mental Health Outcomes Strategy for People of All Ages* (DH, 2011), takes mental health provision along a different trajectory and is underpinned by an alternative ideological perspective. As the title implies, the report includes 'people of all ages' and that certainly should include people with dementia. It outlines a new government approach towards mental health that is committed to 'achieving change by putting more power into people's hands at a local level'. It also draws on the idea of the Big Society and asserts that a stronger and more cohesive society can only be achieved when people and communities are able to take more responsibility for their own wellbeing.

No Health Without Mental Health seeks to address the following outcomes that relate to:

- lifting the burden of bureaucracy;
- promoting empowerment;
- the personalisation of the production and delivery of services and support;
- increasing local control of public finances;
- diversifying the supply of public services;
- opening up the government to public scrutiny;
- promoting social action, social inclusion and human rights;
- strengthening accountability to local people.

While these ideas developed outside dementia care, those within the speciality have moved beyond person-centred care – with its focus on promoting the respect and dignity of people with dementia – to a greater focus on supporting them to have choice and control. These ideas form the basis of the *National Dementia Declaration* which was developed by the Dementia Care Alliance, a collaboration of organisations that support people with dementia. In the *National Dementia Declaration*, a variety of desired outcomes were identified as 'I' statements concerning the sort of services wanted by people with dementia, and comprise:

1. I have personal choice and control or influence over decisions about me.
2. I know that services are designed around me and my needs.
3. I have support that helps me live my life.
4. I have the knowledge and know-how to get what I need.
5. I live in an enabling and supportive environment where I feel valued and understood.
6. I have a sense of belonging and of being a valued part of family, community and civic life.
7. I know there is research going on which delivers a better life for me now and hope for the future.

These developments challenge the mental health nursing of people with dementia and call on mental health nurses to make a dramatic change to the way they work alongside people with dementia and their families. Over the last one hundred years the mental health nursing of people with dementia has passed through two distinct phases. The first was concerned with taking people with dementia out of mainstream society and placing them in long-stay care, and the second was concerned with maintaining people with dementia wherever possible at home. However, health and social policy to people with dementia is moving swiftly and mental health nursing now needs to enter a third phase that focuses on supporting people with dementia to have choice and control over their life within the context of creating supportive social networks and communities. This focus is associated with the idea of 'personalisation' and that of 'dementia-friendly communities'. These ideas are new to mental health nursing and very different from those within institutionalisation. This radical understanding of the way people should be offered support was seen in the recent government White Paper, *Caring for our Future: Reforming Care and Support* (DH, 2012a) which again relates to all people and of course includes people with dementia.

The key principles of the White Paper are:

- The health, wellbeing, independence and rights of individuals are at the heart of care and support; timely and effective interventions help to ensure a good quality of life for longer.
- People are treated with dignity and respect, and are safe from abuse and neglect; everyone must work to make this happen.
- Personalisation is achieved when a person has real choice and control over the care and support they need to achieve their goals, live a fulfilling life, and be connected with society.

- The skills, resources and networks in every community are harnessed and strengthened to support people to live well, and to contribute to their communities where they can and wish to.
- Carers are recognised for their contribution to society as vital partners in care, and are supported to reach their full potential and lead the lives they want.
- A caring, skilled and valued workforce delivers quality care and support in partnership with individuals, families and communities.

There is thus a considerable need for the mental health nursing of people with dementia to adapt to the ideas developed in recent health and social policy. Two new and important ideas are 'personalisation' and 'dementia-friendly communities'.

PERSONALISATION

Personalisation is a new way of thinking about supporting people, and starts with the person as an individual who has particular strengths, preferences and aspirations, putting them at the centre of service provision by helping them identity their needs and make choices about how and when they want to be supported to live their own life. A key idea in nursing over the last thirty years has been the nursing process which sought to identify clients' problems and seek an effective solution for each of these. But the orientation of the nursing process was to the nurse identifying 'the problem' and deciding on possible solutions rather than giving that responsibility to the client. In this way the nurse was at the centre of the nursing process, not the client.

Personalisation offers a radical alternative to the nursing process that places the client at the centre of the decision-making process. Mental health nurses who work alongside people with dementia need to adjust how they engage with people who have dementia and seek new ways of helping them make worthwhile choices.

It is important to note that 'personalisation' is not the same as 'person-centred care' as developed by Tom Kitwood. While personalisation incorporates elements of person-centred care such as those developed by Carl Rogers (for example, giving people with dementia unconditional regard by means of positive person work), it is focused on helping people make worthwhile choices and have optimal control. Some writers have voiced concern with 'hearing the voice of people with dementia', although this has not been fully incorporated within recent approaches towards person-centred care such as the VIPS approach developed by Dawn Brooker. Personalisation is therefore a much stronger concept than person-centred care that not only offers people with dementia respect and dignity but also the ability to choose.

The idea of personalisation developed outside services for people with dementia and within those for disabled people, their families and support organisations. People increasingly wanted to have increased choice and control of the resources that were available for their support – whether these were publicly or privately funded. They wanted what they considered was best for them, rather than finding their having to accept a 'one size fits all' approach. This approach was applied to people with learning difficulties in the government document *Valuing People* (DH, 2001) which is based on four key principles: civil rights, independence, choice and inclusion. *Valuing People* takes a life-course approach that offers an integrated approach to disabled children and their families and offers new opportunities for a full and purposeful adult life. This approach was later applied to all people, including those with dementia, in the government document *Putting People First* (DH, 2007) which outlined a shared vision and commitment to finding new ways of improving social care in England by enabling people to live independently and have complete choice and control in their lives.

Realising that person-centred care is only the first step towards personalisation, it is now appropriate to consider how support to people with dementia can be fully personalised. It is however important that mental health nurses take a pragmatic and realistic approach that fully recognises that while many people with dementia are quite able to make choices many will have lost the ability to do so. Nurses should be careful to note the degree to which people with dementia are able to make decisions and give them increased support as their ability to make decisions declines. In addition, it should be recognised that when a person develops dementia it is not just they who are affected but other family members will also suffer the consequences from this, and that as such they should also be part of the decision-making process.

A specific area of practice within personalisation is concerned with supporting people to develop personal budgets. While this is generally not seen as a task within the remit of mental health nurses, they do need to develop ways of helping people with dementia make worthwhile choices. Various tools are now available to mental health nurses that will enable them to assist people with dementia to make worthwhile choices about what they want (Adams, 2010b). Approaches like these should be offered by mental health nurses seeking to offer personalised support to people with dementia.

DEMENTIA-FRIENDLY COMMUNITIES

While advocating personalisation, *Caring for our Future: Reforming Care and Support* also supports the creation of local communities that are 'dementia friendly'. These communities offer environments that welcome, and are inclusive of, people with dementia. The idea of dementia-friendly communities draws on communitarian ideas that highlight the value of local networks within community and voluntary action that builds up the 'social capital' available within the community and supports people with dementia. The mobilisation of social networks and voluntary action was a key feature of the Prime Minister's Challenge on Dementia in March 2012, when David Cameron asserted that what was required was a 'sustained and concerted effort from all parts of society' to make 'a real difference' with respect to people with dementia.

Due to the newness of the idea and also the lack of research, dementia-friendly communities are difficult to define. One study however has identified the aims of dementia-friendly communities. These were to:

- reduce stigma;
- increase understanding and awareness about dementia and how to support people with dementia;
- support people with dementia to remain active and included members of their communities;
- support people with dementia in maintaining their independence for as long as possible.

The Joseph Rowntree Foundation Report (2012), *Creating a Dementia-Friendly York*, went further and developed the 'The Four Cornerstone Model' of developing dementia-friendly communities. The report asserted that the voices of people with dementia were at the heart of the process, and argued that dementia-friendly communities should develop the afore-mentioned four 'cornerstones':

- *Place* – how does the physical environment, housing, neighbourhood and transport support people with dementia?
- *People* – how do carers, families, friends, neighbours, health and social care professionals and the wider community respond to and support people with dementia?
- *Resources* – are there sufficient services and facilities for people with dementia and are these appropriate to their needs and supportive of their capabilities?
- *Networks* – do those who support people with dementia communicate, collaborate and plan together sufficiently well to provide optimal support and use people's own 'assets' well?

Dementia-friendly communities pose a challenge for mental health nurses working alongside people with dementia that stems from their individualistic approach which allows little understanding of 'the community'. This is once again an area that they must address to make sure they are able to deliver practice that reflects government policy on people with dementia.

MAKING A DIFFERENCE IN DEMENTIA: NURSING VISION AND STRATEGY

In March 2013, the Department of Health launched *Making a Difference in Dementia: Nursing Vision and Strategy* (DH, 2013) which built on its earlier document *Compassion in Practice* (DH, 2012b) and sought to maximise the contribution of nursing to high quality compassionate care and support for people with dementia and their family carers. The document developed a broad understanding of 'dementia nursing' which saw this undertaken not only by mental health nurses but also by any nurse and finding themselves alongside people with dementia and/or their family members. The document also developed a continuum of promoting well-ness and awareness raising/reducing social stigma; early identification, diagnosis and support; maintaining wellbeing and living well with dementia; managing acute and complex conditions with dementia; and end-of-life care and bereavement. To make this happen nurses, including those working in care homes, are commended to take the lead in the following areas:

- Maximising health and wellbeing.
- Helping people to stay independent.
- Supporting a positive staff experience.
- Working with people to provide a positive experience.
- Building and strengthening leadership.
- Ensuring we have the right staff, with the right skills and attributes in the right place.
- Delivering care and measuring impact.

The document outlines three key areas that are incumbent on all nurses – the so-called six C's: Care, Communication, Compassion, Courage, Confidence and Com-mitment. It also argues that there are three levels of expertise that nurses can offer dementia nursing, ranging from 'dementia awareness' for all nurses, through to 'dementia skilled' for all nurses working directly with people who have dementia, to 'dementia specialists' who are experts in the field of dementia care. The docu-ment sees the end result of dementia nursing as the development and delivery of seamless services for people with dementia within a person's own home, commu-nity, hospital settings and between these.

The appearance of a Department of Health vision document on dementia nursing was probably due a long time ago, though it is good that this has now appeared. The idea that dementia nursing is undertaken by all types of nurses is appropriate and something that has been developed in *Dementia Care Nursing* (Adams, 2010a) following the report, *Everyone's Business* (Gillard, 2007). However, the idea that dementia nursing is something that is not restricted to one group of nurses raises a contentious question, namely 'Where does specialism lie in dementia nursing?' I would suggest that mental health nursing is the natural source of specialism in dementia nursing. While Admiral Nurses undoubtedly have expertise supporting family carers, their focus is not the people with dementia but family carers. Admiral Nurses cannot justifiably claim they have a speciality in anything other than support-ing family carers, though their work will indirectly affect the people they support. The problem has always been the need for Admiral Nurses to carve out a new and distinctive role within service provision. There are presently nurses – mental health nurses – working within dementia services, and Admiral Nurses need to justify their existence as they can easily be seen as redundant, expensive, and merely duplicating the work of community mental health nurses. One way out of this dilemma would be for Admiral Nurses to claim they are specialist dementia nurses, but this has been discussed and is probably not appropriate. Mental health nurses are in a much better place to claim they have expertise in dementia nursing, as they employ a dual focus on people with dementia *and* their families.

To conclude, I would like to say that I have been associated with nursing people with dementia for over thirty years, and it has not escaped my notice that I too am getting old and one day soon may develop dementia. When that day occurs I hope the nurses supporting me will not treat me as though I am an object, or worse still, as though I am not there. I hope that instead they will take the trouble to ask me what I want, listen to what I say, and do everything they can to include me in this world before I go on to the next. I hope they do this, but I have to warn you that it could be YOU!

Reflective Exercise

1. How has mental health nursing positioned itself in a 'new era' of dementia care?
2. Can mental health nursing move effectively into this era of cautious optimism and if so how?
3. Are we able to articulate the distinctive contribution mental health nurses can make to the care of people with dementia?
4. Can we see the value of and influence a concept such as 'recovery' in this arena?

BIBLIOGRAPHY

Adams, T. (1996) Kitwood's approach to dementia and dementia care, a critical but apprecia-tive review, *Journal of Advanced Nursing*, 23: 948–953.

Adams, T. (2010a) *Dementia Care Nursing*. Basingstoke: Macmillan Palgrave.

Adams, T. (2010b) The applicability of a recovery approach to nursing people with dementia, *International Journal of Nursing Studies*, 47: 626–634.

Anthony, W.A. (1993) Recovery from mental illness: the guiding vision of the mental health service system in the 1990s, *Psychiatric Rehabilitation Journal*, 16: 12–23.

Audit Commission (1986) *Making a Reality of Community Care*. London: Audit Commission.

Department of Health (1983) *The Management Inquiry, National Health Service*. London: DH.

Department of Health (1989) *Caring for People: Community Care in the next Decade and Beyond*. London: DH.

Department of Health (1996) *Working in Partnership: Chief Nursing Officer's Review of Mental Health Nursing*. London: DH.

Department of Health (2001) *Valuing People*. London: DH.

Department of Health (2007) *Putting People First*. London: DH.

Department of Health (2009) *Living Well With Dementia: A National Dementia Strategy*. London: DH.

Department of Health (2011) *No Health Without Mental Health: A Cross-Government Mental Health Outcomes Strategy for People of All Ages*. London: DH.

Department of Health (2012a) *Caring For Our Future: Reforming Care and Support*. London: DH.

Department of Health (2012b) *Compassion in Practice*. London: DH.

Department of Health (2013)*Making a Difference in Dementia: Nursing Vision and Strategy.* London: DH.

DHSS (1981)*Growing Older.* London: HMSO.

Gillard, J. (The Care Services Improvement Partnership) (CSIP) (2007) 'Everybody's business', *A Life in the Day*, 11 (1): 26–7.

Health Advisory Service (1982) *The Rising Tide: Developing Services for Mental Illness in Old Age.* London: HMSO.

Houliston, M. (1961) *The Practice of Mental Nursing*, 3rd edition. Edinburgh: E. & S. Livingstone.

Joseph Rowntree Foundation (2012) *Creating a Dementia-Friendly York*. London: Joseph Rowntree.

Keady, J., Page, J. & Hope, K. (2009) The person with dementia. In I. Norman, and I. Ryrie (eds) *The Art and Science of Mental Health Nursing*. Buckingham: Open University Press. pp. 550–575.

Robb, B. (1967) *Sans Everything: A Case to Answer.* London: Nelson.

Scottish Executive (2006) *Rights, Relationships and Recovery: The Report of the National Review of Mental Health Nursing in Scotland.* Edinburgh: Scottish Executive.

Whitehead, T. (1970) *In the Service of Old Age.* Harmondsworth: Penguin.

Zarit, S., Todd, P. & Zarit, J. (1986) Subjective burden of husbands and wives as caregivers: a longitudinal study, *The Gerontologist*, 26 (3): 260–266.

7 PERSONALITY DISORDER

Karen M. Wright

Chapter Overview

The care and treatment of those labelled with a personality disorder has puzzled both practitioners and policy makers for some considerable time. Long considered a 'diagnostic dustbin', there have been vexed conversations about whether mental health services can offer any optimistic or evidence-based interventions at all. Many of those who reside in the criminal justice system (as this chapter will show) have received or meet the criteria for a personality disorder. The common, complex and at times challenging presentation of individuals who consume a disproportionate amount of services has given some cause to advocate the presence of specific targeted services for this client group.

Whilst there has been a successful transition from an 'illness' model to one of 'disorder' there still remains debate about the issue of detention and compulsion in the area of treatment. This debate has been focused by high profile events undertaken by those who carry the label. These events when high in profile and characterised by episodes of violence can create a sense of social unease. This sense of unease and a tradition of 'therapeutic nihilism' in the care and treatment (or management) of individuals has been challenged by two significant issues that are discussed in this chapter.

Firstly, there has been the voice of people who have the label of personality disorder where they acknowledge the difficulties they present, but also the poverty of interventions traditionally offered.

Secondly, as will be discussed in the chapter, there have been significant and influential policy documents that have challenged the traditional negative approaches to this client group. This is a clear example of how policy can shape the services provided and change the discourse in relation to a traditionally devalued group.

INTRODUCTION

In the past ten years or so, we have moved from a position where personality disorder (PD) lived within the realms of *'somebody else's problem'* through *'no longer a diagnosis of exclusion'* to a position where we have acknowledged the prevalence and impact of this disorder: we have some dedicated services; 'personality disorder' is an integral part of undergraduate programmes; and there is a national directive for enhanced understanding and provision of care and treatment for people with a personality disorder (DH, 2009).

There is little doubt that people with a diagnosis of personality disorder have often fallen between two stools for several reasons. The diagnosis has often been differentiated from mental illness, (Kendell, 2002), thus creating a rationale for the exclusion of individuals diagnosed with a personality disorder from mental health services by those who have believed that their remit is caring for those who are 'ill' as opposed to 'disordered'. But more worryingly, services have been unprepared to care for people with a personality disorder so the quality of service received may indeed be questionable (Wright et al., 2007). Furthermore, until very recently personality disorder education was not routinely included in pre-registration nurse education and post-qualifying education was at best limited and frequently unavailable. Hence, the capacity to meet directives to provide appropriate care and treatment for a group of people whose needs are largely misunderstood has been a challenge on a number of levels.

Although it is difficult to quantify, the Psychiatric Morbidity Survey (PMS) attempted to measure personality disorders in the UK, and recently Coid et al. (2006) have analysed these data. It is thought that the total number of people with personality disorders is estimated to be 2.46 million. Of this total 53 per cent are male. By 2026 the projected number is 2.69 million. In 2007 the annual service costs were estimated to be £704 million for those in contact with primary care, with this figure projected to be £1.1 billion by 2026. With the inclusion of lost employment costs the figures are £7.9 billion and £12.3 billion respectively (Kings Fund, 2008). Currently, between 5% and 13% of people with a personality disorder are living in the community, and 40% and 50% are inpatients, whilst between 50% and 78% of prisoners are diagnosable with a personality disorder.

WHAT IS MEANT BY THE TERM 'PERSONALITY DISORDER'?

There is some utility in firstly considering what is meant by the term 'personality disorder' which is now commonly used but also frequently misunderstood. Despite experts on the subject referring to PD as a 'fuzzy concept' (Livesley, 2001), the frequency of this diagnosis is increasing, often as a co-occurring condition. Parker and Schneider (2007), writing from a social policy perspective, suggested that personality disorder was sited 'uncomfortably' within the remit of mental health services and that it was not a mental health problem at all, its treatability had been disputed, and that it was actually an enduring feature of an individual's character.

Within the *DSM* and *ICD*, PD has been identified as being different and separate from 'mental illness', with this first becoming apparent in *DSM III*, published in 1980, which placed 'personality disorders' on a separate axis (axis II) to mental disorders (Tyrer & Simonsen, 2003). The *DSM IV* and the *ICD 10* both seem to define PD in terms of a disease model, with the problems associated with PD clearly located within the individual. Both the European and American diagnostic definitions of personality disorder are used in the UK, not least because so much of the personality disorder literature is published in the USA and it is helpful to reconsider the level of severity required to acquire a diagnosis.

The World Health Organization defines personality disorder as:

> A severe disturbance in the charactereological condition and behavioural tendencies of the individual, usually involving several areas of the personality, and nearly always associated with considerable personal and social disruption. (WHO, 1992: 202)

The WHO describe nine different personality disorders ('subtypes') as well as that which is 'unspecified' and provide guidelines for diagnosis.

> The American Psychiatric Association's definition is slightly different and includes the cultural context as an important factor: *"An enduring pattern of inner experience and behaviour that deviates markedly from the expectations of the individual's culture, is pervasive and inflexible, has an onset in adolescence or early adulthood, is stable over time, and leads to distress or impairment."* (APA, 1994: 633)

They identify ten different personality disorders (plus 'personality disorder not otherwise specified') which they group into three 'clusters'.

Both systems highlight the deviation from what is considered to be the norm within a given culture. Crowe (2000: 70) argued *'that the way in which the DSM IV constructs mental disorder effectively constructs normality'*, and yet when Kendell (2002: 100) sought to provide a distinction between personality disorder and mental illness he concluded that it was *'impossible to conclude with confidence that personality disorders are, or are not, mental illnesses'*.

Thus the term PD, as defined by the current classification systems, infers that the individual diagnosed has something inherently wrong, i.e. 'disordered', within their personality. Furthermore, it suggests that the individual falls outside what is considered to be the norm. In recent years there has been criticism made of these systems and their associated practices, most notably by Bentall (2003) in relation to diagnoses of schizophrenia and their reliability and validity. The development of a personality disorder can usually be traced back to childhood and experiences of 'growing up', often rooted in childhood abuse, deprivation neglect or trauma, and these experiences then impact on the person's interpersonal relationships both as an individual or in society. The complex and multifaceted nature of the disorder presents many challenges not only to health, social and criminal justice services but also to society as a whole, as people with PD may present with a range of physical, mental health and social problems such as substance misuse, depression and suicide risk, housing problems, offending and long-standing interpersonal problems (DH, 2009).

Arguments regarding the utility of diagnosis abound, with Livesley (2005) concluding that personality disorders do not exist in discrete neat boxes or categories. The *ICD 10* and *DSM IV* are polythetic categorical systems of classification, depicting specific diagnostic rule-based criteria (Kendall & Jablensky, 2003). Polythetic systems require that only a small number of the identified 'symptoms' or abnormalities are needed to acquire a diagnosis. Such systems are based on set theory, which sees the separation of those that belong in the set and those that don't, thus perpetuating the idea that one is either 'normal', and outside the diagnosis set, or 'abnormal', and inside the diagnostic set. Such a judgement is bestowed on the clinician who is required to observe whether behaviours fit with a certain diagnosis. Judgements are based upon clinicians' values and beliefs which are shaped by the clinical and professional culture within which they work (Crowe, 2000).

THE POLICY FOR DIAGNOSING

Few people diagnosed with PD actually receive a comprehensive assessment ensuring the accuracy or certainty of their diagnosis, and in the main a diagnosis is made using the guidelines provided in *ICD-10* which ask for only a limited number of the traits or behaviours identified in the subtypes to be present. Therefore, before we consider mental health policy in relation to the care and treatment offered to sufferers of personality disorder, we need to acknowledge that the policy for diagnosis may itself be inadequate.

Many authors (Blashfield & Livesley, 1997; Livesley, 2001; Pilgrim, 2001; Kendall & Jablensky, 2003) have written extensively on the basic premise of these classification systems in terms of the reliability and validity of PD, even suggesting that the diagnosis of personality disorder is *fundamentally flawed* (Pilgrim, 2001). The very nature of the human condition is one of immeasurable complexity. Disorders such as depression, anxiety, and to a lesser extent psychosis, are very rarely simple and concise in their make-up and manifestations, and often blur into one another to create a picture where one approach or over-riding treatment will never fit with all of these. If we look at personality disorders, the overall landscape of an individual's illness can be seen to mutate even more. Additionally, co-occurring conditions have led both theorists and clinicians to, if not wholly dismiss the categorical systems of assessment, then to use them in conjunction with dimensional systems (Leibing et al., 2008).

Livesley (2005) suggests that an alternative to the categorical approach is the dimensional model of classification which comprises two components: firstly, a definition of personality disorder and any associated terms; and secondly, a system for tapping into the individual nuances of personality pathology. Thus, moving away from the clustering of disorders towards a system which is more relevant, clinically usable and facilitates the creation of unique information about the service user. The trait theorists who believe dimensional systems to be the future of assessment and treatment planning base such an idea on personality existing along a continuum, and that the continuum works as a measure as to where and for what reasons an individual will occupy a certain place along it. This allows us to view personality in both its 'normal' and 'abnormal' presentation, and in doing so allows for individualised planning towards recovery and improved functioning amongst service users.

Despite the complexities of diagnosis and the prerequisite disabling features of a personality disorder, Coid et al. (2006) suggest that patients diagnosed with PD may not retain that diagnosis and that opinions may differ over time: this fits with recent naturalistic studies of the course of PD indicating that personality psychopathology improves over time, and that the maturation process has a significant impact on the level of distress and disability.

HOW DO WE KNOW HOW TO CARE FOR A PERSON WITH PERSONALITY DISORDER?

The most significant document published in the last ten years has been the policy implementation guide *Personality Disorder: No Longer a Diagnosis of Exclusion* (NIMHE, 2003a), which prompted the emergence of dedicated services for personality disorder. This was based on the premise that the existing provision was inadequate, training and education were inaccessible, and services were unprepared to care for and treat people with PD. Later the same year, a further document (*Breaking the Cycle of Rejection: The Personality Disorder Capabilities Framework*) was published in recognition that health-care workers were being asked to care for people without the requisite skills, knowledge and understanding. Both documents provided guidance for good practice when developing services in general adult-community mental health settings and forensic settings. More recently, a review of the Mental Health Act (2007) has removed the treatability test, thus preventing practitioners using this as a way to deny services to people with personality disorder and so addressing the criticism that *many people with PD have felt disempowered and excluded by services in the past* (DH, 2009: 13).

A number of policy documents and guidance have been published since 2003, demonstrating significant progress in the care, treatment and social inclusion of people with a personality disorder and these are as follows:

- 2003 *Personality Disorder: No Longer a Diagnosis of Exclusion.* Policy implementation guidance published January 2003. Available at www.nimhe.org.uk
- 2003 *Breaking the Cycle of Rejection: The Personality Disorder Capabilities Framework.*

- 2004 Chief Executive's letter to NHS organisations on personality disorder services and issues for commissioners, *Chief Executive's Bulletin*, issue no. 239, 1–7 October 2004.
- 2004 The Department of Health and the Home Office commission NIMHE to deliver a National Workforce and Training Programme. Educational and training programmes on personality disorder through NIMHE Regional Development Centres (RDCs).
- 2005 Local commissioners and stakeholders developed capacity plans for personality disorder services.
- 2005 *Forensic PD Medium Secure and Community Pilot Services: Planning and Delivery Guide DSPD Programme*, and also *DSPD High Secure Services for Men*.
- 2005 *Standards for the Commissioning of NHS Therapeutic Communities*.
- 2006 'Delivering for Mental Health', the mental health delivery plan for Scotland.
- 2007 Reform of the Mental Health Act.
- 2007 National survey of personality disorder training issued by the Institute of Mental Health, the London-based Tavistock and Portman NHS Trust, Borderline UK (now named Emergence), and the Open University.
- 2008 *Beyond Local Services: Commissioning and Providing Services for People with Complex and Severe PD*.
- 2009 *Recognising Complexity: Commissioning Guidance for Personality Disorder Services*.
- 2009 Bradley Report: Lord Bradley's review of people with mental health problems or learning disabilities in the criminal justice system published by the DH.
- 2009 NICE developed clinical guidelines for borderline personality disorder (CG78).
- 2009 NICE developed clinical guidelines for antisocial personality disorder (CG77).
- 2010 *Women with Borderline Personality Disorder in Prison* published by the Centre for Mental Health.
- 2011 Response to the Offender Personality Disorder Consultation by the DH/Ministry of Justice.

IS INCLUSION A REALITY?

In many ways, the promise of specialist services may reinforce the misguided belief that only specially trained workers can care for people with a personality disorder. In the past a lack of knowledge and misguided practice have consistently led to the marginalisation of the client group and the reinforcement of negative attitudes towards them. Those living in the community and using generic services are thought to make heavy demands upon health services, and are viewed by primary care services as '*difficult*' or '*heart-sink*' patients (Macmanus & Fahy, 2008). Similarly, this negative perception of 'dangerousness' has been exaggerated by the development of 'dangerous and severe personality disorder' (DSPD) units within high secure institutions and media portrayals of high profile cases, and is intended to be applied to those offenders with a severe personality disorder.

Yet despite all this people are accessing services: in fact people with personality disorder problems tend to be high users of psychiatric outpatient departments, psychiatric inpatient services, crisis services, general practice, Accident and Emergency departments and social services. They may tend to be routed and re-routed between psychological therapies, primary care, CMHTs, day hospital and inpatient psychiatric services with a limited effectiveness of outcome. Their level of functional impairment in daily life can be very high and comparable with those with a psychotic diagnosis (Newton-Howes et al., 2008).

The document most often quoted and intended to create an inclusive acceptance of people with personality disorder into services provides a damning summary:

> What is clear is that people with personality disorders make heavy demands upon local services, which are often ill equipped to deal with these. One of the characteristics of this group is that they often evoke high levels of anxiety in carers, relatives and professionals. They tend to have relatively frequent, often escalating, contact across a spectrum of services including mental health, social services, A&E, GPs and the criminal justice system. They may present to mental health services with recurrent deliberate self harm, substance abuse, interpersonal problems that may include violence, various symptoms of anxiety and depression, brief psychotic episodes, and eating disorders. (NIMHE, 2003a: 12)

ACCESSIBILITY OF INFORMATION FOR THE PUBLIC

Significant progress has been made on a national level. Department of Health (DH) publications relating to 'personality disorder' refer to personality disorder **offenders** (DH, 2011a). The publication of *No Health Without Mental Health* does not mention 'personality disorder' (DH, 2011b) at all, and the publication of *Closing the Gap: Priorities for Essential Change in Mental Health* has only one reference to PD, which is links with a proposal for exploration, rather than a plan.

> We are also exploring how psychological therapies can be used to help with severe mental illness and personality disorders – as part of a wider programme of care – and looking at how they can be integrated into care for people who have depression or anxiety that is related to a long-term physical condition. (DH, 2014: 14)

A determined pursuit of this via the search engine opens up the full range of documents, and clicking on *'offender health'* leads the reader to a section referring to personality disorder:

> Approximately two-thirds of prisoners meet the criteria for at least one type of personality disorder and a high proportion of cases are managed by probation. For a relatively small number of offenders, in its most severe forms, personality disorder is linked to a serious risk of harm to themselves and to others. These offenders have highly complex psychological needs that create challenges in terms of management, treatment and maintaining a safe working environment. (DH, 2011: 8)

There is obviously a strong link made here between PD and offending. Resources are currently being pumped into prisons and forensic services in an attempt to address this much neglected area of health care and thus offer treatment whilst in custody, as this might be the best chance we have of attaining the engagement with treatment. The DSPD programme, despite its focus on DSPD, has offered new NHS forensic personality disorder services (DH, 2008). Furthermore, Fossey and Black (2010) have emphasised the necessity of meeting the needs of women with borderline personality disorder in prison, along with a number of recommendations including better diversion from custodial sentences and increased training for prison staff.

Both the NICE *Guideline for Antisocial PD* (NICE, 2009a) and Department of Health's document *Recognising Complexity* (DH, 2003) make significant recommendations for what have become known as *'high harm offenders'*, as offenders with a severe personality disorder are likely to present a high or very high risk of serious harm (National Probation Service, 2008). NICE recommends that probation should lead the inter-agency case management for this client group, supported by specialist health services and closely linked to Multi-Agency Public Protection Arrangements (MAPPA). It is of note that there are slight differences between the arrangements for MAPPA in England and Wales and Scotland: MAPPA in Scotland is based on the systems in place in England and Wales, with a few minor differences. The most noticeable of these is that in England and Wales the 'responsible authority' is made up of the Probation Service, the Police Service and HM Prison Services, whereas in Scotland they are made up of the Police Service, Social Work Scotland, Scottish Prison Service and NHS Scotland.

STIGMA AND LABELLING

Although a great deal of work has been done in the last ten years, there remains greater stigma applied to personality disorder than to mental illness *per se*. Phelan et al. (2000) suggest that the general public's understanding of the causes of mental illness has broadened thus reducing stigma, however, that same study indicates that attitudes about persons with mental illness have become more stigmatising in terms of dangerousness during the past thirty years as the proportion who described a mentally ill person as being violent increased by nearly two and a half times between 1950 and 1996. In more recent years, the term *'dangerous and severe personality disorder'* (DSPD) has created an inextricable link between personality disorder and dangerousness (Wright et al., 2007).

All mental health service users are subject to stigmatising and stereotypical representation in the discourse of the lay public, in the pages of the print media and on TV and cinema screens. Quite often these accounts fail to differentiate between the various medical categories of mental disorder, with terms such as 'psychotic' and 'psychopathic' used interchangeably in a context of public fear of violent madness. Various commentators have noted the range of media depictions of people with a mental illness, with individuals described as monsters, homicidal maniacs, parasites, mad, bad, or evil. Individuals diagnosed with personality disorder exemplify the notion of the unpopular patient, provoking a range of negative reactions which have been remarked upon in the literature over a significant amount of time (Main, 1957; Blackburn, 1988; Hinshelwood, 1999; Pilgrim, 2001; Bowers, 2002). A dimension of this is the moral judgements that are brought to bear in the appraisal of people and their behaviour, thus labelling and stigmatising them according to Hinshaw et al.'s definition:

> ... a deep, shameful mark or flaw related to being the member of a group that is deval-ued by the societal mainstream ... once the castigation begins the perceiver comes to view those with mental illness as lacking the fundamental qualities of humanity. (2006: xi)

This was never truer than for the person with personality disorder.

Inevitably, the media prescription for policy is for containment: media portrayals are of a group of people who are either dangerous and in need of secure detention, or they present a risk to themselves and are in need of the emotional security of the asylum (Gleeson, 1991; Hyler et al., 1991; McKeown & Clancy, 1995). Individuals with personality disorder frequently engender feelings of frustration amongst health professionals. Nymande and Sikabbubba (2006) state that these clients are a chal-lenge to nurse and to nurse effectively. This fits with a perception that many of those individuals who are considered violent and criminal should rationally be incarcer-ated as a moral and justifiable action to protect a vulnerable and blameless society. Thus, the route through to personality disorder information (via the offender litera-ture) only seeks to reinforce the term *personality disorder* being synonymous with statements of deviance and criminal activity, and thus more likely to be seen as undeserving of care and treatment (Murphy & McVey, 2003). Current research reinforces that negative attitudes exist towards personality disorder and that the task of working with such a client group is deemed onerous and less reinforcing. Murphy and McVey (2003) suggest that the challenges in treating clinically PD patients cluster around five main themes:

- These patients are less reinforcing and more demanding than mentally ill patients.
- Nurse training does not prepare nurses for this work.
- The role of nursing personality disordered patients is high in conflict.
- Personality disordered patient nursing is traumatising.
- Personality disordered patients require specific skills and qualities.

The consequences of such constructions are keenly felt by service users with diag-noses of personality disorder:

> We get stigma from medical professionals – many older psychiatrists still live with the PD as a dustbin diagnosis – we can't get them better therefore let's give them a label that means they are awkward then we can kick them out. Many psych nurses have the same impressions as they are not trained in PDs so they have no idea how to handle us. They accuse us of 'acting out' when we are doing anything that they do

not understand ... as this is some psychobabble word that they have heard but do not understand truly. (Anderson, 2004)

The subsequent exclusion from mental health services is, in the main, attributed to a lack of knowledge and understanding of the disorder, rather than an open expression of dislike for this client group. However an alternative, and rarely expressed view, has been purported by Scanlan and Adlam (2008) who suggest their destructive behaviour is held to be deliberate by workers who see this as offensive and within the control of the individual.

The voices of service users (Stalker et al., 2005: 363) suggest that the diagnosis of PD *'means that there was something fundamentally wrong with them as a person'*, with the label pejorative and a means of medicalising the distress experienced by the individual. Such comments capture the sense of hopelessness that people diagnosed with the label PD may experience and also the view PD is untreatable and lifelong (Lewis & Appleby, 1988; Markham & Trower, 2003). As far back as 1949, Winnicott likened caring for the difficult patient to a mother caring for a demanding baby:

However much he loves his patients he cannot avoid hating them and fearing them, and the better he knows this the less will hate and fear be the motives determining what he does to his patients. (1949: 195)

Although Winnicott regarded this as a 'normal' process he pointed out that it was not the done thing to seek such opinions or attitudes in the workplace as to do so was seen as professionally unacceptable.

MENTAL HEALTH LAW AND PERSONALITY DISORDER

The Mental Health Act 1983, 2007 applies to England and Wales. One of the most notable reasons for amending the 1983 act was due to concerns about the risks to the public posed by people with a serious mental disorder living in the community: this included personality disorder and psychopathic personality disorder (Lawton-Smith et al., 2008). Scotland has had its own Mental Health Act (the Mental Health (Care and Treatment) (Scotland) Act 2003), which came into effect in 2005, and in Ireland, the Mental Health Act 2001 exists.

The Mental Health Act for England and Wales insists that a patient detained in hospital shall receive treatment which is 'likely to alleviate or prevent a deterioration in his condition' to ensure that those people who lose their liberty under mental health law are likely to benefit from such a detention. Prior to the revision of the Mental Health Act, it was often felt that people with a personality disorder could not be detained in hospital since there was limited evidence that this was treatable. The 'treatability test' contributes to a culture in which PD patients are seen as undeserving of mental health care. Appleby believes that the removal of the treatability test *'will do much to ensure that people with PD get the treatment that they need and are not excluded routinely from care'* (Appleby, 2007: 3). Trebilcock & Weaver (2012) also state most emphatically that even a patient with DSPD doesn't have to be treatable to warrant admission either formally or informally.

In Scotland the law is slightly different and based upon the Mental Health (Scotland) Act 1984. The grounds for detention are much the same as in England and Wales, in that the focus is on the person's ill-health, their safety and the safety of others, the availability of treatment, and the refusal for voluntary admission.

High Secure Services in England (previously known as the 'special hospitals': that is, Ashworth, Broadmoor and Rampton) are broadly equivalent to the State Hospital in Scotland and accommodate a much higher proportion of patients with a primary diagnosis of personality disorder. This reflects both differences in mental health law (the Mental Health Act 1983 in England, which has a specific category of psychopathic disorder) and a different tradition within English hospitals. Although the Scottish Mental Health Act 1984 omits the term 'psychopathy' from their legislation, the term 'personality disorder' is used (Darjee & Crichton, 2003). In England and Wales, the act now describes a specialist 'treatment programme' for groups of high-risk offenders with severe personality disorder (MacManus & Fahy, 2008), whilst Scotland have chosen not to implement a programme of preventive detention. In Scotland this comes under the remit of the Risk Management Authority (RMA) which aims to assess and manage offenders (Scottish Executive, 2000, 2004, 2006).

POLICY TO IMPROVE RESPONSES AND UNDERSTANDING OF PERSONALITY DISORDER

'A little knowledge is a dangerous thing'

This phrase is certainly true for those staff who have had little or no specific training in personality disorder, but who can exert considerable influence on prevailing attitudes and decisions. Anecdotally, most practitioners will be aware of the phase 'she's (he's) a PD' being banded about with negative overtones in services. Furthermore it is possible for hostile or critical attitudes to develop in staff of all disciplines who have contact with service users. Hence, in 2007 a survey of 'trainings' available nationally of direct or indirect relevance to the field of personality disorder was conducted by the Institute of Mental Health, the London-based Tavistock and Portman NHS Trust, Borderline UK (now named Emergence) and the Open University.

'Trainings' included courses, workshops, modules of larger programmes and stand-alone courses, and training events with potentially open-access. Commissioned in-house training for specific staff groups and conferences was not included. Training providers were asked to complete a form detailing the characteristics of the course or workshop. This report, published by the Personality Disorder Knowledge Understanding Framework Partnership, provides an analysis of the 94 returns.

The survey identified only one course available at Master's level that was specifically focused on personality disorder and this was at the University of Central Lancashire: it was developed with a view to helping clinicians in the field develop their skills and conduct research in the area of personality disorder. Subsequently, the Department of Health and Ministry of Justice commissioned the development of a national framework of education and training to support people to work more effectively with personality disorder, from awareness-level education to a Master's level programme (MSc). This has been rolled out throughout the country and is a direct response to the *Breaking the Cycle of Rejection: The Personality Disorder Capabilities Framework* (NIMHE, 2003b).

ACCESSIBILITY AND QUALITY OF CARE

There is something very comforting for somebody who is suffering to know that treatment can be offered that will treat their symptoms/difficulties and thus alleviate their distress. So, for those who are acknowledged as complex and at risk to themselves, and possibly others, the sense of despair that is felt at being told that their treatment options are limited must be devastating and rarely acknowledged. However, it is illness that is 'treated' and, as Gwen Adshead rightly says, 'The status of personality disorder as an illness ... remains contentious', but then, as she later adds, 'Treatments may have different purposes, not all of which aim at cure' (Adshead, 2001: 409, 410), and makes the parallel between the treatment of cancer and the treatment of personality disorder.

There are certainly very few pharmacological approaches recommended, with the exception that the many co-occurring conditions might well be treated very effectively with medication. Vulnerability to other mental health problems such as anxiety, depression, eating disorders and self-harm is high, and it is important that these are not over-looked as merely features of the PD. Moran, Walsh and Tyrer et al. (2003) also emphasise the increased risk of suicide and violence when PD co-occurs with psychosis, reinforcing the importance of offering assertive treatment to these individuals.

More recent research and determined efforts to explore the possibility and adaptation of effective talking therapies for personality disorder have demonstrated that treatment is possible and that skills-based treatments such as cognitive–behavioural therapy, cognitive analytical therapy, and dialectical behaviour therapy should be promoted for use with this client group, despite the limited availability and concerns over suitability (Bateman & Tyrer, 2004a; Koekkoek et al., 2010; Evershed, 2011). NICE (2009b) recommend that psychological treatments should be offered for people with both borderline personality disorder and antisocial personality disorder, suggesting that twice-weekly sessions may be considered and for at least three months in duration. Unfortunately, however, there are long waiting lists for psycho-logical treatments (Norton, 2009).

Bateman and Tyrer (2004a) outlined the different clinical approaches applied to this patient group, describing not just the difficulties in treating personality disordered patients, but also the pitfalls into which the differing management prin-ciples can stumble. While there are obvious limitations to the 'sole-practitioner' approach, especially in relation to the matter of the level of specialist knowledge and training these clinicians possess, there is a complex range of issues that may arise in the case of the 'divided functions' approach, as there are in the more 'specialist-team' model.

There is a fundamental price to pay for a division of roles, since it separates treatment of an individual, who is often already psychologically fragmented, into discrete components at a time when the task is to facilitate improved inte-gration within the person and to establish with them a more constructive place within society. Medication becomes split off from psychotherapy, housing and social care from mental health care. The therapeutic alliance may be weakened by being attached to a number of different mental health professionals, and treat-ment provision can develop into uncoordinated pockets of care. The community team and psychiatrist may intervene in crises, admitting the patient to hospital often without discussion with the psychotherapist, who may have been working with the patient to develop a capacity to remain out of hospital. The housing agency may begin an eviction process without discussion with the social support worker. This lack of coordination, however, is not inevitable, with Batemen and Tyrer observing that the model can work well if the different parts of the system or the different practitioner roles are well integrated, there is good collabora-tion between all involved, and a coherent message is given to the patient. While the multi-disciplinary approach of the specialist team, or the well functioning 'divided-functions' model, does not simply avoid problems and offers significant advantages (particularly for patients with severe personality disorder who require frequent risk assessment, have multiple needs, demand continual engagement if they are to remain in treatment and provoke powerful countertransference reac-tions) they are not without their inherent weaknesses.

Individual staff's reactions to patients with personality disorders commonly sub-vert the task of treatment and lead them to take inappropriate actions (Gabbard, 2001). Paying careful attention to countertransference can reduce the likelihood of unprofessional conduct, aid risk assessment (e.g. of the level of dangerousness), and inform treatment intervention. The team approach offers a protection against the over-involvement or malpractice of any one individual. The question about whether, espe-cially in such austere times, practitioners are happy to treat this client group is an issue rarely confronted, but Scanlon and Adlam face this head on, suggesting that whilst practitioners view the manifestations of the disorder as 'intentional' there is also:

> ample documented evidence that when they do receive 'health care' interventions these can often appear more like 'revenge' or 'retaliation' or, at the very least, prejudice and discrimination meted out by practitioners who have become, at best unwitting arbiters

of 'social worth', and at worst agents of social control acting out society's unconscious hatred of 'them'. (Scanlan & Adlam, 2008: 539)

CARE PATHWAYS

NICE (2009a) state that people with a personality disorder should not be excluded from any health or social care service because of their diagnosis or history of antisocial or offending behaviour, despite the phenomenon of being the patients that 'psychiatrists dislike' (Lewis & Appleby, 1988). While issues such as the service framework within which patients are being treated, and the obvious economic concerns therein, have a bearing on the breadth and particular quality of the service provided, in the case of personality disordered patients a number of issues appear to arise that are inherent to their treatment and to the structures of the teams charged with their care.

The personality disorder capabilities framework has been produced to support the guidance developed by NIMHE (2003), which aimed at ensuring that as well as developing both specialist mental health and forensic services for people with a personality disorder, staff would be well equipped with the education and training they required to work effectively with services users who have a diagnosis of personality disorder.

INTEGRATION AND INCLUSION OR MARGINALISATION?

There is no doubt that people with personality disorder have complex needs and that many of those needs, and underpinning difficulties, are seen as challenging and misunderstood by workers and services. However, do we accept that personality disorder is a complex problem in the same way as other severe and enduring mental health problems, or do we devote specific services to a group of people searching for inclusion in the mainstream? This is a dilemma faced by many, but the Royal College of Psychiatrists, in their document *Enabling Recovery for People with Complex Mental Health Needs,* chose to include PD alongside other 'complex' disorders. In many ways finding a service, any service that can provide consistency and constancy (Bateman & Tyrer, 2004b), would be a way forward in such austere times when treatment programmes have been cut to the bone. However, clinicians report a broad spectrum of experience.

Anecdotally, whilst forensic and prison workers report how pleased they are that service users are gaining access to treatment and that they are gaining access to education, many community mental health workers are struggling. One example here is Blackpool, one of the most deprived council wards in Britain, where between 2005 and 2007 there was the worst suicide rate in males, and worst rate across both genders, out of 152 NHS trusts in England (Peckham & Meerabeau, 2007; NHS, 2009). Factors attributed to poor mental health in Blackpool are being unemployed, being homeless, being poor, having a physical illness, and having a drug or alcohol problem.

The rate of hospital admissions for alcohol-specific conditions in Blackpool is above the England average and there is a higher rate of children living in poverty. Compare these factors identified by NIMHE in the policy implementation guide:

> Personality disordered individuals are more likely to suffer from alcohol and drug problems and are also more likely to experience adverse life events, such as relationship difficulties, housing problems and long-term unemployment. (NIMHE, 2003: 11)

The short life expectancy is attributed, amongst other factors, to overdose, poisoning and self harm, factors associated with Borderline Personality Disorder. A mental health nurse told me recently that if a person with a personality disorder is in crisis they can access the Crisis Team and will gain a response but that if they are coping they will be discharged, leading them to conclude that it doesn't pay to cope.

Johnson and Haigh (2011) discuss the need to be socially inclusive and thus to develop more 'psychologically informed environments' (PIEs) for services working with *severely marginalised and excluded individuals*. This largely refers to the homeless, but it cannot be denied that people with a personality disorder have been some of the most marginalised in mental health services. The tide is now shifting, not least because service users have been given a voice and many of those with a personality disorder are making themselves heard. There are many good examples of this, including the group Emergence (formally known as Borderline UK) and regional groups such those developed as a response to the the National Personality Disorder Development Programme, which explicitly required service users' voices to be heard in the design and development of services (Johnson & Haigh, 2011).

Clearly, acceptance that the service user has a voice, and that this is valid, has been a major breakthrough in mental health services, not least for those with a personality disorder. A number of groups, established over recent years, have been established to lobby for better services, services that listen to their users and services that are inclusive of diversity. Probably one of the most well-known personality disorder service user-led groups is Emergence, who state that their vision is *to make a life changing difference for everyone affected by personality disorders (PD) through support, advice and education.* Others, such as the 'Exclusion Link' (in partnership with the Thames Valley Initiative) focus on the exclusion of PD patients from both services and society. They provide information and training and are affiliated to the National PD Development Network.

RECOVERY

The recovery model, which originated from Alcoholics Anonymous and the civil rights movement, gained impetus as a social movement due to a perceived failure by services or wider society to adequately support social inclusion and by studies demonstrating that many can recover. Hence, for people with personality disorder this offers a level of hope and optimism, but current understandings of recovery are changing and the 'recovery model' has been subject to a number of challenges in terms of its usefulness in contemporary society.

As with many things, the initial challenges seemed to focus on the very meaning and definition of the term:

> There is an increasing global commitment to recovery as the expectation for people with mental illness. There remains, however, little consensus on what recovery means in relation to mental illness. (Davidson and Roe, 2007: 450)

Castillo (2010), from the Haven Research Group, has attempted to provide some insight into what participants consider to be the key steps to recovery for someone with a personality disorder diagnosis. She defines the journey of recovery as a series of small steps highlighting recovering as a *process* rather than a *goal*, leading to the emergence of a new concept of Transitional Recovery.

The recent emphasis upon notions of recovery in mental health care has similarly highlighted ideas of common humanity (Townsend & Glasser, 2003), Indeed, Wright et al. (2007) expressed the need to 'reclaim the humanity' for people with personality disorder. The very concept of 'recovery' encompasses the process whereby an individual can reclaim their self-esteem, pride, choice, dignity and meaning, and requires the mental health worker to embrace people's humanity to facilitate this process (Townsend & Glasser, 2003: 83).

Recovery is about the whole person, identifying their strengths, instilling hope, and helping them to function at an optimal level by allowing them to take responsibility for their life.

Laurie Davidson (n.d.), from the Devon Recovery Group, explains that 'People do not recover in isolation. Recovery is closely associated with social inclusion and being able to take on meaningful and satisfying social roles within local communities, rather than in segregated services'.

This perspective is an important one, since recovery cannot occur in isolation and is dependent upon both interpersonal processes, of great significance in personality disorder, and also the environment in which recovery occurs as relationships and the context may well be the crux of our existence. In this chapter we have tended to consider the environment in terms of the culture and communities created by its members, be it within services or within society. Johnson and Haigh (2011: 58) move this forward and discuss the need to put 'the social back in the social determinants of health'. They propose that we develop more 'psychologically informed environments' for services working with severely marginalised and excluded individuals. These will be 'enabling environments' , which are determined by ten core values and standards including 'belonging' as the first 'value', thus stressing the primary importance of the therapeutic relationship and the pivotal nature of a positive connection (Wright & Jones, 2012). 'Boundaries' are listed next, to emphasise the vital requirement of shared expectations, followed by 'communication' (all behaviour is seen as a mode of communication), 'development' and 'involvement'. 'Containment', 'structure', 'empowerment', leadership, and finally, 'openness' are all listed as core issues for the creation of an 'enabling environment'. These may go some way to facilitating engagement with those who are most marginalised and excluded to improve their own health, and reduce the risk and burden on others (DH, 2009).

As mental health nurses we are conditioned to provide care and 'unconditional positive regard' for all (Rogers, 1957). Undergraduate nursing programmes include 'therapeutic engagement' as a necessary field, and we consider promoting adherence to treatment as part of our duty of care. Our role is greater than care provision: we cannot fail to recognise the importance of context of the care and the civil liberty of the person to make their own choices about engagement with is. Many people with personality disorder feel rejected, abandoned or unworthy, whilst others clearly present a danger to others who are most vulnerable by them. As practitioners, there may be many more arguments about the validity of the diagnosis, but a move away from medicalised care, directed by diagnosis, towards a socially inclusive and enabling environment is certainly one way. However, embedding policy is not a straightforward process (Norton, 2009) and for people with a personality disorder a tolerant, educated and understanding perspective would be a great place to start:

> Our plea is for greater tolerance, understanding and interest in the lives of those who, as a result of fearful refusal, have found themselves on the borderlines and liminal spaces of our deeply troubled society, and for a better informed debate between our systems of care and the wider social world about how to introduce the structural and cultural changes that will be necessary in order for us to relate meaningfully to some of the most vulnerable members of our community whether we – whoever and wherever we are – like it or not. (Scanlon & Adlam, 2008: 545)

Reflective Exercise

1. What are my views about people who carry this diagnostic label?
2. If I had to characterise the attitudes of many of my colleagues what would these be?
3. What do I find challenging about people with this label?
4. To what degree do I feel I was prepared to care for this client group in my undergraduate education?

BIBLIOGRAPHY

Adshead, G. (2001) Murmurs of discontent, *Advances in Psychiatric Treatment*, 7: 407–415.

American Psychiatric Association (1994) *Diagnostic and Statistical Manual of Mental Disorders – Fourth Edition 1994 (DSM-IV)*. Washington, DC: APA.

Anderson, P. (2004) *Personality Disorder and Service User Involvement* [cited 17 February 2005]. Available at: www. nimhennorthwest.org.uk

Appleby, L. (2007) Foreword, *Mental Health Review Journal*, 12 (4): 3–4.

Bateman, A.W. & Tyrer, P. (2004a) Psychological treatment for personality disorders, *Advances in Psychiatric Treatment*, 10: 378–388.

Bateman, A.W. & Tyrer, P. (2004b) Services for personality disorder: organisation for inclusion, *Advances in Psychiatric Treatment*, 10: 425–433.

Bentall, R.P. (2003) *Madness Explained: Psychosis and Human Nature*. London: Penguin.

Blackburn, R. (1988) On moral judgements and personality disorders: the myth of psychopathic disorder revisited, *British Journal of Psychiatry*, 153: 505–512.

Blashfield, R. & Livesley, J. (1997) The problem of the unique beginner in the classification of psychopathology, *Clinical Psychology: Science and Practice*, 4: 267–271.

Bowers, L. (2002) *Dangerous and Severe Personality Disorder: Response and Role of the Psychiatric Team*. London: Routledge.

Castillo, H. (2010) The Process of Recovery for People Diagnosed with Personality Disorder, available at: www.thehavenproject.org.uk/Files/Abstract.pdf.

Chief Executive's Bulletin (2004) Chief Executive's letter to NHS organisations on personality disorder services and issues for commissioners, issue no 239.

Coid, J., Yang, M., Tyrer, P. et al. (2006) Prevalence and correlates of personality disorder in Great Britain, *British Journal of Psychiatry*, 188: 423–431.

Crowe, M. (2000) Constructing normality: a discourse analysis of the DSM-IV, *Journal of Psychiatric and Mental Health Nursing*, 7: 69–77.

Darjee, R. & Crichton, J. (2003). Personality disorder and the law in Scotland: a historical perspective, *Journal Of Forensic Psychiatry & Psychology*, 14 (2): 394–425.

Davidson, L. (n.d.) Recovery Devon Group. Available at www.recoverydevon.co.uk (last accessed 7 June 2012).

Davidson, L. & Roe, D. (2007) Recovery from versus recovery in serious mental illness: one strategy for lessening confusion plaguing recovery, *Journal of Mental Health,* 16: 459–470.

Department of Health (2003) *Personality Disorder: No Longer a Diagnosis of Exclusion – Policy Implementation Guidance for the Development of Services for People with Personality Disorder*. London: DH. Available at www.dh.gov.uk/en/Publicationsandstatistics/Publications/PublicationsPolicyAndGuidance/DH_4009546 (last accessed 8 June 2012).

Department of Health (2009) *Recognising Complexity: Commissioning Guidance for Personality Disorder Services*. London: DH. Available at www.dh.gov.uk/en/Healthcare/Mentalhealth/Personalitydisorder/index.htm (last accessed 6 June 2012).

Department of Health (2011a) *A Guide to Working with Offenders with Personality Disorders*. Available at: www.gov.uk/government/uploads/system/uploads/attachment_data/file/215772/dh_124319.pdf

Department of Health (2011b) *No Health Without Mental Health: A Cross-Government Mental Health Outcomes Strategy for People of All Ages*. London: DH.

Department of Health (2014) *Closing the Gap: Priorities for Essential Change in Mental Health*. London: DH.

Department of Health and the Home Office (2005) *Forensic Personality Disorder Medium Secure and Community Pilot Services Planning and Delivery Guide*. London: DH. Available at www.pdprogramme.org.uk/assets/resources/121.pdf (last accessed 8 June 2012).

Department of Health website: www.gov.uk/government/organisations/department-of-health.

DSPD Programme, Department of Health, Home Office, HM Prison Service (October 2005) www.pdprogramme.org.uk/assets/resources/121.pdf

Emergence (n.d.) Available at www.emergenceplus.org.uk/emergence.html (last accessed 26 July 2012).

Evershed, S. (2011) Treatment of personality disorder: skills-based therapies, *Advances in Psychiatric Treatment,* 17: 206–213.

Fossey, M. & Black, G. (2010) *Women with Borderline Personality Disorder in Prison*. London: Centre for Mental Health. Available at www.centreformentalhealth.org.uk/pdfs/under_the_radar.pdf (last accessed 28 August 2012).

Gabbard, G. (2001) Psychodynamic psychotherapy of borderline personality disorder: a contemporary approach, *Bulletin of the Menninger Clinic*, 65: 41–57.

Gleeson, K. (1991) *Out* of our minds: The deconstruction and reconstruction of madness. Unpublished PhD thesis, University of Reading.

Hinshaw, S.P., Cicchetti, D.T. & Sheree, L. (2006) *Mark of Shame: Stigma of Mental Illness and an Agenda for Change*. Oxford: Oxford University Press.

Hinshelwood, R. (1999) The difficult patient, *British Journal of Psychiatry*, 174: 187–190.

Hyler, S., Gabbard, G. & Schneider, I. (1991) Homicidal maniacs and narcissistic parasites: stigmatisation of mentally ill persons in the movies, *Hospital and Community Psychiatry*, 42(10): 1044–1048.

Johnson, R . & Haigh, R. (2011) Social psychiatry and social policy for the twenty-first century – new concepts for new needs: relational health, *Mental Health and Social Inclusion*, 15 (2): 57–65.

Kendell, R. (2002) The distinction between personality disorder and mental illness, *British Journal of Psychiatry*, 180: 110–115.

Kendell, R. & Jablensky, A. (2003) Distinguishing between the validity and utility of psychiatric diagnoses, *American Journal of Psychiatry*, 160: 4–12.

Kings Fund (2008) *Paying the Price: The Cost of Mental Health Care in England to 2026*. London: Kings Fund.

Koekkoek, B., van Meijel, B. & Hutschemaekers, G. (2010) Community mental healthcare for people with severe personality disorder: narrative review, *The Psychiatrist* 34: 24–30.

Lawton-Smith, S., Dawson, J. & Burns, T. (2008) Community treatment orders are not a good thing, *British Journal of Psychiatry*, 193: 96–100.

Leibing, E. et al. (2008) Dimensions of personality – relationship between DSM-IV Personality Disorder Symptoms, The Five-Factor Model, and the Biosocial Model of Personality, *Journal of Psychiatric Disorders*, 22(1): 101–108.

Lewis, G. & Appleby, L. (1988) Personality disorder: the patients psychiatrists dislike, *British Journal of Psychiatry*, 153: 44–49.

Livesley, J.W. (2001) *Handbook of Personality Disorders: Theory, Research and Treatment*. New York: Guilford.

Livesley, J.W. (2003) *Practical Management of Personality Disorders*. New York: Guilford.

Livesley, J.W. (2005) Behavioural and molecular genetic contributions to a dimensional classification of personality disorder, *Journal of Personality Disorders*, 19 (2): 131–155.

MacManus, D. & Fahy, T. (2008) Personality disorders, *Psychiatric Disorders*, 36 (8): 436–441.

Main, T. (1957) The ailment, *British Journal of Medical Psychology*, 30: 129–145.

Markham, D. & Trower, P. (2003) The effects of the psychiatric label 'borderline personality disorder' on nursing staff's perceptions and causal attributions for challenging behaviours, *British Journal of Clinical Psychology*, 42 (3): 243–256.

McKeown, M. & Clancy, B. (1995) Images of madness: media influence on societal perceptions of mental illness, *Mental Health Nursing*, 15 (2): 10–12.

Moran, P., Walsh, E., Tyrer, P. et al (2003) Impact of comorbid personality disorder on violence in psychosis: report from the UK700 trial, *British Journal of Psychiatry*. 182: 129–134.

Murphy, N. & McVey, D. (2003) The challenge of nursing personality disordered patients, *British Journal of Forensic Practice*, 5 (1): 3–19.

National Institute for Mental Health in England (2003a) *Personality Disorder: No Longer a Diagnosis of Exclusion*. London: DH.

National Institute for Mental Health in England (2003b) *Breaking the Cycle of Rejection: The Personality Disorder Capabilities Framework*. Leeds: NIMHE. Available at www.spn.org.uk/fileadmin/SPN_uploads/Documents/Papers/personalitydisorders.pdf

National Probation Service (2008) PC21/ *Managing High Risk of Serious Harm Offenders with Severe Personality Disorder*. Available at www.personalitydisorder.org.uk/news/wpcontent/uploads/ProbationCircular_Nov08.pdf

Newton-Howes, G., Tyrer, P. and Weaver, T. (2008) *Psychiatric Services*, 59: 1033–1103.

NHS (2009) Blackpool Joint Strategic Needs Assessment. Chapter 2: Health & well-being in Blackpool, NHS Blackpool. Available at www.blackpool.nhs.uk/images/uploads/JSNA_Chapter_2.pdf (last accessed 8 June 2012).

NICE (National Institute for Clinical Excellence) (2009a) *Guideline for Antisocial Personality Disorder*. Available at: www.nice.org.uk/nicemedia/pdf/CG77NICEGuideline.pdf

NICE (National Institute for Clinical Excellence) (2009b) *Guideline for Borderline Personality Disorder*. Available at http://guidance.nice.org.uk/CG78/NICEGuidance/pdf/English

Norton, K. (2009) Understanding failures of NHS policy implementation in relation to borderline personality disorder: learning lessons and moving towards an authentic person-centred service, *Psychodynamic Practice*, 15 (1): 25–40.

Nyamande, M.M. & Sikabbubba J.M. (2006) Managing patients who have personality disorders, *Nursing Times*, 102 (38): 30–32.

Parker, G. & Schneider, J. (2007) 'Social care', in J. Baldcock, N. Manning & S. Vickerstaff (eds), *Social Policy* (3rd edn). Oxford: Oxford University Press. Chapter 15.

Peckham, S. & Meerabeau, L. (2007) *Social Policy for Nurses and the Helping Professions* (2nd edn). Maidenhead: Open University Press.

Pilgrim, D. (2001) Disordered personalities and disordered concepts, *Journal of Mental Health*, 10 (3): 253–265.

Phelan, J., Link, B., Stueve, A. & Pescosolido, B. (2000) Public conceptions of mental illness in 1950 and 1996: what is mental illness and is it to be feared?, *Journal of Health and Social Behavior*, 41: 188–207.

Rogers C.R. (1957) The necessary and sufficient conditions of therapeutic personality change, *Journal of Consulting Psychology*, 21: 95–101.

Scanlon C. & Adlam, J. (2008) Refusal, social exclusion and the cycle of rejection: a cynical analysis?, *Critical Social Policy*, 28: 529.

Scottish Executive (2000) *Report of the Committee on Serious Violent and Sexual Offenders*, SE/2000/68. Edinburgh: Scottish Executive.

Scottish Executive (2004) The new mental health act: a short introduction. Available at www.scotland.gov.uk/Resource/Doc/26487/0013533.pdf

Scottish Executive (2006) *Delivering for Mental Health*. Edinburgh: Scottish Executive.

Stalker, K., Ferguson, I. & Barclay, A. (2005) 'It is a horrible term for someone': service user and provider perspectives on 'personality disorder', *Disability and Society*, 20 (4): 359–373.

Townsend, W. & Glasser, N. (2003) Recovery: the heart and soul of treatment, *Psychiatric Rehabilitation Journal*, 27: 83–85.

Trebilcock, J. & Weaver, T. (2012) 'It doesn't have to be treatable': Mental Health Review Tribunal (MHRT) members' views about Dangerous and Severe Personality Disorder (DSPD), *Journal of Forensic Psychiatry & Psychology*, 23 (2): 244–260.

Tyrer, P. & Simonsen, E. (2003) Personality disorder in psychiatric practice, *World Psychiatry*, 2: 41–44.

Winnicott, D.W. (1949) Hate in the countertransference, *International Journal of Psychoanalysis*, 3: 69–74.

World Health Organization (WHO) (1992) *The ICD-10 Classification of Mental and Behavioural Disorders: Clinical Descriptions and Diagnostic Guidelines*. Geneva: WHO.

Wright, K., Haigh,K. & McKeown, M. (2007) Reclaiming the humanity in personality disorder, *International Journal of Mental Health Nursing*, 16: 236–246.

Wright, K.M. and Jones, F. (2012) Developing healthy working relationships with people with borderline personality disorder who self-harm: re-adjusting perceptions – the service user's view, *Mental Health Practice*, 16 (2): 31–35.

8 SERVICE USER INVOLVEMENT

Mick McKeown and Fiona Jones

Chapter Overview

This chapter provides a fascinating overview of a revolution that has been quietly occurring in the mental health field. Traditional roles for people with mental health issues when receiving services of passivity have been creatively challenged. It is no longer the case that services are something that are exclusively 'done to' people, rather a gradual momentum has achieved a situation where in many settings they are 'created with'.

This chapter provides an insight as to why this has occurred and places it in a fascinating context of policy and also broader social and political change. The changes such a shift in traditional practices creates can be seen in services where service users (a term effectively created to challenge the notion of 'patienthood') are now in a position to engage with the actual provision of services. The presence of service users can be seen throughout the mental health service landscape from the interviewing, selection and teaching of undergraduate health professionals, to engaging in research as partners with health-care researchers. They have effectively moved from being considered the 'subjects' of research to occupying the position of co-investigators.

Service provision has also seen recognition of the concept of 'peer support worker' and specific educational programmes established in 'recovery colleges' to facilitate that purpose. Overall it can be seen that there has been a significant shift not only in the way that services are being provided but also in the power dynamics that inform them. This chapter, itself an example of coproduction, exemplifies that process in real terms.

INTRODUCTION

The recent history of mental health services in the developed world has witnessed a proliferation of policy rhetoric that urges increasing levels of involvement by service users in almost all aspects of the organisation and delivery of services. This policy forms part of a much broader set of governance principles concerned with democratic participation and consumer rights that extend their reach across the public sphere. Involvement policies have intersected with other progressive developments in mental health care and resulted in a wave of practices that are replete with ideals of empowerment and more egalitarian relationships between care providers and care recipients, latterly framed in the language of co-production. These practices are now to be found in various places and spaces spanning institutional and community settings and operating at different levels: strategic involvement, right up to participation in policy formulation; involvement in the day-to-day transaction of care provision, for instance co-produced care plans or examples of peer support; and involvement in the education and training of nurses and other practitioners. The idea of service user involvement is now an important part of the lexicon of policy makers and practitioners alike, and has undoubtedly become part of an ongoing process of change in mental health services that ought to support other initiatives aimed at humanising care and promoting recovery (Shepherd et al., 2007).

Despite these interesting developments, the very nature of psychiatry, its underpinning theoretical models and legal structures that legitimate compulsion and coercion into care are subject to a vigorous external critique marshalled by service users who often prefer to describe themselves as survivors. Associated with this has been a parallel development of independent advocacy practices which similarly aim to ensure that the voice of service users is heard in a meaningful way (Newbigging et al., 2012). The criticisms furnished by the survivor movement can call into question the extent to which services can become democratised, and they contemplate much more radical transformations. Such critical perspectives have historically found support from politicised elements of the practitioner and nursing workforce, and have occasionally resulted in interesting alliances or visions of different, more relational and less oppressive service configurations. In the extreme, these voices challenge the very legitimacy of the caring professions and whether, indeed, disciplines such as nursing are needed at all.

Depending upon one's perspective, the overall policy prescription for public participation either heralds a significant shift in the balance of power from government to citizens or is an illusory smokescreen for a more invidious application of social control. Arguably, any such tensions might be most obviously at play in the context of mental health, where the relationships between individual behaviour and expression, social expectations and norms, and the subtle surveillance of the psy-professions are worked out complexly (Rose 1985, 1989). In this chapter, we review the policies and practices of participation and involvement in the mainstream before turning to consider the more radical challenges to mental health services and the potential for conjoint emancipation of both service users and practitioner staff; in alliances that seek more progressive services, solidaristic and self-reliant communities, and, ultimately a better world. In doing so, we make the case for both strong, empowered service user groupings *and* nursing representative bodies, co-operation between the two, and consideration of a new politics of mental health. The relational and organisational challenges of achieving such ideal formations will be faced up to in the course of making the case for the alternative.

THE LONG ROAD TRAVELLED: UK POLICY FOR SERVICE USER INVOLVEMENT

Mental health services account for a significant proportion of the NHS budget and any relevant policy changes always need to be considered in the context of fluctuations in funding and the wider political economy. It has been estimated that mental ill-health represents £105 billion cost to the economy and the spending on treatment alone will double in the next twenty years (DH, 2011). Government spending on adult mental health services grew significantly in the decade up to 2011, with an increase of 59% in real terms after allowing for inflation. Current spending now stands at a total of £6.629 billion, with an additional £2.859 for older persons' mental health services. The amount spent has now begun to shrink, falling by 1% in real terms for adult services and 3.1% for older people, between 2010/2011 and 2011/2012. Around 25% of the total for adult services funds independent providers, 19% is allocated to secure services, and around 7% to psychological therapies. Growth in previously defined target areas such as assertive outreach, crisis resolution and early intervention has fallen for the first time since being prioritised. Older people's mental health services are commissioned using a mixture of PCT (62%) and local government (38%) arrangements. The non-statutory sector accounts for 43% of investment in older persons' mental health care. The overall spending figures mask substantial differences across regions in the amounts spent per capita on mental health services which points up key questions for commissioners concerned with addressing these inequalities (all spending figures DH 2012a, 2012b).

Gorsky (2007) notes a 200-year history in the UK for some sort of patient or public involvement contribution within the organisation of health-care services. This has been in the form of voluntary sector governance of General Practitioner and hospital services or examples of local government control: for example, within the internal democratic workings of mutual friendly societies who administered forms of medical insurance before the emergence of national insurance systems in the early years of the twentieth century, or aspects of local government control of hospitals prior to the advent of the NHS. Despite such possibilities for service user involvement, this is a history of fairly limited democratic reach into the management and operation of services, and more substantial efforts have really only emerged in relatively recent times with the advent of consumerist approaches to involvement and influence. Gorsky (2007) dates the first flush of consumerism in health care to the establishment of the *Patients Association* in 1963 together with other voluntary sector activity. This was afforded a formal route to having a say in services with the creation of Community Health Councils as part of the 1974 NHS reorganisation, which also introduced new structures for regional and local health authorities.

A number of recent publications have outlined the social policy events in the subsequent three decades or so that have set the context for developments in user involvement across the UK. This period is significant for forming something of a consensus around the value of consumerist notions of public participation, despite various changes of government. The relevant policy territory is also notable for the impact of slightly different pieces of legislation across the devolved countries and the fact that mental health law also differs in this regard, and in relation to Scotland has always done so. For simplicity's sake, we will mainly draw on policy originating in the English parliament but will also note key developments from the devolved nations to support the more general arguments we make. We outline major policy documents and other noteworthy events relevant to service user involvement in Figure 8.1 (pp. 157–163). General policy for involvement and participation is included alongside policy that is particular to the mental health field.

Barnes and Cotterell (2012) offer a detailed and up-to-date review of relevant initiatives and also stress the advent of Community Health Councils as a key milestone in the historical record of user involvement policy. Arguably, this minor realisation of a democratic impulse harked back to the immediate post-war planning for the creation of the NHS, when Bevan offered a vision of direct community control of local services via elected bodies (Foot, 1973). However, to satisfy the objections of doctors this local accountability was sacrificed, prefiguring a long-term tension between public participation ideals and the exercise of medical power. An alternative perspective is that the universalism and state power embodied in the birth of the new NHS actually stifled the nascent forms of public participation that were associated with local government and voluntary sector governance (Gorsky, 2007).

The notion of service user involvement as we know it is strongly bound to policies that reflect the aforementioned consumerism. Most observers of policy developments date the first notable impact of consumerism to the privileging of individualism and personal choice grounded in the New Right political philosophies that were massively influential on the course of Margaret Thatcher's period in office and subsequent administrations. Later this consumerist turn was to remain a central feature of New Labour's modernisation agenda post 1997 (Tait & Lester, 2005). A pivotal policy statement in this regard was the 1988 report written by Roy Griffiths which in turn led to the NHS and Community Care Act 1990. This legislated for the first introduction of an internal market in the NHS, in tandem with specific provisions for public consultation and service user involvement in relation to the planning and delivery of community care. Contemporary critics of the proposals were lukewarm about the genuineness of any commitment to service user involvement. Despite plentiful references to consumers in the document, service users were not central to the recommendations, and their envisaged role was largely passive; relating to reactive services, rather than being truly at the centre of planning and organising those services (Walker, 1989). However, for Barnes and Cotterell (2012) the 1990 Act was the catalyst for a number of local authorities to attempt to place service users at the centre of community care, and best practice initiatives were reviewed and promoted in the Goss and Miller (1995) publication *From Margin to Mainstream*.

Throughout the 1990s and the first decade of the twenty-first century various policies have strengthened the view that service user involvement and other public voices are to be increasingly respected and listened to in the planning and provision of health services. To this end, successive governments have convened reference panels or working groups inclusive of service user perspectives to help frame the formulation of health policy or associated workforce planning, and policy drafts or possible future directions have been circulated for mass consultation. Key policy instruments in this regard have included efforts to insist on certain rights and the accountability of services to patients enshrined in *The Patient's Charter* (1991) and much later in *The NHS Constitution* (2009b) (both with subsequent revisions), and make service user involvement central to a mission to improve the nation's health as set out in *The Health of the Nation* (1992) and numerous other later policies where the direction of travel is towards personal control, self-determination and support for individuals and communities to become more responsible for their own health and wellbeing. The focus on individual rights and entitlements has been criticised in some quarters for a relative neglect of collective concerns or, the classic liberal dilemma, how to decide whose rights are more important in any particular circumstance (McKeown & Mercer, 1995).

At the tail-end of eighteen years of Conservative governments, the NHS Executive (1996) published a *Patient Partnership Strategy* which emphasised the importance of involvement in clinical decision making supported by the provision of high quality information for service user consumers of health care. In the same year the Standing Advisory Group on Consumer Involvement in the NHS Research and Development Programme was formed, later to become the influential INVOLVE. Other important arm's length agencies with a strong stake in service user involvement in the research context are the National Institute for Health and Clinical Excellence (NICE) and the Social Care Institute for Excellence (SCIE), respectively founded in 1999 and 2001. An important route for service users to try and influence policy can be through direct involvement in research partnerships or in organised activity to appraise and disseminate research evidence (Barber et al., 2012).

The whole idea of patient and public involvement gathered apace with the New Labour governments of Blair and Brown. The 2001 Health and Social Care Act legislated for a patient and public involvement duty to fall on the NHS and later policy statements continued in this vein (DH, 2004a, 2004b, 2005). Programmes of peer involvement such as the Expert Patient approach in chronic health conditions reflected this commitment as did a number of important institutional developments. The latter included the establishment of the Commission for Patient and Public Involvement in Health and the NHS Centre for Involvement, based at Warwick University. There have been numerous NHS reorganisations and structural reforms in this period, and alongside these formal mechanisms for public engagement have been serially reorganised over the years, with Community Health Councils replaced by PALS and PPI Forums, in turn giving way to LINKs, and now to be overtaken by Healthwatch.

The process of devolved government offers the possibility of reflecting upon different approaches to the management and organisation of healthcare within the NHS and social services and some subtle differences in language and terminology across policy statements. Indeed, Barnes and Cotterell (2012) point out that the efforts of the Welsh Office to develop consumer involvement practices in a context of learning disability at different levels in the administration of services predate both the aforementioned 1990 Community Care Act and devolution. There is some evidence from comparing public attitude surveys between England and Scotland, where the purchaser-provider split was jettisoned after devolution, discounting the proposition that market forces must inevitably lead to higher quality (Taylor-Gooby, 2008). Scotland's government has a broad policy objective to make their's *a more successful country*; improving the nation's health is one of five strategic arms of achieving this (Scottish Government, 2007) and there is a strong emphasis on the NHS workforce (Scottish Government, 2009). The Scottish Health Council, now hosted by Healthcare Improvement Scotland, was established by the Scottish Executive in April 2005 to promote patient focus and public involvement in the NHS in Scotland. This is to be achieved by ensuring that Scottish NHS boards respond to the views of service users working in partnership to bring about a *mutual* NHS. The SHC uses the term 'service users' to encompass all patients, carers and the public. They issued a comprehensive *Strategy For User Involvement and Person Centredness* in 2011. The Welsh Assembly Government espouses a policy of putting citizens first and at the heart of governance arrangements for the NHS in Wales. To this end they undertook a lengthy review of governance processes and have produced a series of good practice guides to render this transparent to the public. Adherence to the relevant principles will be monitored as part of a ministerial annual performance review of NHS organisations (see WAG, 2010). Of course this is not necessarily at odds with the general consumerist ideology more visible elsewhere, but the choice of terminology focused on citizenship is interesting as it perhaps suggests a stronger commitment to rights, responsibilities and accountability.

One of the later policy acts for New Labour was to initiate and receive the report of the NHS Next Stage Review undertaken by the Health Minister Lord Darzi (DH, 2008). The espoused intention was to move beyond the previous commitment to expanding resources and capacity and turn to refining quality and taking forward the agenda for more personalised health-care services. Implicit in some of the supporting rhetoric, and unfortunately resonating with public revulsion at some scandalous failures in care provision (see Francis, 2010), the nursing profession in particular was implicated in calls for services to show more compassion to patients and their relatives. With this in mind, Gordon Brown set up an expert panel chaired by the ex-nurse and celebrated agony aunt, Clare Rayner, to examine the way forward for nursing (Prime Minister's Commission on the Future of Nursing, 2010). This was hardly a moment of great influence, as the commission had the misfortune to report near to the time of a change of government. The content, however, is of interest for nurses and raises a number of important points. Compassionate nursing care is not presented merely as flowing from the personal qualities of individual nurses; it exists in a context of team working and effective caring alliances with service users, and within a political economy of health that was already feeling the effects of austerity. Darzi had argued that nurses ought to be in the forefront of progressive changes in health services. The commission concurred with this but also remarked that nurses had historically been left in the role of passively implementing other people's policy ideas, many of which they might have disagreed with, or could have offered more innovative ideas themselves if anyone had cared to ask. The vision for nursing includes the assertion that if service users are to be at the centre of excellent nursing care, then the nursing workforce also needs to be looked after:

> Workplace cultures will create positive practice environments for delivering high quality care, providing development and support, and nurses and midwives will care better for others because they themselves are valued and cared for. (Prime Minister's Commission on the Future of Nursing, 2010: 32)

Moving to the present, the principles of user involvement and public participation remain at the heart of general health reforms and have particular resonance within specific proposals for future mental health services. The 2010 White Paper *Equity and Excellence: Liberating the NHS,* which laid the ideological foundations for the most recent Health and Social Care Act (2012), was replete with the language of involvement and participation and looked forward to an NHS 'genuinely centred on patients and carers' that 'gives citizens a greater say in how the NHS is run'. Part of this promise was to be grounded in the adoption of a principle of 'shared decision-making' with empowered patients at the centre of decisions about their care with the support of clinicians equally committed to conjoint assessment and planning. This has been presented as part of a blueprint for a future NHS that has been freed from stifling bureaucracy and is hence much more patient centred.

Whichever organisations actually end up delivering care, these services will be legally mandated to:

- put service users and carers at the centre of the NHS;
- focus on continually improving things that really matter to patients;
- empower and liberate clinicians to innovate, with the freedom to focus on improving health-care services.

USER INVOLVEMENT POLICY FOR MENTAL HEALTH SERVICES

Service user involvement principles and practices have been vigorously promoted in policy where there is a specific focus on mental health. This social policy territory includes bespoke policy instruments that singularly address mental health services and more generic policy that has a mental health component. Mental health law is a significant part of this policy landscape and other legislation is also important, such as that dealing with equalities and human rights. Also of note are changes to the regulatory frameworks for professionals and how they are trained into professional roles. Furthermore, a number of landmark public inquiries into failings in mental health services and the wider public sector have had a telling impact and opened up debate or initiated practices that are relevant to user involvement.

The aforementioned Griffiths Report focused upon community care was mostly concerned with the process of deinstitutionalisation and as such was heavily influential in the shaping of mental health services. Associated subsequent policy, such as Building Bridges (DH, 1995) attempted to improve case management processes and inter-agency and inter-disciplinary working and, amongst other things, introduced the Care Programme Approach to community mental health services. The policy commitment to enhance user involvement extended into the *National Service Framework for Mental Health* which was published in 1999 near the start of New Labour's modernisation programme. A key part of New Labour's later mental health policy can be seen as a response to service user demands, with a focus on increasing access to psychological therapies and enabling the growth of *personalisation* of services towards the adoption of a policy of *direct payments* or user-held *personal budgets*. A number of agencies were influential in refining these policies and advising on implementation, including the Sainsbury Centre for Mental Health, which undertook research and staff training, and the National Institute for Mental Health England (NIMHE). The latter quango was formed in 2002 to assist with the implementation of the National Service Framework and spawned a number of regional development centres. Strategic thinking, the dissemination of mental health policy, and action on race equality initiatives (see below) were taken up by the National Mental Health Development Unit, established in 2009.

In the Welsh context, service user involvement figured strongly in *Raising the Standard: The Revised Adult Mental Health National Service Framework an Action Plan for Wales* (WAG, 2005). Thomas and colleagues (2010) took stock of efforts by the Welsh Assembly Government to promote public participation and user and carer involvement in relation to Welsh mental health services. The starting point was a number of policy commitments from the WAG to ensure service users and carers were afforded opportunities for genuine and empowered involvement (WAG, 2004, 2005, 2008). Focus groups for service users and carers inquired into current views on the state of play for involvement in Wales and explored the possibilities for future arrangements for national level involvement and consultation. The authors concluded that despite a range of involvement opportunities, service users and carers mainly felt that their voice was not heard within inefficient structures for supporting involvement, and that the full potential for genuine partnership working was as yet unrealised. They made a case for a new mechanism to support involvement at a national level.

In Northern Ireland, service user involvement has to be seen in the context of the particular circumstances of devolution which meant that efforts were made to legislate that certain groups or categories of person would not suffer discrimination and policy should seek full citizenship for all amongst other equality and social justice objectives; these aspirations were enshrined in the 1998 Northern Ireland Act. The history of civil conflict has arguably had a significant impact upon the mental health of the population in Northern Ireland, not least in terms of social exclusion (Heenan, 2009). The Bamford Review (2005), which was a comprehensive analysis of mental health services in Northern Ireland, eventually delivered *A Strategic Framework For Adult Mental Health Services*. The review was notable for emphasising partnership with service users in the planning, development and evaluation of services and also in the various aspects of assessment and therapy. Interestingly, in the course of the review, service users objected to being invited to be involved only at a late stage of the proceedings, and commentators have noted negligible changes to the extent of involvement in areas such as service level planning (Heenan, 2009). To date, however, there has been little research on service user involvement in Northern Ireland. In a recent study of user involvement in Northern Irish health and social care services, Duffy (2008) concluded that slow and uneven progress had been made.

Going back to the early years of devolved responsibility, the Scottish parliament has also been concerned to formulate policy that seeks the active participation of service users to shape or influence mental health services (Scottish Office, 1997; Scottish Executive, 2000, 2001, 2003a, 2003b). For example, *Delivering for Mental Health* (Scottish Executive, 2006) makes commitments to involve service users in the delivery and design of services. Implementation of policy relevant to user involvement has been assisted by the establishment of the Scottish Development Centre for Mental Health (2001) which merged with the Mental Health Foundation for Scotland in 2011, and has increasingly been involved with the Scottish Recovery Network in taking forward policy initiatives relating to recovery practices and peer support. The Mental Health (Care and Treatment)(Scotland)Act 2003 came into force in 2005, two years before England and Wales, and is arguably a more rights-based approach, though very similar tensions exist between the social control function of the act and the rhetorical commitment to empowerment in other policy (Lewis, 2005).

The grand period of consumerism also witnessed two major reviews of mental health nursing, the first led by Tony Butterworth which made numerous recommendations relevant to service user involvement and partnership working (Report of the Mental Health Nursing Review Team, 1994), and the second led by Neil Brimblecombe on behalf of the Chief Nursing Officer, which stressed the importance of nursing actions being predicated on clear values with service user-centred care being key (DH, 2006a). These nursing reviews linked up with other policy activity focused on workforce and wider strategic thinking and service users and carers were involved in relevant DH workforce planning and strategy activity, including the Workforce Action Team. Associated with this, the NIMHE document *Ten Essential Shared Capabilities* and the *National Mental Health Education Continuous Quality Improvement Tool* (Northern Centre for Mental Health, 2003) were influential in framing practitioner competencies for mental health practice common to all disciplines (Brooker et al., 2005). NIMHE also worked with the Mental Health in Higher Education network, led by Jill Anderson, to produce an important guide to involving service users in practitioner education and training (Tew et al., 2004).

Indeed the whole teaching and learning agenda for mental health professionals has been another important locus for the development of policies and practices to make the most of the contribution of service users and carers. There is a growing literature on service user and carer involvement in the education of the health and social care workforce, and this contribution extends beyond face-to-face teaching to involvement in curriculum planning, course validation and evaluation (see Wykurz & Kelly, 2002; Felton & Stickley, 2004; Bassett et al., 2006; Beresford et al., 2006; Lathlean et al., 2006; Repper & Breeze, 2007; Brown & Young, 2008; Morgan & Jones, 2009; McKeown et al., 2010; Towle et al., 2010). Alongside this there has been a simultaneous demand for service user involvement at all levels of the research process (see Church, 2005; Hanley, 2005; INVOLVE, 2007; Frankham, 2009), so much so that levels of participation are now typically evaluated as part of research grant approval processes and user involvement is thoroughly appraised in the quality assurance of teaching and learning programmes.

Service user involvement can now be found in the training of all disciplines of mental health staff. It is commonplace for service users to be involved in the pre-qualification and post-registration education of mental health nurses and social workers, and also for clinical psychologists (Harper, 2003; BPS, 2008) and occupational therapists, especially in a context of inter-professional learning (Barnes & Carpenter, 2006). Mental health service users were thoroughly involved in the planning and implementation for new staff roles such as Support Time and Recovery Workers and Primary Care Graduate Mental Health Workers; many people with relevant lived experience have successfully completed this training and taken up these posts. Service users are involved in medical schools teaching psychiatrists, for example focusing on the development of a therapeutic alliance and knowledge of psychological processes, interviewing and formulation skills. In one evaluation, the involvement of service users in such training was largely positively received and it was remarked that an effective articulation of the service user perspective helped the doctors to develop their empathy and understand differences between their views and those of service users. On the negative front, some of the trainees failed to appreciate the value of having service user input, precisely because it was grounded in personal experience, accusing them of holding the wrong views and, in one case, 'overly democratic values'! (Ikkos, 2005: 142).

Policy that addresses equality issues is of importance, as inequality can be a significant barrier to authentic user involvement, and the value placed on interdependence rather than simple individualism in certain communities is of no little consequence (Rai-Atkins et al., 2002). Together with responding in a general way to the challenges thrown up by the public inquiry into the death of Stephen Lawrence (Macpherson, 1999) the government found itself needing to respond to a number of longstanding anomalies in the care and treatment of ethnic minorities in British mental health services. Various commentators, researchers and institutional audits had demonstrated that black men in particular were over-represented across a range of diagnoses of mental disorder and were more likely to be coercively introduced into health-care services, less likely to receive psychotherapies rather than physical treatments, and much more likely to be concentrated at higher levels of security (Keating et al., 2002; Bhui et al., 2003; Healthcare Commission, Mental Health Act Commission & National Institute for Mental Health England, 2005, 2007). Furthermore, a number of accusations of racism and deaths of black men whilst under psychiatric detention, including famously David 'Rocky' Bennett, led to increasing external calls for reform and a concerted effort to address a range of equality issues in mental health policy formulation (Committee of Inquiry, 1992; Prins, 1993; Blofeld, 2003). The result was the Delivering Race Equality Programme which was instigated in and delivered an action plan in 2005 and was formerly reviewed after five years (Wilson, 2009).

Notable recent mental health policy includes *New Horizons: A Shared Vision for Mental Health* in 2009 at the end of the New Labour tenure, to be superseded by the incoming government's *No Health Without Mental Health* (2011). The former makes much of developments in thinking around recovery and user involvement remains significant as one means for ensuring holistic care is to be delivered. A changing landscape in provision of services is looked forward to with better partnerships urged between central and local government, the voluntary sector and professional interests. The coalition government's first policy statement on mental health takes forward these ideas and is interesting in the way that some of the language and aspirations of service user and disability movements are clearly co-opted. Personalisation is a key objective and the movement's slogan *'nothing about me without me'* is prominently aired at the start of the document. There is also a heavy emphasis on the desirability of measurable outcomes, undoubtedly bound up with the direction of travel within commissioning towards systems for payment by results.

BEST PRACTICE IN SERVICE USER INVOLVEMENT

Far too many examples of innovation and best practice exist to detail all of these, but a number of noteworthy initiatives are worthy of mention for illustrative purposes. In a study of our own, we found that the Yorkshire and Humber Specialist Secure Services Commissioning Team has supported service users and professional staff to work in partnership to enact numerous examples of good practice in user involvement in secure mental health settings (McKeown et al., 2012). The most notable of these in terms of its scale and the quality of shared decision making is their Involvement Strategy Group, which is a forum that brings together staff and service users for strategic thinking in a non-secure community setting and conducts its business using creative approaches to inclusion and deliberative styles of communication. This group has instigated various examples of collaborative local policy and practice, including user-led standards for the conduct of CPA meetings, a participatory film-making project, and a model service for women at Garrow House, York, based upon effective relational principles (Forensic Catchment Group, 2007; Secure Commissioning Team, 2010).

At a national level, the Scottish government have made substantial efforts to involve service users and third sector groups in the development of policy and practices aimed at promoting a cultural shift in services to a recovery focus, including an expansion of peer worker roles. This has involved supporting the work of the Scottish Recovery Network, which has produced a range of supportive materials and tools and is beginning to systematically influence staff training (e.g. Smith & Bradstreet, 2011). There has also been a national strategy to fight stigma which has involved a successful Scottish Arts and Film Mental Health Festival. The Oor Mad History group has supported involvement and advocacy by narrating its history, in its own words and on its own terms (CAPS, 2010). This activity is mirrored in the work of the Survivors History Group (2012) in England.

Mersey Care NHS Trust have a positive reputation for involving service users in different aspects of their work, including representation to board level, the selection of staff and an evaluation of service quality. An interesting dimension of this work has been a focus on introducing a framework for care based upon human rights principles, including work to develop involvement practices in risk assessment (Greenhill & Whitehead, 2011). This has led to the Trust's Director for Service Users and Carers, Lindsey Dyer, taking the lead role in the NHS Human Rights in Healthcare programme.

Our own Comensus project at the University of Central Lancashire is a good example of a systematic and comprehensive approach to service user and carer involvement in the university education of mental health and other practitioners. This initiative was grounded in a process of community engagement and has made a significant difference to teaching and learning and research at the university, and also the way in which the university is perceived by its community has changed for the better (Downe et al., 2007; McKeown et al., 2010). Julia Terry (2011), as part of a Florence Nightingale travel scholarship, has effectively mapped examples of good practice in involvement for mental health education across the UK.

There is a range of examples of user involvement supporting research in mental health with organisations such as SCIE and INVOLVE doing much to promote involvement at all stages of the research process. For instance, the National Institute For Health Research as part of the UK Mental Health Research Network operates the Service Users in Research Group, England (SURGE). User-led research is not so common, but groups such as Shaping Our Lives are making a positive contribution to the field, and there is a growing demand within the user movement for more influence or control over research, what questions are posed and how studies are conducted (Lowes & Hulatt, 2005; Sweeney et al., 2009).

Keeping alive the connection between the present and critical user movement politics of the past is *Asylum: The Magazine for Democratic Psychiatry*, which is produced by a collective that includes service user activists, mental health practitioners and academics. The September 2012 issue focused on connections between user movement politics and the broader struggle to defeat neo-liberalism (see below).

THE PATH OF INVOLVEMENT DOES NOT ALWAYS RUN SMOOTH

Despite a now longstanding policy commitment supportive of service user involvement, the actual practice of involvement at strategic level has seldom been without challenges. From a critical perspective, if service user involvement is to move beyond tokenism and realise genuine empowerment or autonomy for participants some significant hurdles must be surmounted (Downe et al., 2007; McKeown et al., 2010).

Many commentators have been critical of government policy on service user involvement, including in mental health services. The language and key concepts of involvement and participation are contested, and the terminology and ideas are criticised as being vague or poorly defined, such that the very idea of involvement can mean different things to different people (Beresford, 2005). In the Scottish context, but offering a general critique of policy, Lewis (2005) bemoans the concept of service user involvement for conceiving of people solely in terms of pathology, thereby neglecting other aspects of diversity. She also remarks on how this language constructs people as universally disempowered to start with. Similarly, there is a raft of criticisms about the failure of policy to articulate in detail how involvement is to be put into practice (Duffy, 2008), to deliver what services users consistently ask for from services (Connor & Wilson, 2006), or that apparently systematic approaches continue to reinvent tokenistic involvement (Horrocks et al., 2010). These short-comings include a fetishisation of a requirement for representativeness and a failure to always value service user views as a valid commentary on services, with some voices being too easily discounted or ignored altogether (Beresford, 1994). Such concerns have prompted efforts to account for different levels of participation, valuing authentic partnerships over more tokenistic forms (Arnstein, 1969; Tew et al., 2004; Tritter & McCallum, 2006).

More fundamentally, questions have been raised as to whether service users' goals can ever be fully achieved when faced with incorporated systems of involvement or services dominated by psychiatric models of understanding people's needs (see Beresford, 2002; Lewis, 2005; Pilgrim, 2005; Carr, 2007), and it has been argued that this policy agenda can be viewed as propping up wider strategies of governance and social control (Cooke & Kothari, 2002). Hopton and Nolan (2003) wryly, and presciently as it turned out, suggested the policy aspirations of involvement seemed to be jarringly contrary to the actualities of Mental Health Act reforms, which arguably saw an increasing focus on compulsion and detention which few service users would explicitly want more of.

Diamond and colleagues (2003) noted some discrepancies between staff reports of the extensiveness of involvement and the actualities of observable practice; also that some of the changes needed for more inclusive practices were solely in the hands of staff to initiate. Studies of user involvement within services flag up limitations where service users have to insinuate themselves into meetings that they have not had a say in organising and can only respond to other people's agendas, or some important topics are not up for discussion (Hodge, 2005a, 2005b, 2009; Godin et al., 2007). Such problems can lead to fractious relations. For example, service user members of the expert panel advising on the preparation of the *National Service Framework for Mental Health* resigned over the issue of compulsory treatment orders being non-negotiable (Tait & Lester, 2005) and there have also been service user resignations from NICE committees, for example in relation to the development of guidelines on the treatment of self-harm (Smith & Pembroke, 2005). Similarly, groups such as the Alzheimer's Society (2007) have criticised NICE committees for giving insufficient weight to patient perspectives. In a largely positive account of the experiences of being involved in the development of NICE guidelines there were some misgivings about the relative lack of weight given to experiential perspectives when they clashed with findings from quantitative research (Harding et al., 2010).

Shifting from a shared voice to the first person for a moment, Fiona, a service user and co-author of this chapter, offers her mixed experiences of user involvement:

> When it has worked well, it has been a rewarding and fulfilling experience. For me, it is all about the quality of relationships. Encounters with a particular nurse in secure settings felt like they were about me as a person and focused upon my needs as we worked them out together. This felt a lot like the sort of compassion that I've since found out David Brandon (1976) wrote so eloquently about. I felt cared for for the first time in my lengthy stay in

services. It felt like a friendship. Unfortunately, this was not typical of most other relationships I had with staff, much of these not worth even calling relationships.

I have been involved in a number of different involvement opportunities, inside and outside services, and have taken a lead role in a self-organised user group. There is often a different quality to discussions inside and outside of services, with much more open communication within the user forum, where staff only attend, if at all, on our terms. My experience of formal involvement within services has often been frustrating, especially when big efforts to make a contribution appear to make no difference to the end results of consultation exercises. There is limited scope on what we can actually be involved in. We don't really care about some of the things we are allowed to influence if we're not allowed to say the things that are important to us, good or bad. We know that the food budget is set, we expect to see the fabric sample books whenever a new unit is built. What we haven't got, is the chance to really change things and shake up the system, to speed people's journey's through the system and to bring humanity into services. We have half a say, the rest is done to us by 'responsible' clinicians and others who we may never meet or have a chance to talk to.

Scrutiny of the timeline of involvement policy highlights some of the contradictions between democratising and incorporation tendencies. For example, the serial reorganisations of bodies set up to facilitate public participation in health services (CHCs, PALs and PPI, LINKS and Healthwatch) appear to represent swings from organising involvement forums in ways that smack of attempts to manage it from the inside, to valuing the contribution of external voices, and back again (Barnes & Cotterell, 2012).

The notion of service user involvement cannot be thought of in isolation from other significant policy changes and related ideologies. For example, policies originating in other government departments can undermine the objectives of mental health policies or the personal agency of service users; witness the opposition from the service user movement, the Royal College of Psychiatrists and others to the current policy on incapacity benefit (Farmer et al., 2011). In a broad sense, the headlong rush to embrace markets in the delivery of healthcare is clearly at odds with the ideal of maximising patient choice which it purports to be focused upon. Directing the allocation of healthcare resources via the mechanism of contracting between purchaser and provider organisations, regardless of whether the purchasers are clinicians, transparently overlooks the idea of patient choice all together. Neither are the reforms necessarily about ensuring a more efficient delivery of health care, as the costs of organising the various systems of contracting and administration to support a market in health are enormous.

POLICY IN A CONTEXT OF NEOLIBERALISM

Any social policy can be seen as an attempt at social change, to make things different, to alter the order of things (Baldock et al., 2003), though the messy and complicated end results of the application of policy do not always reflect a rational purpose (Adams, 2002). Actual policy and its real-world implementation can reflect a complex and often contradictory amalgam of theory and practice with all the appearance of a cock-up or conspiracy, depending on your particular viewpoint. Critics of the evolution of health-care policy from Thatcherism, through New Labour to the present coalition government have remarked upon various continuities but also inconsistencies and limits to the extent that grand objectives can actually be realised in practice (see Taylor-Gooby, 1989; Paton, 2001, 2006; Clarke, 2004; Correia, 2012). Despite some nuances of difference with regard to equality, there are clear lines of consensus in the adoption of neo-liberal goals to decentralise authority and shrink the state, especially the welfare state, yet many of the iterative reforms over the years have actually concentrated power back to the centre. Similarly, managerialist objectives to wrest power away from the vested interest of clinicians appear to sit oddly at ease with the valuing of clinical control over supposedly more bureaucratic models of commissioning. Furthermore, privileging the concept of competition at the organisational level seems inconsistent with the spirit of co-operation envisioned in shared decision making at the sharp end of care.

This tension within neoliberal policies as they extend to service users and the threat posed to welfare services was apparent from the start (Morris, 2011). Alan Walker's (1989: 29) early review of the seminal Griffiths Report was prescient in highlighting the retreat from the state as problematic if the espoused objectives also included increased user choice and involvement:

> The report's recommendations are not likely to promote better quality community care, increase choice or extend user participation. In fact the dynamic of further privatisation underlying the Griffiths report would be likely to have the opposite effects, especially the increased exclusion and marginalisation of the most vulnerable users.

If neo-liberalism and its attendant social policies are the bogey, it would be easy for opponents to be cowed into inertia or pessimism in the face of its seeming ascendancy and endurance, despite telling evidence that as a political and economic philosophy it has, at the very least, significant shortcomings. Quiggin (2010) entertainingly likens the survival of ought-to-be-redundant economic tenets, such as faith in markets or de-regulation, to the spooky immortality of zombies. Similarly, Colin Crouch (2011) suggests that the strange non-death of neoliberalism is counter-intuitive, but on deeper reflection not surprising. He makes a compelling argument that the durability of neo-liberalism is predicated on its concern not merely with the free operation of markets but in establishing its dominance by weaving an incestuous and relatively impregnable relationship between global corporations, the political classes and the mass media.

Addressing the increasingly precarious potential for privatisations and market forces to threaten the relationship between the public and public services, Clarke (2007) poses the question of what is not neo-liberal. He does so to open up the possibilities for challenging the self-defeating assumption that neo-liberalism is omnipresent and omnipotent. He identifies the neo-liberal objective of transform-ing citizens into consumers as an important site where all is not yet lost and resist-ance, or in his terms, recalcitrance, is alive and kicking. Similarly, Holloway (2010) argues that people must find new ways of doing social relations other than those defined by capitalism. Clarke (2007) insightfully sees the complexity which hides in the working spaces of public institutions that might explain a so-called 'imple-mentation gap'; when government aims to re-invent us as customers of services are frustrated. At least two recalcitrant groups might be involved here. First, the service users or patients who make claims of their own:

> ... to take the social democratic welfare state and say: it's not enough; it fails to address not just diversity but relations of structured difference that produce inequality; it fails to transform and enable people's lives; it fails to really redress the inequalities of market relations; and it fails to deliver anything but the barest minimum of poverty protection. (Clarke, 2007: 243)

They may also assertively question the power of professionals in a context of clinical decision making, but in complex ways that defy simplistic reduction to a notion of consumerism. Interestingly, a second group who may show resistance might be recalcitrant professional staff, amongst whose numbers will undoubtedly be individuals who range from conservatives who would resist any change to those with allegiances to allegedly outmoded principles of public service or, indeed, may be characterised by more radical interest in the future of the NHS as a bastion of collectivism.

For Clarke (2007) a feature of the neoliberal project, exemplified by New Labour, but also echoed in the softer presentations of the present coalition, is to attempt the co-option of various interest groups (for instance those with a stake in equalities or community issues) by talking up progressive aims, couched in user-friendly language. Witness the Blairite rhetoric on social inclusion or indeed, Cameron's Big Society. The threat that co-option or incorporation might water down the radicalism of the mental health service user/survivor movement is a perennial issue of concern for informed commentators (see Pilgrim, 2005). There is also a parallel discursive tactic to reframe opposition and alternative viewpoints as apparently dated or outmoded. New Labour's very title is an attempt to locate itself in time, underscoring their *new-ness* as a virtue and implicitly denigrating oppositional political ideas:

> In this discussion of New Labour and neo-liberalism, I want to emphasise how 'telling the time' is a distinctive and potent discursive strategy, locating alternative conceptions of how the future might be constructed as 'residual', 'out of time', 'nostalgic' or the product of 'old ways of thinking'. (Clarke, 2007: 246)

Importantly, however, any co-opted ideas must, of necessity, remain subordinate to the grand neo-liberal project. This both aids the survival of the more naked neo-liberal objectives by neutralising some opposition and softens some of the rougher edges of the dominant force, leaving open the space for more recalcitrant voices to emerge. Arguably, it is in these interstices that user involvement has thrived and the survivor movement has tried to pragmatically make the most of opportunities to seek change framed in terms of consumerism.

MOVEMENT POLITICS AND THE POTENTIAL FOR CONSTRUCTIVE ALLIANCES

Various scholars have seen mental health service users as constituting a social movement seeking changes in services and wider society. As such, they are part of a panoply of movements that include disability rights movements and other groups organised around progressive political objectives (see Crossley, 2006; Spandler, 2006; Beresford & Branfield, 2012). Typically, a distinction has been drawn between so-called new social movements and older movements, like political parties or trade unions, with the latter being criticised for bureaucratisation and hierarchical leadership structures, squeezing out the democratic influence of the grassroots membership. European political philosophers such as Jurgen Habermas (1981) have argued that it is just this sort of democratic deficit that led to the emergence of a plurality of issue or identity focused social movements, service user or survivor movements being prominent amongst them. It can be argued that the debate about the differences between new and old social movements is a distraction, and the strategic imperative ought to be about forging alliances between the two (Cresswell & Spandler, 2009).

Seen from a perspective of movement politics, service user involvement practices are bedevilled with ideological contradictions, as consumerism comes up against social movement radicalism (Brown & Zavetoski, 2005; Crossley, 2006; Spandler, 2006; Stickley, 2006; Cowden & Singh, 2007; Williamson, 2008). For example, movement activism is focused on movement goals grounded in a common cause rather than being motivated by personal reward; in this context, a desire to make a positive difference to services is prominent (McKeown et al., 2010). Interestingly, despite often having quite radical objectives or making potentially transformative demands upon services, it took a consumerist turn in policy to open up the possibility for services to connect with the dynamism of these patient-led collectives. The involvement of service users inside mental health services and within policy bureaucracies raises the possibility of engaging with the politics of the wider user movement, mainly externally situated,but now infiltrating the places where care is transacted. From this perspective, public participation and involvement strategy have opened a door through which more progressive transformational forces might slip. As such, viewing involvement activity through the lens of service user movement politics opens up certain possibilities. Amongst these is the potential for alliances between service users and critically-minded staff or groups that represent staff interests. Such alliances would, by definition, be political alliances, and would also be fraught with perils as well as possibilities (Cresswell, 2009).

One of the possibilities for trade unions that organise nurses and other health-care staff is that alliances with service user groups can be one means by which they might solve some problems of their own. Furthermore, the neo-liberal threats to the future of welfare might represent a jumping-off point for finding a common cause between staff and service user interests. It has been argued that trade unions across the board are caught up in a distinct legitimacy crisis; they struggle to get the public at large to understand their role and purpose and, hence, face pressing problems with regard to the recruitment and retention of members. Furthermore, their internal relations have become denuded to the point that they appear to have become hollowed out, losing sight of any sense of the collective, with individuals having a seemingly private relationship to the union based upon servicing rather than organising principles (Wills & Simms, 2004; Jarley, 2005; Simms & Holgate, 2010). This means they rely on the union for a basket of services including formal representation should they need it, but need not necessarily play any part in activism toward union objectives: indeed for many being in the union amounts to little more than regularly paying a subscription. This is so much the case that there is a distinct focus within trade unions on strategies for union renewal, and public sector unions are in the vanguard of this. In the nursing context, the effectiveness of unions is further undermined by divided membership between traditional unions and professional bodies (Hart, 2004).

The mental health service user movement has a legitimacy crisis of its own. The most obvious grounds for questioning the legitimacy claims for service users are the previously highlighted process of co-option and incorporation which threaten the vitality of the movement. Radical demands on services risk being watered down, or being pulled away from the territory of protest and activism into more formal structures. This is akin to what Brown (2000: 230) has referred to as the peril of 'the transposition of venue from the streets to the courtroom', where collective action becomes neutralised into an individualised and legalistic form (Cresswell, 2009).

One solution for the legitimacy crises facing service user and trade union activists can be found in models of community organising. Numerous examples of effective community organising have been enacted in different parts of the world, informed by ideals of participatory democracy, collective self-resilience, and building social capital amongst members of the community (see Alinsky, 1971; Freire, 1971; Sennett, 2012). In a similar way, one inward-looking strategy for union renewal is to make strenuous efforts to build relationships and networks of mutual support within the union (Hoerr, 1997; O'Halloran, 2006). Another, perhaps of more interest and utility, is the idea of reciprocal community unionism which looks to build alliances and solidarity reaching out to the local community. One example of this is the way in which the broadly-based coalition London Citizens has campaigned for a living wage for people in precarious employment in London. From time to time, usually in defence of services, similar coalitions have been forged between unions and service user groups. Scholars of community union organising have remarked upon the necessity of establishing relationships and solidarity in advance of the need to rely on these and the challenges faced by trade union activists seeking alliances with service users who might blame them for perceived failings in services (Wills & Simms, 2004). Any actual alliance would have to be grounded in both an organising model of trade unionism and a collectivised view of mental health service user movement activism. The fruits of such an alliance could be a revitalisation of union *and* user movement activism and the overarching struggle not just to defend the NHS from the ravages of austerity, but also to look forward to transforming it towards more egalitarian goals.

Arguably, trade unions don't always fully appreciate the politics of mental health, to the detriment of solidarity with the survivor movement. For example, the reproduction of negative stereotypes is often part of the media coverage of health and social care disputes. Typically these portray service users as potentially dangerous and in need of psychiatric containment or alternately as passive and uncritical recipients of expert care: there is also usually a framing of mental health in singularly psychiatric terms, with an uncritical acceptance of the notion of mental illness. It is a short step to make the case that cuts in services might render the public vulnerable to such dangerous individuals, and that the incompetent and personally vulnerable sufferers of mental illness might be lost and abandoned without adequate services. Plainly, if an industrial dispute involves the defence of service, then this sort of media coverage can serve the interests of trade unions or striking workers, as they can make a case for the continuance of service provision and the necessity of professional care (McKeown, 2009). This sort of happenstance, where progressive values are subverted in the pursuance of instrumental goals, has been referred to elsewhere as 'imperfect solidarity' (Millon-Delsol, 2000).

Undoubtedly, exemplars of significant alliances of this sort are few and far between, and those that have occurred more often than not expose the tensions in relations between activists as much as any achievement of deeper solidarity. Nevertheless, a couple of UK examples illustrate some of the specific perils and possibilities at stake. First, and most notably, was the establishment of the Mental Patients Union in the 1970s, emerging from an alliance to oppose the closure of the Paddington Day Hospital therapeutic community. Helen Spandler (2006) makes a persuasive case that the democratising features of the therapeutic community approach were an important foundation for the solidarity that grew between staff and service users and that key staff were instrumental in eventually supporting service users to launch their own radical organisation. Purposively modelled on the idea of a trade union for patients, the MPU was nevertheless largely ignored by the wider labour movement. In a second example, Mark Cresswell (2009), a mental health nurse and now sociologist, was involved as a NALGO shop steward in a lengthy social services' strike in Sheffield in 1991. In the course of the industrial action the local service user movement organised an occupation of one of the day hospitals in support of the strikers but also keeping the venue open for service users to make use of. Interestingly, relationships of solidarity forged in the dispute affected subsequent relations after its resolution. The service users made demands of their own: they had fought in defence of a service and now wanted more of a say in the actual *type of service* delivered. This resulted in the eventual use of the premises at weekends for user-led, user-only space. Such a state of affairs highlights the importance of a constructive strategic dialogue between mental health workers and service users, raising questions about the most appropriate form this might take. Arguably, there is a need to enhance the democratic characteristics of our communication both inside services and within any alliances (McKeown, 2012).

DIFFERENT FORMS OF DEMOCRACY FOR INVOLVEMENT?

Habermas (1986, 1987) has argued that it is the act of communication itself which ultimately makes a difference in attempts to transform society. He urges better forms of democracy within which communication is as free as it can possibly be, unconstrained by prejudice or unequal power relationships. Such social relations can be prefigured in the political deliberations of movement groups, old or new, and could, with a concerted effort, be brought into arenas such as those for service user involvement. For Habermas, taking the time to talk things through carefully, respectfully and deliberatively, whilst always holding open the possibility of changing one's own positioning on any issue if so persuaded, is the surest way of ensuring that better ideas will emerge in the long run. Beresford (2010), for example, highlights the use of *deliberative structures* as one means of moving beyond simplistic notions of partnership or one-off consultation in a context of formal user involvement. Hodge (2005a, 2005b, 2009), however, has bemoaned the fact that most user involvement opportunities, as presently constituted, do not reach the ideals of unconstrained communication necessary for transformative action.

Other critics of Habermasian ideas call into question their value or utility in a mental health context. Largely this amounts to a critique of the premium he places on rationality as a key aspect of communicative action. This poses a number of problems, not least the ways in which mental health service users have historically had their voices discounted or even silenced because under psychiatry they are defined as irrational (O'Hagan, 1986; Bracken & Thomas, 2001; Hornstein, 2002; Campbell, 2009). Habermas is also criticised for relying on particular psychological framings of what would constitute disordered communication or a perceived neglect of other dimensions of communication which may be important in this context, such as emotionality and non-verbal physicality (Crossley, 2004; Lewis, 2009; Clifford, 2009). Revisions of communicative action theory which take account of this critique contextualise the persuasive power of reasoned argument whilst reaffirming the utility of these ideas for those who would seek progressive change and more democratic deliberations in the field of disability movement activism (Gardiner, 2004). In any event, the user/survivor movement has long established its credentials as being able to offer a trenchant, sustained and rational critique of psychiatry (Coleman, 2008).

Church (1995) remarks that the social relations between critically engaged staff and service users who wish to work together for change will always be both unsettled and unsettling. This is not a bad thing, it just should not be taken for granted that co-operation or alliance building will be accomplished smoothly. Spandler (2009) has noted different forms of social space within mental health services. A convergent space might be where consensus around a particular view or strategy is easily achieved. More likely there will be paradoxical spaces where solutions or strategies are imagined, and result from creative interaction and communication arising from the very tensions between different views or perspectives.

CONCLUSION

The possibilities for service user alliances with representative staff groups are demonstrably real and offer at least one route by which the progressive framing of demands for change made by activists can be actioned in services. The solidarity that grows in political alliances can be extended into therapeutic alliances, but perhaps the latter need to be modelled in services that are a step-change away from those we currently have, necessitating a shift from a singular biological psychiatry to more relational approaches to organising care. For Lewis (2005) the major flaw in user involvement policies is that they take for granted the dominance of the psychiatric model to the exclusion of more social understandings of mental distress. A number of crucial factors are germane to finding out whether any transformative possibilities can trump the perils. Past examples of productive alliances include those social spaces wherein key, politicised individuals have been present in circumstances which for various reasons have potentiated more democratic social relations between staff and service user participants. Public attitudes and media coverage of mental health issues are crucial, especially on how these might reproduce or challenge prevailing pejorative stereotypes. Our reflections pose some serious questions about the preparedness of trade unions and mental health movements to take up the various opportunities for establishing effective alliances. Ultimately, however, we offer an optimistic analysis which sees possibilities in even the perils and always considers the implicit creativity of community campaigning, political and industrial action in defence of welfare, and how this might connect with other imaginative acts of insurgency elsewhere (Hyman, 1989).

Clearly, there are different possibilities for framing our relationship to mental health and the politics of delivering wholesome and consensual caring services. Alternatives such as Soteria (Calton et al., 2008) are available and supported by elements of the survivor movement, or existing services could be radically transformed if more democratic and co-operative styles of communication were the norm. These might intersect with other forms of resistance to the neo-liberal political project (Spandler, 2014). We could perhaps imagine a reconnection with older forms of collectivism held to by the traditional labour movement, or we might see more hope in the newer projects embodied in social movements, or we may find even newer forms in alliance and the synthesis of ideas:

> Such imaginaries could be either residual or emergent – but they are certainly active forces in the present and may yet underpin other futures. (Clarke, 2007: 247)

Once such novel imagining could be in the direction of a new politics of mental health, connecting the interests of workers and service users alike. Cresswell and Spandler (2009) offer one such vision, reworking the ideas of Peter Sedgwick for modern times. These ideas must include a reframing of the very idea of service user involvement away from the current favouring of individualised needs towards more collective concerns or remedies in the arena of social justice (Lewis, 2005). More completely democratising the social relations of caring services holds out the opportunity to maximise expressions of compassion and dismantle the alienating features of more traditional services, offering greater rewards and fulfilment for staff as well as service users. Despite the undoubted progress that has been made already in mental health services, this requires much more in the way of transformation than the limited manifestations of user involvement and contradictory policy ideologies we have at present.

In a celebration of international involvement initiatives, Kathryn Church and David Reville (2010) quoted Robbie Robertson, famously of The Band, who said *'The thing you've got to learn is not to be afraid of it'*. There is perhaps no better advice for nurses wishing to be part of the progressive change that is needed in mental health services if service users are to become truly fully respected, active and empowered partners in their own care.

Establishment of Community Health Councils	1974	Created as part of a wider restructuring of NHS services to provide a voice for patients and the public in the NHS in England and Wales. They were to remain the mainstay of public involvement for 25 years.
The Griffiths Report *Community Care: Agenda for Action* Roy Griffiths London: HMSO	1988	Influential White Paper from Conservative government introduced New Right ideology to NHS strategy and the idea of patients as consumers.
NHS and Community Care Act	1990	Took forward ideas from Griffiths and brought internal market into NHS with the purchaser-provider split. Established the concept of user involvement in community care assessments.
The Patient's Charter London: DH, HMSO.	1991 Revised 1995 & 1997	Charter of rights, including right to named nurse. Attempt to increase accountability of services to users; associated with the introduction of published league tables.
The Health of the Nation: A Strategy for England London: DH, HMSO.	1992	Service user involvement encouraged in the context of a strategic approach to improving the health of the whole population, with mental illness as one of the key target areas.

(Continued)

Figure 8.1   (Continued)

Local Voices: The Views of Local People in Purchasing for Health National Health Service Management Executive London: DH.	1992	Urged Health Authorities to consult service users over the planning and monitoring of services.
Guidelines for Empowering Users of Mental Health Services. Read, J. & Wallcraft, J. MIND/COHSE.	1992	Best practice guidelines for empowerment and user involvement aimed at union members. Co-authored by influential user activists Jim Read and Jan Wallcraft in conjunction with national officers in the nursing section of COHSE the health service union, later merged into UNISON. The collaboration continued and resulted in later Unison guides for supporting advocacy and equal opportunities in a context of mental health services.
Report of the Mental Health Nursing Review Team [The Butterworth Report] *Working in Partnership: A Collaborative Approach to Care.* London: DH, HMSO.	1994	Encouraged a commitment from nursing profession to user involvement with a central focus on the relationships between nurses and service users. Recommended that service users take a role in nursing education and curriculum development.
Building Bridges: A Guide to Arrangements for Inter-agency Working for the Care and Protection of Severely Mentally Ill People. London: DH.	1995	Service user involvement encouraged in the context of community mental health care case management processes.
Patient Partnership Strategy National Health Service Executive Leeds: NHSE.	1996	Focus on involvement in clinical decision making. Stressed the role of information provision in enabling service users to exercise informed choices about care.
Establishment of the *Standing Advisory Group on Consumer Involvement in the NHS Research and Development Programme*. Later to become *INVOLVE*.	1996	Official recognition of the value of service user involvement in research. Later developments extended this to social care research.
Patient and Public Involvement in the New NHS London: NHS Executive, DH.	1999	New Labour government carries on with consumerist policies. Restates the aims of the Patient Partnership programme, and builds upon the 1997 establishment of *Health Action Zones*. Extends involvement principles to new NHS structures (Primary Care Groups, later to become Primary Care Trusts) and urges new action to further develop service user and public involvement.
National Service Framework for Mental Health: Modern Standards and Service Models. London: DH.	1999	Overarching commitment to user involvement in care, planning for services, and evaluation of services. Involvement highlighted as one mechanism for delivering equalities. Little direct reference to involvement, however, in the actual standards.

The NHS Plan: A Plan for Investment, A Plan for Reform London: DH.	2000	Identified patient disempowerment as a problem for the NHS. Carries on the commitment to patient involvement at different levels and looks forward to the creation of PALS and PPI forums.
Involving Consumers in Research and Development in the NHS: Briefing Notes for Researchers. Hanley, B. et al. Winchester: Consumers in NHS Research Support Unit, Help for Health Trust.	2000	Best practice guide for service user involvement in research and development in the NHS.
The Expert Patient: A New Approach to Chronic Disease Management for the 21st Century London: DH.	2001	Established the *Expert Patient Programme* which has gone on to involve people with lived experience in supporting a range of self-management initiatives.
Health and Social Care Act	2001	Enshrined patient and public involvement as a duty for NHS organisations. Led to the demise of Community Health Councils and the establishment of a system of PPI forums in every Health Trust.
NHS Reform and Health Care Professions Act	2002	Created the Commission for Patient and Public Involvement in Health.
General Social Care Council accreditation of social worker training	2002	All pre-qualification social work courses must have user and carer involvement for curriculum to be accredited. HEIs receive ring fenced monies to support user involvement in teaching and learning.
Building on the Best: Choice, Responsiveness and Equity in the NHS London: DH.	2003	Delineation of the government's choice agenda following a national consultation. A commitment to listen to patients and develop respectful relationships with clinicians. Looks forward to service user control over information and health records and systems for choosing services and booking appointments. Patient Tsar appointed.
Involving the Public in NHS, Public Health and Social Care Research: Briefing notes for researchers Hanley, B. et al. Eastleigh: INVOLVE.	2003	Second edition of the earlier guidance, 2000.
The Mental Health Service User Movement in England Wallcraft, J. & Bryant, M. London: The Sainsbury Centre for Mental Health (SCMH).	2003	Results of a survey of mental health user groups. Demonstrated extensiveness of self-organised groups but insecurity of funding highlighted. Gender and ethnicity issues were not always well served in established groups nor were BME individuals well represented in the groups. The SCMH was influential in the New Labour years, both in terms of policy research and education.

(Continued)

Figure 8.1   (Continued)

Establishment of Foundation Trusts	2004	One aim was to improve local accountability via patient and public presence as members or elected governors.
The Ten Essential Shared Capabilities: A Framework for the Whole of the Mental Health Workforce The National Institute for Mental Health (England) Leeds: NIMHE.	2004	Describes the essential capabilities for practitioners working in mental health, intended to guide education and training. Grounded in extensive consultation with service users. Working in partnership, empowerment and user involvement are stressed as key dimensions of the stated capabilities.
A Good Practice Guide: Learning from Experience. Involving Service Users and Carers in Mental Health Education and Training Tew, G. et al. Nottingham: Mental Health in Higher Education/NIMHE.	2004	Lays out best practice for service user involvement in teaching and learning for mental health practitioners. Offers a revised version of Arnstein's Ladder for evaluating the quality of involvement. Supported by the influential *mental health in higher education* network, established by the Higher Education Academy. *MHHE* also set up a network to support development workers for establishing user and carer involvement in university settings (DUCIE).
Delivering Race Equality in Mental Health Care: A Summary: An action plan for services a model for reform Melba Wilson London: DH.	2005	Raft of initiatives aimed at addressing insititutionalised racism and inequalities in mental health services. An emphasis on models of community engagement to better understand diverse needs and improve cultural sensitivity of services.
From Values to Action: The Chief Nursing Officer's Review of Mental Health Nursing. London: DH.	2006a	Service user involvement is central to this review of mental health nursing. A number of best practice examples presented.
Our Health Our Care Our Say: A New Direction for Community Services London: DH, The Stationery Office.	2006b	White paper introducing the concept of personalisation and aiming that citizens have a stronger voice in shaping service improvements. Mental health framed in terms of wellbeing and access to psychological therapies is highlighted. Informed by mass consultation process including *citizen summits* listening events.
Launch of NHS Centre for Involvement	2006	Established to support service user involvement and public engagement in the NHS. Based at the University of Warwick. Began with a strong interest in democratic accountability in services and together with INVOLVE launched the book *Healthy Democracy*. Ceased to exist in 2009.
Local Government and Public Involvement in Health Act	2007	Abolished PPI Forums to be replaced by Local Involvement Networks – LINKs.

Mental Health Act	2007	Amended the 1983 Act and emerged after lengthy consultation and revision process which saw significant contribution from the Mental Health Alliance. Arguably a disappointment for the user movement because of the main focus on public safety and risk containment. Did result in statutory right to advocacy for patients subject to compulsion.
Putting People First: A Shared Vision and Commitment to the Transformation of Adult Social Care London: HM Government.	2007	Introduces plans for personal budgets, a longtime goal for the disability movement. Self-determination and user control over services is stressed. Service user involvement described as part of a statement of values and vision for reforming adult social care. Placed in a context of joint planning between central and local government, social care professionals, provider organisations and the regulators.
User Involvement in Research by Nurses: RCN guidance London: RCN Research Society, Royal College of Nursing.	2007	Guidance for best practice in user involvement in research undertaken by nurses. Archived in 2012 because overtaken by plethora of writing on the subject. RCN members now directed to the book: Morrow et al. (2011) *Handbook of Service User Involvement in Nursing and Healthcare Research*. Wiley, Chichester.
User Involvement in Social Work Education Branfield, F. & Shaping Our Lives. London: Social Care Institute for Excellence (SCIE). *Common Aims: A Strategy to Support Service User Involvement in Social Work Education.* Branfield, F., Beresford, P. & Levin, E. London: SCIE/Shaping Our Lives.	2007	Two influential publications for guiding involvement practices in relation to social work education. Shaping Our Lives is an important user-led group involved in research and education. Peter Beresford is an influential academic with lived experience of service use himself. SCIE are an important body for the marshalling and dissemination of evidence relevant to social care.
User Involvement in Public Services London: Public Administration Select Committee House of Commons.	2008	Reviewed progress on service user involvement in public services. Re-emphasised desirability of user involvement as a force for democracy and contemplated different forms, including models for user control of services. Makes the case that public sector staff have to be prepared to face up to the challenge of user involvement. Hints at some potential hazards, such as introducing inequalities or being too risky or costly in certain circumstances.

(Continued)

Figure 8.1   (Continued)

The Darzi review 'High quality care for all: NHS next stage review final report' London: DH.	2008	In a context of promoting health as opposed to just treating illness this report looks forward to the introduction of notion of personalization in health care, with piloting of personal health budgets. Also a new right to choice will be enshrined in an NHS Constitution. Dignity, respect and compassion are highlighted as key expectations of patient care, with compassion in nursing particularly emphasised.
Good Practice Guidelines: Service User and Carer Involvement within Clinical Psychology Training. Leicester: British Psychological Society (BPS)	2008	Guidance for service user involvement in the teaching and learning of clinical psychologists.
Primary Care and Community Services: Personal Health Budgets: First steps. London: DH.	2009a	Makes the case for personal health budgets and reviews the piloting process. Foregrounds the idea of co-production as key component of implementing the Next Stage Review. Highlights the aim of personal health budgets to give service users or families more control over their own care so that it better meets holistic needs. Suggests that the introduction of these measures might make practitioners more likely to engage in detailed discussions with service users about their views on their own care and hence drive wider change in the NHS.
The NHS Constitution London: DH.	2009b Revised 2010, 2012	Enshrines the values of the NHS and sets out rights, responsibilities and pledges for patients and the public and also staff. One of its stated goals is to protect the NHS into the future so that it continues to service the public and be free at the point of use.
New Horizons: A Shared Vision for Mental Health London: HM Government, DH.	2009	One of the last health policy acts for New Labour. Makes recovery a central theme and service user involvement continues to figure significantly as a route to more holistic care. Makes the case for alliance between central and local government, the professions and the voluntary sector. Superseded by *No Health Without Mental Health* (see below).
No Health Without Mental Health: A Cross-government Mental Health Outcomes Strategy for People of All Ages London: DH.	2011	The coalition government's new mental health policy extends the approach taken up in *New Horizons*. The policy rhetoric is strong on self-determination and personalisation. A connection is made with the wider commitment to a Big Society ideal. A concomitant stress on measurable outcomes is cross-referenced to another document: *Delivering Better Mental Health Outcomes*.

Health and Social Care Act	2012	Legislation brought in by Conservative-Liberal Democrat coalition government in face of large-scale public and trade union protest. Arguably opens up the possibility for increasing levels of marketisation and privatization. Major structural reforms of NHS. Creates Clinical Commissioning Groups to replace PCTs as commissioners of services, privileging the notion of clinicians at the heart of purchasing. LINKs to be replaced by Healthwatch. New commissioning groups will be obliged to make plans to incorporate public engagement into the commissioning process.

Figure 8.1   Key policy events relevant to service user involvement in health and social care, England

Legislation

NHS and Community Care Act 1990
Northern Ireland Act 1998
NHS Reform and Health Care Professions Act 2002
Mental Health (Care and Treatment)(Scotland) Act 2003
Local Government and Public Involvement in Health Act 2007
Mental Health Act 2007
Health and Social Care Act 2011
Health and Social Care Act 2012

Reflective Exercise

1. How has this social movement been undertaken?
2. Does it have parallels with other social movements based on issues of equality?
3. How much do you feel that issues of power (both professional and personal) under-pin the issues in this chapter?
4. What changes to your practice does this discussion ask of you?

BIBLIOGRAPHY

Adams, R. (2002) *Social Policy for Social Work*. Houndmills: Palgrave.
Alinsky, S. (1971) *Rules for Radicals: A Pragmatic Primer for Realistic Radicals*. New York: Random House.
Alzheimer's Society (2007) Inquiry into the National Institute for Health and Clinical Excellence: The Alzheimer's Society submission to the Health Committee inquiry into aspects of the work of the National Institute for Health and Clinical Excellence (NICE). London: Alzheimer's Society.

Arnstein, S. (1969) A ladder of citizen participation, *Journal of the American Institute of Planners*, 35: 216–224.

Baldock, J., Manning, N. & Vickerstaff, S. (eds) (2003) *Social Policy* (2nd edn). Oxford: Oxford University Press.

Barber, R., Boote, J., Parry, G., Cooper, C. & Yeeles, P. (2012) Evaluating the impact of public involvement on research. In M. Barnes and P. Cotterell (eds), *Critical Perspectives on User Involvement*. Bristol: Policy. pp. 217–233.

Barnes, D. & Carpenter, J. (2006) The outcomes of partnerships with mental health service users in interprofessional education: a case study, *Health and Social Care in the Community*, 14: 426–435.

Barnes, M. & Cotterell, P. (2012) Introduction: from margin to mainstream. In M. Barnes and P. Cotterell (eds), Critical Perspectives on User Involvement. Bristol: Policy. pp. xv–xxvi.

Basset, T., Campbell, P. & Anderson, J. (2006) Service user/survivor involvement in mental health training and education: overcoming the barriers, *Social Work Education*, 25: 393–402.

Beresford, P. (1994) Disabled people, service users, user involvement and representation, *Disability & Society*, 9: 315–325.

Beresford, P. (2002) User involvement in research and evaluation: liberation or regulation?, *Social Policy & Society*, 1 (2): 95–105.

Beresford P. (2005) 'Service user': regressive or liberatory terminology?, *Disability & Society*, 20: 469–477.

Beresford, P. (2010) Public partnerships, governance and user involvement: a service user perspective, *International Journal of Consumer Studies*, 34: 495–502.

Beresford, P. & Branfield, F. (2012) Building solidarity, ensuring diversity: lessons from service users' and disabled people's movements. In M. Barnes and P. Cotterell (eds), *Critical Perspectives on User Involvement*. Bristol: Policy. pp. 217–233.

Beresford, P., Branfield, F., Taylor, J. et al. (2006) Working together for better social work education, *Social Work Education*, 25: 326–331.

Bhui, K., Stansfeld, S.A., Holt, S. et al. (2003) Ethnic variations in the pathways to and use of specialist mental health services, *British Journal of Psychiatry*, 182: 105–116.

Blofeld, J. (2003) Independent inquiry into the death of David Bennett report. Norwich: Norfolk, Suffolk and Cambridge Strategic Health Authority.

Bracken, P. & Thomas, P. (2001) Postpsychiatry: a new direction for mental health?, *British Medical Journal*, 322: 724–727.

Brandon, D. (1976) *Zen and the Art of Helping*. London: Routledge & Kegan Paul.

Branfield, F. & Shaping Our Lives (2007) *User Involvement in Social Work Education*. London: Social Care Institute for Excellence.

Branfield, F., Beresford, P. & Levin, E. (2007) *Common Aims: A Strategy to Support Service User Involvement in Social Work Education*. London: SCIE/Shaping Our Lives.

British Psychological Society (2008) *Good Practice Guidelines: Service User and Carer Involvement within Clinical Psychology Training*. Leicester: BPS.

Brooker, C., Curran, J., James, A. & Readhead, E. (2005) Developing and piloting an audit tool for mental health education and training: The National Mental Health Education Continuous Quality Improvement Tool, *Journal of Interprofessional Care*, 19: 280–293.

Brown, K. & Young, N. (2008) Building capacity for service user and carer involvement in social work education, *Social Work Education: The International Journal*, 27 (1): 84–96.

Brown, P. & Zavestoski, S. (eds) (2005) *Social Movements in Health*. New York: Blackwell.

Brown, W. (2000) Suffering rights as paradoxes, *Constellations*, 7: 230–241.

Calton, T., Ferriter, M., Huband, N. & Spandler, H. (2008) A systematic review of the Soteria paradigm for the treatment of people diagnosed with schizophrenia, *Schizophrenia Bulletin*, 34: 181–192.

Campbell, P. (2009) The service user/survivor movement. In J. Reynolds, R. Muston, T. Heller et al. (eds), *Mental Health Still Matters*. Basingstoke: Palgrave/Open University Press.

CAPS (the Consultation and Advocacy Promotion Service) (2010) *Oor Mad History: A Community History of the Lothian Mental Health Service User Movement*. Edinburgh: Living Memory Association/CAPS.

Carr, S. (2007) Participation, power, conflict and change: theorizing dynamics of service user participation in the social care system of England and Wales, *Critical Social Policy*, 27: 266–276.

Church, K. (1995) *Forbidden Narratives: Critical Autobiography as Social Science*. London: Routledge.

Church, K. (2005) Conflicting knowledge/s: User involvement in the field of knowledge. In S. Tilley (ed.), *Field of Knowledge of Psychiatric and Mental Health Nursing*. Oxford: Blackwell. pp. 181–185.

Church, K. & Reville, D. (2010) Foreword: Strike up the band! In M. McKeown, L. Malihi-Shoja and S. Downe (eds), *Supporting The Comensus Writing Collective*. Oxford: Wiley. pp. ix-xiv.

Clarke, J. (2004) Dissolving the public realm? The logic and limits of neo-liberalism, *Journal of Social Policy*, 33: 27–48.

Clarke, J. (2007) Citizen-consumers and public service reform: at the limits of neo-liberalism?, *Policy Futures in Education*, 5: 239–248.

Clifford, S. (2009) *Disabling Democracy: How Disability Reconfigures Deliberative Democratic Norms*. American Political Science Association 2009 Annual Meeting, Toronto, September 3–6, published proceedings. Available at http://papers.ssrn.com/sol3/papers.cfm?abstract_id=1451092 (last accessed 30 August 2012).

Coleman, E. (2008) The politics of rationality: psychiatric survivors' challenge to psychiatry. In B. Da Costa and K. Philip (eds), *Tactical Biopolitics: Art, Activism, and Technoscience*. Cambridge, MA: The MIT Press. pp. 341–363.

Committee of Inquiry (1992) Report of the Committee of Inquiry into complaints about Ashworth Hospital (Blom-Cooper report). London: HMSO.

Connor, S. & Wilson, R. (2006) 'It's important that they learn from us for mental health to progress', *Journal of Mental Health*, 15: 461–474.

Cooke, B. & Kothari, U. (2002) *Participation: The New Tyranny?* London: Zed.

Correia, T. (2012) Debating the comprehensive basis of western healthcare systems in the light of neo-liberalism. CIES Working Paper 124/2012. Centro de Investigacao e Estudos de Sociologica, Instituto Universitario de Lisboa.

Cowden, S. & Singh, G. (2007) The 'user': friend, foe or fetish?: a critical exploration of user involvement in health and social care, *Critical Social Policy*, 27: 5–23.

Cresswell, M. (2009) Deeply engaged relationships? Community trade unionism and mental health movements in the UK. Lead Address to Fringe Meeting: Unison in the Community: Mutuality and Solidarity. Unison Health Conference, Harrogate, April 20–22.

Cresswell, M. & Spandler, H. (2009) Psychopolitics: Peter Sedgwick's legacy for the politics of mental health, *Social Theory and Health*, 7: 129–147.

Crossley, N. (2004) On systematically distorted communication: Bourdieu and the socio-analysis of publics, *The Sociological Review (Special Issue), After Habermas: New Perspectives on the Public Sphere*, 52, s1: 88–112.

Crossley, N. (2006) Contesting psychiatry: social movements. In *Mental Health*. London: Routledge.

Crouch, C. (2011) *The Strange Non-death of Neoliberalism*. Cambridge: Polity.

Department of Health (1991) *The Patient's Charter*. London: HMSO.

Department of Health (1992) *The Health of the Nation: A Strategy for England*. London: HMSO.

Department of Health (1995) *Building Bridges: A Guide to Arrangements for Inter-agency Working for the Care and Protection of Severely Mentally Ill People*. London: DH.

Department of Health (1999) *National Service Framework for Mental Health: Modern Standards and Service Models*. London: DH.

Department of Health (2000) *The NHS Plan: A Plan for Investment, A Plan for Reform*. London: HMSO.

Department of Health (2001) *The Expert Patient: A New Approach to Chronic Disease Management for the 21st Century*. London: HMSO.

Department of Health (2003) *Building on the Best: Choice, Responsiveness and Equity in the NHS*. London: DH.

Department of Health (2004a) *NHS Improvement Plan: Putting People at the Heart of Public Services*. London: DH.

Department of Health (2004b) *Patient and Public Involvement in Health: The Evidence for Policy Implementation*. London: DH.

Department of Health (2005) *Creating a Patient-Led NHS: Delivering the NHS Improvement Plan*. London: DH.

Department of Health (2006a) *From Values to Action: The Chief Nursing Officer's Review of Mental Health Nursing*. London: DH.

Department of Health (2006b) *Our Health Our Care Our Say: A New Direction for Community Services*. London: HMSO.

Department of Health (2008) *High Quality Care For All: NHS Next Stage Review: final report* (the Darzi review). London: DH.

Department of Health (2009a) *Primary Care and Community Services: Personal Health Budgets: first steps*. London: DH.

Department Of Health (2009b) *The NHS Constitution*. London: DH.

Department of Health (2011) *No Health Without Mental Health: A Cross-government Mental Health Outcomes Strategy for People of All Ages*. London: DH.

Department Of Health (2012a) *2011/12 National Survey of Investment in Adult Mental Health Services*. London: DH.

Department Of Health (2012b) *2011/12 National Survey of Investment in Mental Health Services for Older People*. London: DH.

Diamond, B., Parkin, G., Morris, K. et al. (2003) User involvement: substance or spin?, *Journal of Mental Health*, 12: 613–626.

Downe, S., McKeown, M., Johnson, E. et al. (2007) The UCLan Community Engagement and Service User Support (Comensus) project: valuing authenticity, making space for emergence, *Health Expectations*, 10: 392–406.

Duffy, J. (2008) *Looking Out from the Middle: User Involvement in Health and Social Care in Northern Ireland*. London: SCIE.

Farmer, P., Jenkins, P., Grove, B. et al. (2011) Fatal consequences of benefit changes [Letters and e-mails], *The Guardian*, 1 June, p. 31.

Felton, A. & Stickley, T. (2004) Pedagogy, power and service user involvement, *Journal of Psychiatric and Mental Health Nursing*, 11: 89–98.

Foot, M. (1973) *Aneurin Bevan: A Biography*, Volume 2 (1945–1960). London: Davis-Poynter.

Forensic Catchment Group (2007) *Women's Involvement Project: Full report*. NHS Forensic Catchment Group Yorkshire.

Francis, R. (2010) *Independent Inquiry into Care provided by Mid Staffordshire NHS Foundation Trust, January 2005 – March 2009*. London: HMSO.

Frankham, J. (2009) Partnership research: a review of approaches and challenges in conducting research in partnership with service users. ESRC National Centre for Research Methods Review Paper. NCRM/013. London: ESRC.

Freire, P. (1971) *Pedagogy of the Oppressed*. Harmondsworth: Penguin.

Gardiner, M. (2004) Wild publics and grotesque symposiums: Habermas and Bakhtin on dialogue, everyday life and the public sphere, *The Sociological Review (Special Issue), After Habermas: New Perspectives on the Public Sphere*, 52, s1: 28–48.

Godin, P., Davies, J., Heyman, B. et al. (2007) Opening communicative space: a Habermasian understanding of a user led participatory research project, *Forensic Psychiatry & Psychology*, 18 (4): 452–469.

Gorsky, M. (2007) Memorandum submitted to the Health Select Committee inquiry into Public and Patient Involvement in the NHS January 2007: History and Policy. London: London School of Hygiene and Tropical Medicine/Centre for History in Public Health.

Goss, S. & Miller, C. (1995) *From Margin to Mainstream: Developing User and Carer Centred Community Care*. York: Joseph Rowntree Foundation.

Greenhill, B. & Whitehead, R. (2011) Promoting service user inclusion in risk assessment and management: a pilot project developing a human rights-based approach, *British Journal of Learning Disabilities*, 39: 277–283.

Griffiths, R. (1988) *Community Care: Agenda for Action* (The Griffiths Report). London: HMSO.

Habermas, J. (1981) New social movements, Telos, 49: 33–37.

Habermas, J. (1986) *The Theory of Communicative Action, Volume 1: Reason and the Rationalization of Society*. Cambridge: Polity.

Habermas, J. (1987) *The Theory of Communicative Action, Volume 2: The Critique of Functionalist Reason*. Cambridge: Polity.

Hanley, B. (2005) *Research as Empowerment? User Involvement in Research: Building on Experience and Developing Standards*. York: Toronto Seminar Group/Joseph Rowntree Foundation.

Hanley, B., Bradburn, J., Barnes, M. et al. (2003) *Involving the Public in NHS, Public Health and Social Care Research: Briefing Notes for Researchers* (2nd edn). Eastleigh: INVOLVE.

Hanley, B., Bradburn, J., Gorin, S. et al. (2000) *Involving Consumers in Research and Development in the NHS: Briefing Notes for Researchers*. Winchester: Consumers in NHS Research Support Unit, Help for Health Trust.

Harding, E., Brown, D. & Pettinari, C. (2010) Service user perceptions of involvement in developing NICE mental health guidelines: a grounded theory study, *Journal of Mental Health*, 19: 249–257.

Harper, D. (2003) Involving users of services in clinical psychology training, *Clinical Psychology*, 21: 14–19.

Hart, C. (2004) Nurses and Politics: The Impact of Power and Practice. Basingstoke: Palgrave Macmillan.

Healthcare Commission, Care Services Improvement Partnership, National Institute for Mental Health in England (2007) *Count Me In: Results of the 2006 National Census of Inpatients in Mental Health and Learning Disability Services in England and Wales*. London: Healthcare Commission.

Healthcare Commission, Mental Health Act Commission, National Institute for Mental Health in England (2005) *Count Me In: Results of a National Census of Inpatients in Mental Health Hospitals and Facilities in England and Wales*. London: Healthcare Commission.

Healthcare Improvement Scotland and Scottish Health Council (2011) *User Involvement and Person Centredness: Strategy for Healthcare Improvement Scotland and the Scottish Health Council*. Edinburgh: NHS Scotland.

Heenan, D. (2009) Mental health policy in Northern Ireland: the nature and extent of user involvement, *Social Policy and Society*, 8: 451–462.

HM Government (2007) *Putting People First: A Shared Vision and Commitment to the Transformation of Adult Social Care*. London: HM Government.

HM Government (2009) *New Horizons: A Shared Vision for Mental Health*. London: DH.

Hodge, S. (2005a) Participation, discourse and power: a case study in service user involvement, *Critical Social Policy*, 25: 164–179.

Hodge, S. (2005b) Competence, identity and intersubjectivity: applying Habermas's theory of communicative action to service user involvement in mental health policy making, *Social Theory & Health*, 3: 165–182.

Hodge, S. (2009) User involvement in the construction of a mental health charter: an exercise in communicative rationality?, *Health Expectations*, 12: 251–261.

Hoerr, J. (1997) *We Can't Eat Prestige: The Women Who Organized Harvard*. Philadelphia: Temple University Press.

Holloway, J. (2010) *Crack Capitalism*. London: Pluto.

Hopton, J. & Nolan, P. (2003) *Mental Health Practice*, 6 (7): 14–18.

Hornstein, G. (2002) Narratives of madness as told from within. *Chronicles of Higher Education*. January 25 2002. Available at: www.freedom-center.org/pdf/narrativesofmadnesshornstein.pdf (accessed 30 January 2014).

Horrocks, J., Lyons, C. & Hopley, P. (2010) Does strategic involvement of mental health service users and carers in the planning, design and commissioning of mental health services lead to better outcomes?, *International Journal of Consumer Studies*, 34: 562–569.

Hyman, R. (1989) *Strikes* (4th edn). Basingstoke: Macmillan.

Ikkos, G. (2005) Mental health service user involvement: teaching doctors successfully, *Primary Care Mental Health*, 3: 139–144.

INVOLVE (2007) *Good Practice in Active Public Involvement in Research*. Eastleigh: INVOLVE.

Jarley, P. (2005) Unions as social capital: renewal through a return to the logic of mutual aid?, *Labor Studies Journal*, 29 (4): 1–26.

Keating, F., Robertson, D., McCulloch, A. & Francis, E. (2002) *Breaking the Circles of Fear: A Review of the Relationship between Mental Health Services and African and Caribbean Communities*. London: Sainsbury Centre for Mental Health.

Lathlean, J., Burgess, A., Coldham, T. et al. (2006) Experiences of service user and carer participation in health care education, *Nurse Education in Practice*, 6: 424–429.

Lewis, L. (2005) User involvement within Scottish mental health policy: locating power and inequality, *Scottish Affairs*, 51: 79–107.

Lewis, L. (2009) Politics of recognition: what can a human rights perspective contribute to understanding users' experiences of involvement in mental health services?, *Social Policy & Society*, 8: 257–274.

Lowes, L. & Hulatt, I. (eds) (2005) *Involving Service Users in Health and Social Care Research*. London: Routledge.

McKeown, M. (2009) Alliances in action: opportunities and threats to solidarity between workers and service users in health and social care disputes, *Social Theory and Health*, 7: 148–169.

McKeown, M. (2012) Linking the academy and activism: from constructed subjectivities to participatory, communicative agency. PhD, University of Central Lancashire, April.

McKeown, M. & Mercer, D. (1995) Is a written charter really necessary? Human rights in secure mental health settings, *Psychiatric Care*, 1 (6): 219–223.

McKeown, M., Jones, F., Wright, K. et al. (2012) *An Evaluation of Service User Involvement in Secure Mental Health Services across Yorkshire and Humber.* Preston: UCLAN.

McKeown, M., Malihi-Shoja, L. & Downe, S. (2010) *Supporting The Comensus Writing Collective: Service User and Carer Involvement in Education for Health and Social Care.* Oxford: Wiley.

Macpherson, W. (1999) *The Stephen Lawrence Inquiry: Report of an Inquiry by Sir William Macpherson of Cluny.* London: HMSO.

Millon-Delsol, C. (2000) Barbarity and solidarity, *Znak*, 543: 51–59. English translation available at http://tischner.org.pl/thinking_pliki/thinking_1/tischner_6_delsol.pdf (last accessed 30 August 2012).

Morgan, A. & Jones, D. (2009) Perceptions of service user and carer involvement in healthcare education and impact on students' knowledge and practice: a literature review, *Medical Teacher*, 31: 82–95.

Morris, J. (2011) Rethinking disability policy. Joseph Rowntree Foundation, *Viewpoint*, November.

Morrow, E., Boaz, A., Brearley, S. & Ross, F. (2011) *Handbook of Service User Involvement in Nursing and Healthcare Research.* Chichester: Wiley.

National Health Service Management Executive (1992) *Local Voices: The Views of Local People in Purchasing for Health.* London: DH.

National Institute for Mental Health in England (2004) The Ten Essential Shared Capabilities: A Framework for the Whole of the Mental Health Services. Leeds: NIMHE.

Newbigging, K., Ridely, J., McKeown, M. et al. (2012) The Right to Be Heard: Review of the Quality of Independent Mental Health Advocate (IMHA) Services in England. Research report, University of Central Lancashire, Preston. Available at www.uclan.ac.uk/schools/school_of_health/files/review_of_independent_mental_health_advocate_research_report_190612.pdf (last accessed 30 August 2012).

NHS Executive (1996) *Patient Partnership Strategy.* Leeds: NHSE.

NHS Executive (1999) *Patient and Public Involvement in the New NHS.* Leeds: DH.

Northern Centre for Mental Health (2003) *National Continuous Quality Improvement Tool for Mental Health Education.* York: Northern Centre for Mental Health.

O'Hagan, M. (1986) From taking snapshots to making movies, *Community Mental Health in New Zealand*, 3 (1): 31–49.

O'Halloran, L. (2006) *Relational Organising: A Practical Guide for Unionists.* Available at www.newunionism.net/.../organizing/O'Halloran (last accessed January 2012).

Paton, C. (2001) The state in health: global capitalism, conspiracy, cock-up and competitive change in the NHS, *Public Policy and Administration*, 16: 61–83.

Paton, C. (2006) *New Labour's State of Health: Political Economy, Public Policy and the NHS.* Farnham: Ashgate.

Pilgrim, D. (2005) Protest and co-option: the recent fate of the psychiatric patient's voice. In A. Bell and P. Lindley (eds), *Beyond the Water Towers: The Unfinished Revolution in Mental Health Services 1985–2005.* London: Sainsbury Centre for Mental Health. pp. 17–26.

Prime Minister's Commission on the Future of Nursing and Midwifery in England (2010) *Front Line Care: Report of the Prime Minister's Commission on the Future of Nursing and Midwifery in England.* London: DH.

Prins, H. (1993) *Report of the Committee of Inquiry into the Death in Broadmoor Hospital of Orville Blackwood and a Review of the Death of Two Other Afro-Caribbean Patients: Big, Black and Dangerous?* London: Special Hospitals Service Authority.

Public Administration Select Committee (2008) *User Involvement in Public Services*. HC 410. London: HMSO.

Quiggin, J. (2010) *Zombie Economics: How Dead Ideas Still Walk Amongst Us*. Princeton: Princeton University Press.

Rai-Atkins, A., Jama, A., Wright, N. et al. (2002) *Best Practice in Mental Health: Advocacy for African, Caribbean and South Asian Communities*. York: Joseph Rowntree Foundation.

RCN Research Society (2007) *User Involvement in Research by Nurses: RCN Guidance*. London: Royal College of Nursing.

Read, J. & Wallcraft, J. (1992) *Guidelines for Empowering Users of Mental Health Services*. London: MIND/COHSE.

Report of the Mental Health Nursing Review Team (1994) *Working in Partnership: A Collaborative Approach to Care*. London: HMSO.

Repper, J. & Breeze, J. (2007) User and carer involvement in the training and education of health professionals: a review of the literature, *International Journal of Nursing Studies*, 44: 511–519.

Rose, N. (1985) *The Psychological Complex: Psychology, Politics and Society in England, 1869–1939*. London: Routledge & Kegan Paul.

Rose, N. (1989) *Governing the Soul: The Shaping of the Private Self*. London: Routledge.

Scottish Executive (2000) *Our National Health: A Plan for Action, A Plan for Change*. Edinburgh: Scottish Executive.

Scottish Executive (2001) *Patient Focus and Public Involvement*. Edinburgh: Scottish Executive.

Scottish Executive (2003a) *Sustainable Patient Focus and Public Involvement*. Edinburgh: Scottish Executive.

Scottish Executive (2003b) *Partnership for Care: Scotland's Health White Paper*. Edinburgh: Scottish Executive.

Scottish Executive (2006) *Delivering for Mental Health*. Edinburgh: Scottish Executive.

Scottish Government (2007) *Better Health, Better Care: Action Plan*. Edinburgh: Scottish Government.

Scottish Government (2009) *A Force for Improvement: The Workforce Response to Better Health, Better Care*. Edinburgh: Scottish Government.

Scottish Office (1997) *A Framework for Mental Health Services in Scotland*. Edinburgh: Scottish Office.

Secure Commissioning Team (2010) *Reaching Joint Solutions 2007–2010, Regional Forensic Involvement Strategy* (Yorkshire and the Humber), Yorkshire Secure Commissioning Team.

Sennett, R. (2012) *Together: The Rituals, Pleasures and Politics of Cooperation*. London: Allen Lane.

Shepherd, G., Boardman, J. & Slade, M. (2007) *Making Recovery a Reality*. London: Sainsbury Centre for Mental Health.

Simms, M. & Holgate, J. (2010) Organising for what? Where is the debate on the politics of organising?, *Work Employment & Society*, 24: 157–168.

Smith, A. & Pembroke, L. (2005) Diatribe, *Mental Health Today*, June: 35.

Smith, L. & Bradstreet, S. (2011) *Experts by Experience: Guidelines to Support the Development of Peer Worker Roles in the Mental Health Sector*. Glasgow: Scottish Recovery Network.

Spandler, H. (2006) *Asylum to Action: Paddington Day Hospital, Therapeutic Communities and Beyond*. London: Jessica Kingsley.

Spandler, H. (2009) Spaces of psychiatric contention: a case study of a therapeutic community, *Health & Place*, 15: 672–678.

Spandler, H. (2014) Letting madness breathe? Critical challenges facing mental health social work today. In J. Weinstein (ed), *Critical and Radical Debates in Social Work*. Bristol: Policy Press.

Stickley, T. (2006) Should service user involvement be consigned to history? A critical realist perspective, *Journal of Psychiatric and Mental Health Nursing*, 13: 570–577.

Survivors History Group (2012) Survivors History Group takes a critical look at historians. In M. Barnes and P. Cotterell (eds), *Critical Perspectives on User Involvement*. Bristol: Policy. pp. 7–18.

Sweeney, A., Beresford, P., Faulkner, A. et al. (2009) *This is Survivor Research*. Ross-on-Wye: PCCS.

Tait, L. & Lester, H. (2005) Encouraging user involvement in mental health services, *Advances in Psychiatric Treatment*, 11: 168–175.

Taylor-Gooby, P. (1989) Welfare, hierarchy and the 'New Right': the impact of social policy changes in Britain, 1979–1989, *International Sociology*, 4: 431–446.

Taylor-Gooby, P. (2008) Trust and welfare state reform: the case of the NHS, *Public Policy and Administration*, 42: 288–306.

Terry, J. (2011) The pursuit of excellence and innovation in the implementation of service user involvement in nurse education, Florence Nightingale Scholarship Report, Swansea University.

Tew, J., Gell, C. & Foster, F. (2004) *A Good Practice Guide: Learning from Experience: Involving service users and carers in mental health education and training*. Nottingham: Mental Health in Higher Education/NIMHE.

Thomas, P., Wilson, C. & Jones, P. (2010) Strengthening the voice of mental health service users and carers in Wales: a focus group study to inform future policy, *International Journal of Consumer Studies*, 34: 525–531.

Towle, A., Bainbridge, L., Godolphin, W. et al.(2010) Active patient involvement in the education of health professionals, *Medical Education*, 44: 64–74.

Tritter, J. & McCallum, A. (2006) The snakes and ladders of user involvement: moving beyond Arnstein, *Health Policy*, 76: 156–168.

Walker, A. (1989) Managing the package of care: implications for the user. In I. Allen (ed.), *Social Services Departments as Managing Agencies* [PSI Discussion Paper 23]. London: Policy Studies Institute.

Wallcraft, J. & Bryant, M. (2003) *The Mental Health Service User Movement in England*. London: The Sainsbury Centre for Mental Health.

Welsh Assembly Government (2004) *Stronger in Partnership: Involving Service Users and Carers in the Design, Planning, Delivery and Evaluation of Mental Health Services in Wales* (Policy Implementation Guidance). Cardiff: WAG.

Welsh Assembly Government (2005) *Raising the Standard – The Revised Adult Mental Health National Service Framework and An Action Plan for Wales*. Cardiff: WAG.

Welsh Assembly Government (2008) *Stronger In Partnership 2: Involving Service Users and Carers in the Design, Planning, Delivery and Evaluation of Mental Health Services in Wales*. Cardiff: WAG.

Welsh Assembly Government (2010) *Citizen Centred Governance Principles: Making Sense of Them: A governance good practice guide*. Cardiff: WAG.

Williamson, C. (2008) The patient movement as an emancipation movement, *Health Expectations*, 11: 102–112.

Wills, J. & Simms, M. (2004) Building reciprocal community unionism in the UK, *Capital & Class*, Spring, 82: 59–84.

Wilson, M. (2009) *Delivering Race Equality in Mental Health Care: A Review*. London: DH/NMHDU.

Wykurz, G. & Kelly, D. (2002) Learning in practice – developing the role of patients as teachers: literature review, *British Medical Journal*, 325: 818–821.

9 EQUALITIES IN MENTAL HEALTH NURSING

Ann Jackson and Lindsey Ambrose

Chapter Overview

The assertion of rights and the insistence of being seen as an individual who is more than an ascribed label has been an ongoing struggle for many who use mental health services. This chapter deftly demonstrates how such assertions have been listened to and addressed by means of policy and law. The authors show how recognition of the growing diversity of the United Kingdom and the relatively poor experience of certain groups receiving services has driven an awareness of the need for change.

Some of these drivers of change have come as a result of tragic events, and also others at the behest of groups no longer to contentedly adopt the role of 'patient'. This chapter can be very helpfully read in conjunction with the chapter on service user involvement. The assertion and claiming of granted rights and the responsibilities of others to meet them are a key factor in the changes that have made this chapter content a reality.

INTRODUCTION

Getting things right in relation to equalities, diversity and human rights (EDHR) has become more important – and more complex – in recent years. Today evidence-based practice requirements involve everyone working in mental health from senior managers to mental health nurses. Equality has to be a central consideration to the role of the contemporary mental health nurse.

There are two key reasons why equality, diversity and human rights have steadily risen in the mental health agenda. Firstly, there is the increasing diversity of our service users, with often immediate challenges in language barriers, and also a plethora of cultural and social differences that play their part in the presentation of the whole person, their mental health difficulties and needs. Secondly, there has been recognition of:

- the social and health inequalities experienced by people with mental health problems;
- the relationship between stigma and discrimination and inequality;
- the role that social inequality plays in causing mental ill-health.

In addition, increasing public awareness of human rights in all areas of social living creates additional opportunities and challenges to tackle inequalities and promote equality and social inclusion. As the requirements of the Equality Act 2010 become embedded in healthcare, in 2012 numerous equalities compliance publications show progression in developing the health and equalities datasets of NHS Trusts, the equalities objectives and measures of regulators such as the Care Quality Commission and the Department of Health.

It seems however that some mental health nursing texts have not kept up with these fundamental and rapid changes in care provision. A number of high profile cases around specific inequalities and poor practice – for example, David 'Rocky' Bennett – led to the development of specific initiatives such as the Delivering Race Equality Programme (DRE). This programme, along with other equality initiatives, has had varied success and shall be discussed more fully later in this chapter.

This chapter will draw on current legislative frameworks relevant to equality in the UK, particularly for England and Wales, including the NHS Equality Delivery System (EDS). It will also highlight some specific inequalities experienced by people with mental health problems in an overview of each of the protected characteristics. Mental health nurses need to have a good understanding of these and also the common shared issues and broad concepts to meet the needs of people who use mental healthcare services. Opportunities for mental health nursing that supports and promotes equality will be outlined, together with issues to consider for personal professional reflection.

LEGAL FRAMEWORK AND EVIDENCE-BASED PRACTICE

The Equality Act 2010: the duties and who they apply to

Over the years equalities laws became inconsistent and confusing – challenging the ability of organisations to work meaningfully and improve equalities outcomes. Old law was simplified and replaced by the Equality Act 2010, which today co-exists with the Human Rights Act. Case law from before 2010 continues to apply.

The Equality Act 2010 brought together the legal requirements for private, public and voluntary organisations to follow including in relation to the provision of services and workplace law. This act replaces, amongst others, the Equal Pay Act 1970, The Sex Discrimination Act 1975, the Race Relations Act 1976 and the Disability Discrimination Act 1995. Public bodies and organisations providing a public function have to meet certain general and specific 'duties' which oblige them to evidence looking to improve equality outcomes for staff and people who use their services, including in services they commission from charities etc.

The general public sector equality duty has three components which require public bodies and others providing public functions to have due regard in the provision of their services to the need to:

- eliminate discrimination, harassment, victimisation and any other conduct that is prohibited by or under the act;
- advance equality of opportunity between persons who share a relevant protected characteristic and persons who do not share it;
- foster good relations between persons who share a relevant protected characteristic and persons who do not share it (adapted from Section 149 of the Equality Act 2010).

The Equality Act 2010 introduces 'protected characteristics' which relate to a person's identity and which everyone has to some extent (e.g. everyone has an age). The protected characteristics are:

- age;
- disability;
- gender reassignment;
- marriage and civil partnership;
- race;
- religion or belief;
- sex (gender);
- sexual orientation;
- maternity, including breastfeeding.

Learning Point

Equalities is not just about 'minority groups'. Everyone is protected by the law.

Evidence-based practice: equalities analysis

Although there is no requirement for services to publish an equality impact assessment, the rapidly emerging body of case law from the courts underlines the important need for public bodies and organisations of all kinds providing public functions to evidence consideration of equality implications when designing policy or service delivery. There has to be a meaningful and evidenced process to support equality analysis.

Like equality impact assessment, equality analysis highlights the potential negative impact (or 'harm' – intended or unintended) on specific equality groups and the actions taken to mitigate against unjustified negative impact. The process encourages services to identify opportunities to promote equality. The aim is to ensure that different perspectives are explicitly taken into account based on good information and effective consultation. This leads to action planning to remove barriers to accessing services and ensure protected groups do not experience poorer outcomes.

Equality analysis has to be documented to demonstrate that legal duties are being met. EHRC (2011a) cite the case of *R (Kaur and Shah) v London Borough of Ealing [2008]*:

> The process of assessments should be recorded ... records contribute to transparency. They serve to demonstrate that a genuine assessment has been carried out at a formative stage. They further tend to have the beneficial effect of disciplining the policy-maker to undertake the conscientious assessment of the future impact of [his/her] proposed policy.

Organisational equality objectives and accountability

Public bodies are also required to develop and publish organisational equality objectives every four years, to outline how equality will be advanced in support of the three general duties. These objectives should be specific and measurable, with annual reporting to show improvements on equalities are taking place. The objectives should be reviewed at least every four years.

Public bodies must also publish data, for example in annual reports about their workforce in relation to the protected characteristics of the staff. Such reports should help to show that efforts are made to reflect communities served through the make-up of the workforce, that there is fair distribution of opportunity for progression and training within the organisation, that bullying and harassment are managed, and that regard is given to equal pay and the gender pay gap. Issues such as the workforce not reflecting the people an organisation serves have, in the past, been among findings of institutionalised racism – such as in the David Rocky Bennett Inquiry (2003).

Learning Points

Equalities is not about 'tick box approaches'. Good practice approaches have been developed with the ambition of improving outcomes for everyone – the workforce, patients and other users of services, the communities we serve, the reputation of service providers, and through improved cost-effectiveness, even the taxpayer.

Relevance and proportionality

Organisations need to be realistic for improvements to happen. Actions to improve outcomes should be reasonable and proportionate.

The following questions, suggested by the Equality & Human Rights Commission in its revised guidance, *Meeting the Equality Duty in Policy and Decision-making* (2011b), are helpful in establishing the relevance of policy/practice to equality:

- Does the policy affect service users, employees or the wider community? The relevance of a policy to equality depends not just on the number of those affected but on the significance of the impact on them.
- Is it likely to affect people with particular protected characteristics differently?
- Is it a major policy, significantly affecting how functions are delivered?
- Will the policy have a significant impact on how other organisations operate in terms of equality?
- Does the policy relate to functions that engagement has identified as being important to people with particular protected characteristics?
- Does the policy relate to an area with known inequalities?
- Does the policy relate to any equality objectives that have been set?

The above outlines the requirements of public bodies to protect certain individuals, groups and communities who have known inequalities. The act serves to protect the rights of these groups in the workplace and in services.

Learning Points

In order to plan appropriately, equalities risks and relevance need to inform priorities for action. Solutions should avoid 'treating everyone the same' and 'one size fits all' approaches, but should actively consider how particular needs may be reasonably met.

MENTAL HEALTH POLICY AND INEQUALITY

Healthy Lives, Healthy People (DH, 2010) showed that almost one in five adults experiences *mental ill-health* at any one time and there is evidence that this prevalence has been rising over the last two decades. Mental ill health can have a very significant impact on overall health and accounts for a considerable share of the overall burden of disease. It tends to be concentrated amongst disadvantaged groups, including older people, those who are already sick, and those who are at risk of other poor public health equalities outcomes.

Mental ill-health is linked to increased mortality from cardiovascular disease, cancer, respiratory disease, metabolic disease, nervous system diseases, accidental death and mental disorders. Another risk factor is that poor mental health is associated with poor compliance with treatment for health problems.

It has never been better documented how social inequality leads to health inequality. The Marmot Review's *Fair Society, Healthy Lives* (2010) states that:

People with higher socioeconomic position in society have a greater array of life chances and more opportunities to lead a flourishing life. They also have better health. The two are linked: the more favoured people are, socially and economically, the better their health. This link between social conditions and health is not a footnote to the 'real' concerns with health – health care and unhealthy behaviours – it should become the main focus.

Marmot goes on throughout his review to outline the many aspects there are to mental health and inequality, making evident the links between poor childhood opportunities for education, low education attainment, unemployment and poor housing to poor mental health and wellbeing. At the same time, the review outlines the evidence base of poor mental health experienced by people with mental health illness. This is particularly significant as it is now well accepted that people with mental health problems experience worse morbidity and mortality than the general population. This is a core theme within *No Health Without Mental Health* (DH, 2011b) in an attempt to redress the imbalance and tackle inequality through giving mental health a 'parity of esteem' with physical health. For commissioners of health and social care, there is a clear 'equality case' to reduce a 'prior discrimination' for minority groups. There is heavy criticism of the lack of equity when it comes to health resources for mental health provision in spite of the wealth of data highlighting the burden of disease from mental health (see for example the Centre for Economic Performance, 2012).

Anyone seeking the evidence base for health inequalities would also be recommended to look at the *First Triennial Review* of the Equalities and Human Rights Commission, published in 2010.

Chapter 6 of *No Health Without Mental Health* (DH, 2011b) highlights three key areas when looking at reducing inequalities in mental health:

- Tackling the inequalities that lead to poor mental health.
- Tackling the inequalities that result from poor mental health – employment rates, poor housing, education and physical health.
- Tackling the inequalities in service provision – access, experience and outcomes.

Each of the protected groups can be described separately in relation to the specific inequalities that are experienced within mental health, in addition to the shared and general inequalities that commonly co-exist. For contemporary mental health and nursing practice to achieve a good promotion of equality, diversity and human rights in practice nurses must understand the documented experiences of protected groups. Many initiatives focus on diversity without an informed analysis of the equality issues. It is still evident that equality is wrongly misinterpreted as 'treating everybody the same', without any recognition of the specific issues.

The assessment of the impact on equality of *No Health Without Mental Health* outlines three key issues around inequality:

- People who experience inequality or discrimination in social or economic contexts have a higher risk of poor mental wellbeing and of developing mental health problems.
- People may experience inequality in access to, and experience of, and outcomes from, services.
- Mental health problems result in a broad range of further inequalities.

Taking the protected groups (except marriage and civil partnerships) in turn, we can outline key resources and strategies to tackle inequality and promote fairness and equity across mental health services.

Age and mental health

No Health Without Mental Health has taken a life-span approach to the overall strategy, ensuring that all ages have their mental health and wellbeing needs met. The Age Review of 2009 emphasised the existing level of age discrimination in mental health services, and provided a useful resource for promoting older adult-age equality. The older adult has been excluded from service design and monitoring, with local strategies often concentrating on either the needs of 'working age' adults or dementia services. A definition of age equality, in support of 'what good looks like', has been developed by the National Development Team for Inclusion (2011) and comprises four components:

- A shared vision of age equality in mental health.
- Better outcomes for and experiences of older people.
- Positive attitudes and mindsets.
- Responsive, personalised services and support.

The priorities in eliminating age discrimination in mental health services will include improving information and data relating to the older adult; improving training in detection and diagnosis in primary mental health for adequate referral into secondary services (particularly drugs and alcohol); and improving access to both physical and psychological services.

Disability and mental health

Equalities law follows the 'social model' of disability, rather than the medical one. This can be a particular challenge in medical contexts, in which the patients are often initially most understood in terms of a medical diagnosis. The social model has value though, particularly as it helps to challenge stigma around certain diagnoses – such as some personality disorders – by inviting medical professionals to take the necessary steps in their approach to challenge themselves and identify ways to remove stigma and other barriers which may lead to unfair treatment of the patient, such as a lack of cultural competence.

The social model also helps to remind us that a diagnosis may affect different people in different ways and that there needs to be focus on identifying what the impacts of an impairment or multiple impairments are on an individual so that these can be removed. Too often people with mental health needs struggle to access health services not only because of written communication barriers (e.g. a lack of Easy Read documents and good techniques in face-to-face interviews) but also due to professionals mistaking mental health problems such as depression for challenging behaviour leading to inappropriate treatment (NMHDU Factfile 5). As recently as 2011, Mencap launched the 'Getting It Right' campaign following A.P. Dinsmore's (2011) research findings on such health inequalities in relation to access to the NHS.

Note that the Adult Autism Act and related statutory guidance reflect the inequalities many people with autistic spectrum disorder experience in accessing all kinds of services.

Gender reassignment and mental health

Although a small (if growing) number of people, the experiences of Trans people may have an impact on their mental health. Research (Notts NHST, 2009) identified that Trans people are often ignored by society, and experience disproportionate levels of discrimination, harassment and violence, including at work and at home, when they disclose their gender issues to colleagues, friends and family. As a result they have distinct social experiences and needs, which the service provided needs to address to create welcoming and sensitive approaches. Many experience violent intimidation on the streets or outside their homes. Unsurprisingly, such suffering has been associated with Trans people being susceptible to depression and at risk of suicide. Such daily experience has also tended to be associated with Trans people being less engaged in health issues at a local or neighbourhood level. Research has highlighted the need for specific LGBTQ engagement opportunities. In 2010 the Brighton and Hove Health and Inclusion Project found that Trans people were less likely to access sexual health services and were unsure where they could go to discuss sexual relationships (LGBT Health and Inclusion Project, n.d.).

NHS Greater Glasgow and Clyde's Transgender Policy recommends that staff appreciate the needs of Trans people to ensure policies and services are appropriate and sensitive. Examples here might include:

- providing a gender neutral public toilet;
- use of preferred titles such as 'Mr' and 'Miss';

- allowing the patient to choose the gender of the practitioner they see wherever possible;
- allocating a ward of the current gender the patient is living in.

Race and mental health

People from ethnic minorities may face particular health equality challenges both within healthcare organisations and in the community.

The National Mental Health Development Unit Factfile 5, 'Equalities in Mental Health' notes that:

> Rates of psychosis are up to nine times higher for people from African Caribbean communities living in the UK than for the White British population, six times higher for people from African communities and also higher, but to a smaller degree, for other Black and minority ethnic (BME) groups in England. Rates in the Caribbean and Africa are comparable to the overall rate in England. Immigrants to the UK are typically at two to eight times greater risk of psychoses than native-born groups. This higher risk extends into the second generations. Factors that explain raised rates in immigrants and their descendants include: stressful life events, discrimination, urban living and socio-economic deprivation.

The inquiry into the death of David 'Rocky' Bennett (2003) identified institutionalised racism as a significant part of his care experience, and made recommendations which are still relevant for services to consider when looking to identify and reduce potential health inequalities in relation to race and culture in their services. These included the following:

- All staff should receive regularly updated mandatory training in cultural awareness and sensitivity. This should include training to tackle overt and covert racism and institutional racism.
- All services should set out a written policy dealing with racist abuse, which should be disseminated to all members of staff and displayed prominently in all public areas under their control. This policy should be strictly monitored and a written record kept of all incidents in breach of the policy. If any racist abuse takes place by anyone, including patients in a mental health setting, it should be addressed forthwith and appropriate sanctions applied.
- Every Care Programme Approach care plan should have a mandatory requirement to include appropriate details of each patient's ethnic origin and cultural needs.
- Where appropriate, active steps should be taken to recruit, retain and promote black and minority ethnic staff to ensure the workforce is reasonably diverse and reflective of the communities served.
- All medical staff in mental health services should have training in the assessment of people from the black and minority ethnic communities with special reference to the effects of racism upon their mental wellbeing.

Sewell and Waterhouse (2012), in *Making Progress on Race Equality in Mental-Health* – a survey of mental health providers – identified four areas suggested by the services as 'enablers' to making progress:

- Developing capacity and capability in commissioning mental health for BME groups.
- Improving accountability in the system through better measurement of outcomes for BME service users (commonly referred to as 'performance management').
- Development of national guidance and best practice guides to spread evidence and knowledge about what works to improve outcomes for BME service users.
- Establishment of organised networks to allow professionals to learn from each other.

Sewell and Waterhouse stated:

> Providers should consider how they currently measure and monitor information relating to access, experience and outcomes for BME mental health service users and how this forms part of regular board level reporting and discussion. Boards may want to consider receiving a composite race equality (taking other protected characteristics into account) report at least once a year on the organisation's progress against identified objectives and priorities.

Religion or belief and mental health

In 2009 *Religion or Belief: A Practical Guide for the NHS* (DH, 2009) sought to respond to research which showed that the needs of patients and service users can contribute to their wellbeing and, for instance, reduce their length of stay in hospital.

Most religious and belief systems prescribe a 'way of life' and 'values'. Such factors may influence attitudes and behaviours around contraception, abortion, perceptions of mental ill-health (for example as 'demonic' or a 'spiritual event'), diet and nutrition, end-of-life care, blood transfusions, signing consent forms, willingness to accept porcine-based treatments (such as insulin) and more. The use of spiritual needs assessment tools with individual patients can help direct care to their particular needs and support recovery.

Sex (gender) and mental health

Men's mental health has become increasingly more considered, although still has fallen behind the level of critique of failings of mental health services in relation to the specific needs of women (see for example Philips and Jackson, 2012).

The following are some of the important statistics from *Untold Problems* (Wilkins, 2010) and put the challenges for men's social development, health and wellbeing in context:

- Almost three quarters of people who kill themselves are men.
- 73% of adults who 'go missing' are men and 90% of rough sleepers are men.
- Men are three times more likely than women to become alcohol dependent and more than twice as likely to use Class A drugs, and 79% of drug-related deaths occur in men.

- Men make up 94% of the prison population and their co-morbidity with mental health is well-documented.
- More than twice as many male psychiatric inpatients are detained and treated compulsorily.
- Over 80% of children permanently excluded from school are boys, and boys generally perform less well than girls at all levels of education.

It is a startling fact that men are significantly more likely to commit suicide but only half as likely to be diagnosed with depression. It is well known that men do not present at GP surgeries for support with mental health problems, and the indicators for depression in men are ill-defined (MIND, 2009). This is illustrated well by Addis (2008, cited in Wilkins, 2010):

> The existing clinical and research literature on depression in men has provided widely varying answers to these questions, and it is safe to say that there is currently no unifying conceptual framework guiding clinical research or practice. Nor have the assumptions underlying different theoretical frameworks been outlined in detail.

Health professionals need to be able to understand the social and health experience of men as different from women, and plan interventions and services accordingly. *Delivering Male*: *Effective Practice in Male Mental Health* (Wilkins and Kemple, 2011) discusses seven 'big ideas' to develop best practice for male mental health:

- Treating men as individuals.
- Inter-agency working in the early years.
- Stigma.
- Promoting services.
- The role of third parties.
- Joined-up approach.
- Profession training and an improved knowledge base.

Women's mental health has been well addressed through major policy. The *Into the Mainstream* consultation document (2002) and the subsequent implementation strategy Mainstreaming Gender and Women's Mental Health in 2003 drew together for the first time a cohesive and thorough evidence-base underpinning women's needs and preferences for mental health services. Importantly, the social experiences of women, particularly as victims and survivors of all forms of violence and abuse, were put at the centre of understanding women's mental health. Three thousand women were involved in the study that concluded the following as services wanted by women in addition to being safe:

- Promote empowerment, choice and self-determination.
- Place importance on the underlying causes and context of women's distress.
- Address issues relating to roles as mothers and the need for work and accommodation.
- Value women's strengths and abilities and potential for recovery.

Of course, 'safe' services are difficult to achieve as highlighted through, amongst others, *Safety in Mind* (Scobie et al., 2006) and policy continues to emphasise the need to completely eradicate mixed sex accommodation in inpatient facilities.

The following principles underpinning mental health nursing were developed with a view to developing anti-oppressive and action-oriented practices, based on the rights of women and nursing values (Royal College of Nursing, 2005):

- Women need gender-sensitive staff and service; nurses have a significant role in raising awareness and influencing gender-sensitive approaches in all staff.
- Women need seamless services where issues affecting their mental health will be taken into account; nurses provide holistic care of women's mental and physical health (i.e. menarche and menopause issues; fertility, breast care, gynaecology and midwifery issues).
- Women need environments that are free from all forms of discrimination; nurses challenge discriminatory language and practices and draw attention to gender-blind policy.
- Women need relationships that are empowering; nurses, through their values and actions, demonstrate and promote anti-oppressive practices.
- Women need access to staff who have regular high-quality supervision; nurses, through the use of supervision, reflect on their own gender-sensitive practice to develop greater self-awareness and contribute to the development of others.
- Women need services that are flexible and respond to individual needs; nurses recognise issues relating to age, ethnicity, physical and mental abilities, faith and sexuality.
- Women need access to staff who identify the signs of physical, sexual and emotional violence and abuse; nurses formally assess and act to prioritise the safety of women.
- Women need staff who are able to recognise specific gender-related risk periods such as menarche, childbirth, menopause and carer roles; nurses recognise the specific risk periods in women's lives and provide care accordingly.

Sexual orientation and mental health

The NMHDU Factfile 5 notes (2009: 8):

Lesbian and bisexual women are at particular risk of suicidal feelings and drug or alcohol dependence. Gay and bisexual men are over four times more likely than heterosexual men to attempt suicide. More than a quarter of gay men and almost a third of lesbians have self-harmed themselves deliberately, compared with one in seven heterosexual people. Of those who self-harm, 65% of gay men and 48% of lesbians attribute this wholly or partially to difficulties associated with their sexual orientation. There is a strong association between homophobic bullying and mental ill health, including low self-esteem, fear, stress and self-harm. Young people who identify themselves as lesbian, gay or bisexual face a higher risk of being bullied at school. Half of all lesbian, gay and bisexual adults who have been bullied at school have contemplated suicide or self-harm.

Stonewall published guidance for the NHS in 2012 which stated that older lesbian, gay and bisexual people do not feel able to access the health services they need:

> Many lesbian, gay and bisexual people report that they have experienced or fear discrimination because of their sexual orientation. They say this creates a barrier to receiving appropriate care and treatment. Additionally, many lesbian, gay and bisexual staff in the NHS experience discrimination and hostility at work because of their sexual orientation. They say this stops them from performing to the best of their ability and reaching their full potential.

Health inequalities may be reduced where health services put up posters about gay equal rights encouraging LGB people to feel welcomed, provide patient experience feedback opportunities, train staff, and take part in the Stonewall Diversity Champions scheme.

Learning Points

Mental health and wellbeing may be impacted on by a number of factors. Sometimes actions by mental health-care providers can help to reduce or remove factors which can lead to, or be associated with, poor mental health. Such actions include taking steps to promote equality, dignity and respect, and to eliminate discrimination and stigma.

MECHANISMS TO ACHIEVE EQUALITY IN SERVICES

The Operation Framework for the NHS in 2012–13 responded to changes in the NHS and reports by the Care Quality Commission and Health Service Ombudsman which found failures in the NHS to provide dignified compassionate care to elderly and vulnerable patients and failures around inclusive communication.

A key theme for 2012–13 was putting patients at the centre of decision making as part of a new outcomes approach to performance also aiming to improve dignity in care. From 2013–14 the NHS Commissioning Board should be held to account using the Outcomes Framework. This is in line with its duty in the Health and Social Care Act 2012 to have regard for the need to reduce inequalities in access to, and outcomes of, healthcare.

The framework draws on the Care Quality Commission's report *Dignity and Nutrition for Older People* in identifying specific actions to improve care for older people, including dementia care (p.11).

Addressing equalities needs includes specific ideas for improvement in relation to carers and military and veterans (p.13) and reference to the mental health strategy *No Health Without Mental Health* (p.16).

The NHS constitution

The constitution sets out the values, principles and responsibilities of the NHS. It draws attention to existing law, including the Equality Act 2010 and the new duties on NHS commissioners to reduce inequalities. It is a binding document for all providers of NHS services. The Health and Social Care Act 2012 placed new duties on NHS commissioners to promote the constitution.

The NHS Constitution should be woven into everything the NHS does, guiding the expectations of people who work for, and people who use, NHS services. In November 2012 the government consulted on amending the constitution from April 2013 so as to give people more ability to use it to hold the NHS to account and have an influential voice that informs continual improvements in patient care.

Liberating the NHS

Recognising the need to ensure organisations do more on their equality obligations (as for example in the implementation framework 2012), proposed changes to the NHS Constitution from 2013 include:

- Patient rights for dignity, respect and compassion.
- An emphasis on using patient contact to help minimise health inequalities.
- Care tailored around the patient's needs and preferences.
- An awareness that patients (and their carers) should be actively involved in shared decision making about their care and treatment.

The constitution puts physical and mental health on a par with one another. This has complete resonance with recovery-oriented practice.

NHS Equality Delivery System

The Equality Delivery System has been developed by the NHS Equality and Diversity council to ensure there is a systemic approach to supporting quality performance and is referenced within *The Operating Framework for the NHS in England 2012/13* (DH, 2011a). It supports organisations to implement both the Equality Act 2010 and human rights laws by self-assessing their achievement of outcomes against particular objectives.

Its five competency areas are:

- To operate from a human rights context.
- To build capacity to respond to diverse community needs.
- To apply a robust equalities and human rights analysis to service planning and improvement.
- To communicate a compelling business case for EDHR and influence strategically.
- To influence and lead change to improve equality outcomes for everyone.

The Department of Health, the Care Quality Commission, NHS Trusts and others have developed their equality plans and strategies around this system.

Learning Points

Information about how well a health-care provider is doing on equalities should be easy to find in its web presence. The consistent use of self-assessment against the EDS system helps to compare one provider against another, the comparative robustness of approaches taken and the outcomes being achieved. Ultimately this could influence patient choice, recruitment and commissioning decisions.

THE MENTAL HEALTH ACT

Importantly, the revised Mental Health Act code of Practice has introduced five guiding principles one of which is the 'respect principle', and this states:

> People taking decisions under the Act must recognise and respect the diverse needs, values and circumstances of each patient, including their race, religion, culture, gender, age, sexual orientation and any disability. They must consider the patient's views, wishes and feelings (whether expressed at the time or in advance), so far as they are reasonably ascertainable, and follow those wishes wherever practicable and consistent with the purpose of the decision. There must be no unlawful discrimination.

HUMAN RIGHTS-BASED APPROACH

As the communities we service become more diverse, taking a human rights approach offers the opportunity for effective, integrated, services which understand the impacts on other people of oppression and distress, rather that attempt to understand the individual needs of each cultural requirement.

The 'dignity agenda' makes us look at people's individual needs, taking into account personal preferences, experiences, and the cultural and spiritual. It keeps the focus on the people using our services, rather than ignoring both their and our values and prejudices, in a flawed attempt to impose 'one size fits all' standardised solutions in the false belief that somehow treating everyone the same will achieve equality in outcomes.

The onus is on public bodies to take practical action that demonstrates due regard, leading to practice that accommodates and balances sometimes apparently conflicting sets of needs (e.g. religious belief versus sexual orientation). The human rights context provides a helpful way to approach such complexities, with its emphasis on dignity and respect, and the acceptance that rights can vary in the extent of their application.

Learning Point

In mental health-care contexts the acronym developed in the Human Rights Inquiry (2009) may be helpful:

Fairness
Respect
Equality
Dignity
Autonomy

MENTAL HEALTH NURSING AND EQUALITY IN PRACTICE

So what does all this mean for the effective practice of mental health nursing? What policy is there to support practice? And what are the levers for services to provide care and services which are fair and address issues of equality in a way that is meaningful at the point of delivery and for those experiencing the services?

All mental health nurses should promote equitable care for all groups and individuals. A suggested way to make this happen is by 'encouraging reporting of inequalities in service provision, and advocating for service users where they may be disadvantaged'.

So how do we ensure that the outcomes are not unequal for different groups? Here I take the social model of disability discussed above (the approach of seeing people disadvantaged by barriers which can often be removed to enable them to be differently-abled and more en-abled than dis-abled).

Taking spirituality as an example, Gilbert and Parkes (2011) suggest that humane and holistic care could be achieved if 'spirituality' included attitudes, beliefs, values, culture and religion. In order to achieve this staff need to be trained and supported to appreciate the different perspectives and deep beliefs of individuals. The links between spirituality, hope and recovery approaches to mental health are key to meeting service user needs. Use of robust and accessible spiritual assessment approaches may help improve recovery for patients, and cumulatively build on the knowledge and understandings of nurses and others providing services.

The qualities and characteristics that make mental health workers effective include the ability to focus on each patient's needs without allowing their values and beliefs to distract from what is required by that patient to support their personal recovery. For example, a nurse's religious belief about sexuality should not impede their ability to support a patient who has just come out as being gay.

Learning Points

As part of your own 'due regard' to relevant issues, consider:

- What is there to support EDHR in your practice (e.g. equality champions, equality groups, policies and procedures, training opportunities, leaders who role model challenging inequality and promoting inclusion, equality monitoring of patients and staff)?
- What gets in the way of you delivering on EDHR (e.g. gaps in knowledge, over-standardised procedures, need for training etc.)?
- What do you need to develop effective EDHR in your practice, context, and organisation?
- How are you going make that happen?

MEASURING UP TO CQC STANDARDS

The Care Quality Commission (CQC) has set out nine organisation equality objectives. They have said that they will monitor whether detained service users have their rights to equality protected. Their objectives and their measures reflect the general and specific duties of the Equality Act 2010. Organisations providing public functions, as well as public bodies, are on notice that they need to ensure they use good practice, including:

- robust equality monitoring and analysis;
- accessible communications e.g. about patients' rights (including to complain and challenge decisions);
- reasonable adjustments;
- evidenced patient feedback (positive and negative about being treated with dignity and respect, their confidentiality and privacy, and their involvement in their care and how services are provided);
- to demonstrate they are reviewing and planning services to take appropriate steps to reduce and remove inequalities in health-care provision.

Providers will need to show staff are adequately trained not just in general diversity but also in being aware of needs across the protected characteristics.

The CQC say they will be 'actively seeking' improvements: this objective is specifically examining the 'respect principle contained within the amended MHA code of practice'.

The mental healthcare market is a competitive one. Staff to patient ratios may be tight. There may be times when bank staff are relied on. It is important that mental health nurses appreciate that as well as safety risks, other considerations in determining appropriate levels of staffing may include ensuring that patients' human rights are not compromised inappropriately. For example, each patient's:

- right to be free from degrading treatment;
- right to liberty;
- right to see family and friends;
- right to take part in community activities e.g. worship.

Could staffing levels or the skills mix mean that people's needs in relation to equality cannot be met?

- Communication needs.
- Maintaining or developing links with their own community.
- Preferred gender of staff for personal care tasks.

Learning Points

Situations may arise in a secure environment which may impact on a patient's human and equal rights if staffing and competency levels are not adequately met. Consider things like taking part in communal worship, laundry processes and the return of clothes, impacts on a patient of moving from one ward or hospital to another, grounds and community leave, and important documents relating to a patient's care and hospital experience. How would you plan to minimise problems and barriers? What would you do if you had concerns that patients' needs were not being met?

There are also a number of other issues to consider here:

Supporting staff, removing barriers to deliver equality, diversity and human rights in the workplace **and** in practice?

- Do we have a reputation for inclusive recruitment and retention practices at all levels?
- Do we handle equality issues transparently, including grievance and complaints, and are the outcomes different for equality groups?
- Do we have data to monitor? Information to manage? Knowledge to act on?
- What would be our equality priorities for objective setting?
- How aligned are we to national drivers for fairness and equality?
- Do any of our outcomes vary by equality characteristics?
- As regards personal challenges, what do these mean for each of us as members of a profession? And what are the specific responsibilities of different professions to challenge discrimination and promote equality?
- What does this mean for each of us as people, both as humans and citizens?
- How do we resolve the many and complex dilemmas using human rights as a framework?
- What do we need to develop judgment skills for agreeing the principles of 'proportionate' and 'reasonable'?
- How do we develop and support the language, the narrative, the humanity, the intellect, and the compassion?

CONCLUSION

If there is to be good implementation resulting in improved care experiences for people with mental health distress, then mental health nurses need to be able to articulate their values, the evidence and policy. There is a set of skills we need to nurture to be effective in the way we develop and influence practice.

The language of anti-oppressive practice would provide us with a clear direction for working with difference and diversity, and allow a language which supports an understanding of the basis of oppression – the workings of structural power – gender, age, race, sexual orientation, religion and disability.

Reflective Exercise

1. Why do people with mental health issues find they need to 'assert' their rights?
2. What institutional obstacles have typically been in their way?
3. Do you find yourself encroaching on human rights in your practice?
4. What legal obligations are upon you in this area of practice?

BIBLIOGRAPHY

British Institute of Human Rights (2006) *Your Human Rights: A Guide for People Living with Mental Health Problems.* London: British Institute of Human Rights.

Care Quality Commission (2012) *Our Equality Objectives.* London: CQC.

Centre for Economic Performance (2012) *How Mental Illness Loses Out in the NHS.* London: LSE.

Department of Health (2008) *Code of Practice, Mental Health Act 1983.* London: HMSO.

Department of Health (2009) *Religion or Belief: A Practical Guide for the NHS.* Available at www.dh.gov.uk/prod_consum_dh/groups/dh_digitalassets/documents/digitalasset/dh_093132.pdf

Department of Health (2010) *Health Lives, Healthy People – Impact Assessments.* London: HMSO.

Department of Health (2011a) *The Operating Framework for the NHS in England 2012/13,* COI. London: DH.

Department of Health (2011b) *No Health Without Mental Health: A Cross-Government Mental Health Outcomes Strategy for People of All Ages.* London: DH.

Dinsmore, A. (2011) A small-scale investigation of hospital experiences among people with a learning disability on Merseyside: speaking with patients and their carers, *British Journal of Learning Disabilities,* 40: 201–212.

Equality and Human Rights Commission (2010) *How Fair is Britain? Equality, Human Rights and Good Relations in 2010, The First Triennial Review.* London: EHRC.

Equality and Human Rights Commission (2011a) *Equality Analysis and the Equality Duty: A Guide for Public Authorities,* Vol 2 of 5, Equality Act 2010 guidance for English public bodies (and non-devolved bodies in Scotland and Wales). London: EHRC.

Equality and Human Rights Commission (2011b) *Meeting the Equality Duty in Policy and Decision-making.* London: EHRC.

Gilbert, P. & Parkes, M. (2011) Faith in one city: exploring religion, spirituality and mental wellbeing in urban UK, *Ethnicity and Inequalities in Health and Social Care*, 4 (1): 16–27.

LGBT Health and Inclusion Project (n.d.) Available at http://switchboard.org.uk/projects/health-and-inclusion-project

Marmot Review (2010) *Fair Society, Healthy Lives: A Strategic Review of Health Inequalities in England Post-2010*. London: The Marmot Review. Available at: http://www.institute ofhealthequity.org/Content/FileManager/pdf/fairsocietyhealthylives.pdf (accessed 13 November 2013).

MIND (2009) *Men and Mental Health: Get It Off Your Chest*. London: Mind.

National Development Team for Inclusion (2011) *A Long Time Coming: Achieving Age Equality in Mental Health Service*. (Part 1). London: NDTI.

National Mental Health Development Unit Factfile 5 (2009) 'Equalities in Mental Health'.

NHS Greater Glasgow and Clyde's Transgender Policy (2010) Available at www.equalitiesinhealth.org/documents/NHSGreaterGlasgowClydeTransgenderPolicy_002.pdf

Norfolk, Suffolk and Cambridgeshire Strategic Health Authority (2003) *Independent Inquiry into the Death of David Bennett*. London: HMSO.

Notts Healthcare NHS Trust (2009) *Briefing Report to Equality and Diversity Committee of the Department of Health*. London: DH.

Phillips, L. and Jackson, A. (2012) Gender specific healthcare. In *Mental Health: Practice and Policy in a Changing Environment*. London: Routledge.

Royal College of Nursing (2005) *Women's Mental Health Group: Eight Principles for Working with Women*. London: RCN.

Scobie, S., Minghella, E., Dale, C., Thomson, R., Lelliott, P. and Hill, K. (2006) *With safety in mind: mental health services and patient safety*. London: National Patient Safety Agency. Available at: http://www.nrls.npsa.nhs.uk/resources/patient-safety-topics/abuse-aggression/?entryid45=59801 (accessed 13 November 2013).

Sewell, H. and Waterhouse, S. (2012) *Making Progress on Race Equality and Mental Health*. London: DH.

Stonewall (2012) *Sexual Orientation: A Guide for the NHS*. Available at www.stonewall.org.uk/documents/stonewall_guide_for_the_nhs_web.pdf

Wilkins, D. (2010) *Untold Problems: A Review of the Essential Issues in the Mental Health of Men and Boys 2010*. London: Men's Health Forum. Available at: www.menshealthforum.org.uk/sites/menshealthforum.org.uk/files/UntoldProblems_dec09.pdf (accessed 13 November 2013).

Wilkins, D. and Kemple, M. (2011) *Delivering Male: Effective Practice for Male Mental Health*. Available at: http://www.mind.org.uk/media/273473/delivering-male.pdf (accessed 13 November 2013).

10 CHILD MENTAL HEALTH POLICY IN THE UK

Tim McDougall

Chapter Overview

This chapter persuasively argues that services have been traditionally designed and operated with scant regard given to the needs of children and young people. Effectively a history is presented that places children in a situation where their needs were considered subservient to adults and where an element of restorative justice was required to elevate their needs to those of others. Within this debate there is of course the voice of the young people themselves, and it also to be noted that the growing emergence of a young person's service user movement has articulated clearly the needs that were to be met.

In these financially straitened times the argument of the cost effectiveness of early intervention or even the notion of preventative mental health services could once again gain traction. This realisation that one can 'spend to save' is as ever compromised by short-term thinking and 'siloed' budgets that compete for scarce resources.

It is also clear that models of distress amongst young people as presented in this chapter have changed over time and have been subject to changing models of explanation. As in many areas of mental health it can be seen that there have been movements and fashions that have shaped policy and services. It is a challenge to consider how services and policy will continue to change in the context of our children and young people.

INTRODUCTION

This chapter is divided into two parts. The first is an historical summary of the key milestones in the development of theory and practice relating to children's mental health from Victorian times until the present day. The second is an account of UK government policy and strategy in the new millennium. How theory and policy have affected the development of services is discussed in both sections.

The chapter does not discuss the causes, prevalence and treatments for specific childhood mental health problems and disorders. Readers are guided to a number of critical and high quality reviews (Roth & Fonagy, 2005; Rutter et al., 2009; Martin & Volkmar, 2012) which summarise the modern psychological, pharmacological and psychosocial treatments for children and adolescents.

As many as 1 in 10 children and young people aged 5–16 years has a diagnosable mental disorder (Green et al. 2005). However, as a recent report by the London School of Economics and Political Science points out, only a quarter receive treatment for problems such as anxiety, depression and conduct disorder (LSE, 2012). This is of concern, since over half of all adults with mental health problems were diagnosed in childhood, and less than half were treated appropriately at the time (Maughan & Kim-Cohen, 2005).

There is no doubt that poorly developed emotional wellbeing in childhood contributes to a range of negative outcomes in adulthood. These include physical ill health, educational failure, family dysfunction, crime and anti-social behaviour (Richards & Abbott, 2009; Sainsbury Centre for Mental Health, 2009). This growing evidence base is increasingly reflected in the UK's mental health policy.

BACKGROUND

Patching together a seamless, linear account of how, when and why mental health services for children originated and evolved is no easy task. The dates of key landmarks often vary, and claims about who was responsible and for what developments are frequently contradictory. Historical accounts tend to be enshrined in wider reports about the nature, prevalence and treatment of childhood mental disorder. Steeped in the discourse of psychiatry, psychology or sociology, there are often parochial differences in how this history is retold. This account is no different. It is just one version of history, woven together from just a few selected sources of information in what is now a worldwide library of knowledge.

PART 1: A HISTORY OF THEORY AND PRACTICE

Individual reports of what might today be recognised as childhood mental disorder go back centuries. Historical influences on modern child psychiatry have been summarised by many writers including Wardle (1991) and Parry-Jones (1998). Thomas Phaer, sometimes referred to as the founding father of British paediatrics, wrote his '*Boke of Chyldren*' in 1545. This addressed problems such as bedwetting and terrible dreams which continue to trouble children who are referred to modern day child and adolescent mental health services (CAMHS).

Earlier still was Sebastian Oesterriecher's account of psychological problems in children which was published in 1540. In this, Oesterriecher advises that good mental habits in children can be corrupted by what they see and hear, including bad music (Walk, 1964).

The nineteenth century

A key milestone in the recognition and treatment of mental health problems in children came with the passage of the Lunacy Act in 1845. This was a confused piece of legislation covering people with mental illness and learning disability. Based on this act, children with a range of difficulties were often removed from workhouses and placed in institutions or county asylums. Gingell (2001) reports that dangerous or suicidal behaviour was frequently recorded as the reason that children were taken from workhouses into the care of asylums. However, closer examination of case records reveals other reasons why children were placed in these Victorian and Edwardian institutions. Case reports refer to children being frightened by dogs or being tossed by cows, the non-appearance of menses and cutting teeth. The available treatments such children received were rarely documented in any detail, but records cite bromide, chloroform, and brandy and eggs for 'private class' patients (Gingell, 2001).

The Royal Albert Hospital in Lancaster was established under the Lunacy Act 1845 and opened in 1870 as an institution for the care and education of children with learning problems aged between 6 and 15. It was named the *Royal Albert Asylum for the Care, Education and Training of Idiots, Imbeciles and Weak Minded Children and Young Person's of the Northern Counties*, which illustrated the rather muddled attitudes to children with problems and the confusion between mental disorder and learning disability. Today, the Royal Albert is an Islamic education centre for girls, which is once again another illustration of how the passage of time sees changes in attitudes towards children.

Another cornerstone in the history of child mental health is Great Ormond Steet Hospital in London which still provides mental health services for children today. Charles West, the founder of the hospital, focused on diseases of infancy and childhood in his lectures between 1845 and 1860. In these he talked of hypochondriasis, night terrors and disorders of the highest function of the brain. Treatment for these conditions affecting children was separation from parents and boarding with a quiet family (Walk, 1964). Today, Great Ormond Street offers treatments for childhood eating disorders and other mental health conditions.

It is important to note that Emil Kraepelin's classification of mental illness, published in 1883, ignored children. It was not until the end of the nineteenth century that professionals began to take a developmental approach to understanding the disorders of childhood and the role of emotional health and wellbeing (Black, 1993). This was assisted by the birth of health visiting at the turn of the nineteenth century in Manchester and surrounding districts (Abbott & Wallace, 1998). Health visiting evolved as a profession from the Ladies Sanitary Reform Association where 'respectable working women' were paid to teach poorer parents the skills of hygiene, child welfare, mental health and social support (While, 1987). However, it was to be another fifty years before attention was paid to maternal mental health which became a key part of the health visitor's role in the UK (DH, 1956).

The twentieth century

At the turn of the twentieth century there was a significant lack of services for children who were suffering from the effects of abuse or mental illness. A number of local government initiatives and charitable organisations existed, but they offered little in the way of medical and psychological expertise (Evans et al., 2008). Much of the research into childhood mental health problems during the early 1900s was funded by philanthropists and charities and led by charismatic and dedicated physicians.

Mental hygiene movement

What was originally known as the field of 'psycho-hygiene' developed into the social or mental hygiene movement of the early 1900s. In many ways mental hygienists were ahead of their time. Instead of mental illness they were interested in mental health promotion, prevention and early intervention. A century on, these same objectives are at the heart of UK government's policy and the latest mental health strategy, *No Health Without Mental Health* (DH, 2012). Mental hygienists invested their resources in children because they believed that mental disorder and maladjustment arose from negative experiences during the early years. They took a public health approach and worked alongside parents and teachers to educate and inform them about advances in child care and illnesses affecting children. These same preventative interventions are today represented in school-based mental health programmes and parenting programmes. Mental hygienists also provided individual psychotherapy for children whose parents were motivated to access help for them.

During 1918, an epidemic of encephalitis lethargica, so-called 'sleepy sickness', swept across the UK. The number of reported cases increased rapidly and peaked in 1924 (Dourmashkin, 1997). Clinicians treating children with the disease noticed a decline in moral standards or behaviour in children who had been infected with encephalitis lethargica, many of whom were referred for psychiatric treatment or institutionalised. Post-encephalitic children were described as disinhibited, impulsive, restless and noisy (Evans et al., 2008). Such difficulties might today be recognised as attention deficit hyperactivity disorder (ADHD).

In another commentary about the epidemic of encephalitis, Wender (1995) describes children who survived the outbreak being left with impaired attention, hyperactivity, a lack of coordination and poor impulse control. This was sometimes labelled as 'post-encephalitic behaviour disorder', the characteristics of which are the same as the modern syndrome ADHD (Adler & Chua, 2002). In the decade that followed, doctors began to use amphetamine to treat hyperactive and brain-damaged children. Terms such as 'minimal brain dysfunction', 'imbecility' and 'idiocy' later came into clinical use due to the similarities shown by patients with central nervous system injuries arising from head injuries, infection and toxic damage (Rafalovich, 2001).

Child guidance clinics

The mental hygiene movement was instrumental in the development of the child guidance clinics of the late 1920s. These were influenced strongly by the Swiss psychiatrist Adolf Meyer who believed that the functioning of the brain was largely unimportant in understanding patients' problems. Meyer proposed that the key to helping deviant children lay not in their constitution, but in understanding the circumstances in which they lived. Meyer was a thorough historian and the modern practice of clinical examination and of taking detailed developmental histories in modern mental health services is often attributed to his work (Gelder, 1991).

Whilst the early child guidance clinics in the United States were associated mainly with juvenile delinquency, they grew in number and expanded their focus to include emotional health and wellbeing during the 1930s. The first child guidance clinic in England opened in 1927 under the leadership of a psychiatrist, psychologist and social worker (Williams & Kerfoot, 2005). The clinics favoured no particular theoretical orientation but adopted several methods of practice. It was around this time that the profession of children's psychiatric social work began to grow (Thom, 1992). Working out of the child guidance clinics, social workers would carry out home assessments in an attempt to understand how family life was impacting on a child's emotional difficulties.

Inpatient care

The history of inpatient care for children and young people originates in the eighteenth-century poorhouses of the USA and workhouses in the UK. It was during the 1940s that the first inpatient psychiatric units for children opened in London (Williams & Kerfoot, 2005). At around the same time inpatient units were being developed, residential communities and reform schools for delinquent children were also created. Parry-Jones (1998) suggests that residential care, confinement and treatment have long been part of society's response to mentally ill, handicapped, homeless and deviant children. The first children's inpatient units in the United States had a mainly custodial and management function and only later became therapeutic agents in themselves (Hersov, 1998). The first English adolescent psychiatric units focused on what Cameron (1949) referred to as 'the socio-psychobiological unity of the child'. Such units grew steadily in number until the 1980s when the concept of 'general purpose' adolescent units was introduced, where children and young people could be admitted for short- and long-term care as well as in an emergency (NHS Health Advisory Service, 1985).

Maternal deprivation

Another key milestone in the history of child mental health is John Bowlby's work on early deprivation. Bowlby trained first as a psychologist and later as a child psychiatrist. His early work focusing on children who were separated from their mothers during the First World War informed our understanding of human attachment, and was to have a major influence on the child guidance clinics of the day. However, Bowlby is best known for his report on the mental health of children displaced after the Second World War (Bowlby, 1951). His thesis was that the child should experience a warm, intimate, continuous attachment with the mother. Without this, Bowlby warned, the child risked serious and irreversible mental health damage.

As well as bringing about wide-scale changes in child care practice, this was a politically controversial claim. Cynics suggested that at a time when servicemen were returning to work and when jobs were scarce, it was convenient that women were discouraged from going to work and leaving their children at home or in child care (Ainsworth, 1962). Bowlby's hypothesis of maternal deprivation was challenged by many, not least Michael Rutter, who pointed to other important variables in determining child maladjustment including family discord (Rutter, 1981). Some commentators suggest that Bowlby's interest in maternal deprivation, separation anxiety and attachment came from his own experience of childhood. It is said that his mother believed that too much parental attention and affection would spoil the child, and thus spent only one hour each day with her son, the rest of his care being provided by nannies (Croates, 2004).

The influence of parenting in the mediation of mental health or disorder began to gain popular support in the 1950s. A theme of blame began to emerge, with the concept of 'refrigerator parents' coming into use and lasting until the early 1970s. This involved parents (usually mothers) being blamed for the difficulties of what were usually labelled schizophrenic or autistic children. Terms like 'infantile schizophrenia' led to conceptual confusion and the finger of blame was pointed at emotionally neglectful parents. It was not until the 1960s that autism was recognised as a separate syndrome, distinguished from schizophrenia or mental retardation, and not until the 1980s that the Austrian pediatrician Hans Asperger's name was associated with the autism spectrum condition recognised today.

The Robertsons' psychoanalytic studies of children in hospital in the early 1950s also shaped the work of the mental health professions. As a psychiatric social worker James Robertson was concerned that the severely restricted visiting times in London hospitals were distressing for children on the wards. Some hospitals banned parents visiting altogether, and others only permitted them to visit once a week for a very short period. Parents were also sometimes only permitted to view their child through a partition (Munroe-Davies, 1949). Together with his wife Joyce, Robertson commented on the despair and detachment of younger children in particular, and their theories later came to influence bonding and attachment theory as well as the modern practice of fostering and adopting children and hospital visiting policies.

The 1970s was a decade of widespread research into childhood mental disorders. The first population study of children's mental health was carried out in the Isle of Wight by Michael Rutter and colleagues. As well as addressing issues such as prevalence rates, important concepts of impairment and adjustment were introduced to the child mental health research world.

A number of reports into the abuse of children during the 1980s changed the way in which children's services were provided. Stephen Wolkind, a psychiatrist who informed the Cleveland Inquiry into the sexual abuse of children during the 1980s, suggested that decisions in children's services had often been motivated less by considered judgement and more by strongly held beliefs and political attitudes (Wolkind, 1991). The reports of the Cleveland Inquiry (Butler-Sloss, 1987) and the abuse of children in care in Wales (DH, 2000) each raised concern about the impact of abuse on children's mental health and called for agencies to work together to safeguard vulnerable children. There was a stronger focus on children's rights resulting in a number of public reviews, including the Staffordshire 'pin-down' Inquiry into the physical restraint of children in residential care settings (Levy & Kahan, 1991). This led to a loss of confidence in the sector and in some areas of the UK children's residential facilities were closed down altogether.

This increased recognition of the rights of the child throughout the 1980s culminated in the passage of the 1989 Children Act. A duty was placed on local authorities to identify children in need and to safeguard and promote their welfare. The concept of 'parental rights' was replaced with that of 'parental responsibilities' (Cottrell & Kraam, 2005), and there followed an increased focus on absent fathers and the impact of separation and divorce on children.

The move away from treatment orientations of the 1970s and 80s which focused exclusively on the child brought systemic and contextual explanations for childhood psychosocial disorders that focused more broadly on families and communities. The 1990s saw the inception of a number of cross-departmental government initiatives to improve outcomes for children.

PART 2: POLICY AND STRATEGY

Since the creation of the National Health Service in 1948, health and welfare policy makers have focused on poverty, social disadvantage, and crime and disorder. Successive governments have given these themes greater or lesser focus in their election manifestos and plans. There are few records of child mental health policy prior to the 1990s.

The 1990s

A landmark in the development of children's mental health services came in 1995 with the publication of guidance on the commissioning, role and management of child and adolescent mental health services (NHS Health Advisory Service, 1995). *Together We Stand* proposed the four-tiered framework that remains the model for planning and organising CAMHS across the four countries of the UK today.

The *United Nations Convention on the Rights of the Child* (1990) raised the expectation that children should be active participants in their own health care, and guidance issued to the NHS at the time was aimed at giving service users a stronger voice in care delivery (NHS Executive, 1995). The first time English government funding was allocated specifically for CAMHS was in 1998 when part of the Mental Illness Specific Grant (later to become the Mental Health Specific Grant) and NHS Modernisation Fund was used to fund a number of CAMHS Innovation Projects (CSIP, 2008).

1998 saw the launch of New Labour's 'Quality Protects' agenda, a programme designed to transform children's services and improve the life chances for Looked After Children. Amongst other things, it placed a requirement on local authorities to collaborate with their health partners to improve the mental health and psychological wellbeing of children in care (DH, 1998). The Crime and Disorder Act led to the creation of Youth Offending Teams with the primary aim of reducing offending.

In 1999 the UK government made mental health one of its three clinical priorities, along with heart disease and cancer. The *National Service Framework for Mental Health* was published in England in 1999 and the government's Sure Start programme was launched the same year. This was modelled on the US 'Head Start' programme and was the Treasury Department's strategy to give children the best possible start in life by improving early education, childcare and family support.

Also in 1999, the Richardson Committee was commissioned by the government to review the 1983 Mental Health Act. The committee's report declared that the law relating to the treatment of children suffering from mental disorder was in need of clarification. The committee was concerned that the multiplicity of legal provisions created a climate of uncertainty, and suggested that professionals were unsure of their authority and of the legal and ethical entitlements of the children in their care (DH, 1999).

The new millennium

Children's policy started to transform at a fast pace at the turn of the century. The Children's Fund was announced in 2000 for children aged between 5 and 13. This was part of the child poverty initiative and was given to local authorities for them to reduce child health inequalities, educational failure, and crime and antisocial behaviour.

It wasn't until 2000 that the UK government set requirements for health authorities and local councils to work together by developing local CAMHS strategies. These were to include early intervention and prevention programmes and targets were set for local services to provide comprehensive CAMHS by 2006.

The most important landmark in the history of CAMHS in Wales came with the publication of the All Wales CAMHS Strategy, 'Everybody's Business' (National Assembly for Wales, 2001). This 10-year comprehensive policy framework embraced the four-tier strategic concept based on the HAS framework, and promoted inclusion, multi-disciplinary working, inter-agency collaboration and user involvement. Wales was the first UK country to have a national CAMHS strategy.

The same year saw publication of the *Health and Wellbeing Survey* in Northern Ireland which showed that people there were at greater risk of mental ill health than those in England and Scotland (DH, Social Services & Public Safety, 2001). This was due to higher levels of socioeconomic deprivation and the ongoing 'Troubles'.

In the year that followed publication of the survey a number of important political and strategic developments in relation to CAMHS in Northern Ireland emerged. The Department of Health, Social Services and Public Safety set planning priorities and actions for health and personal social services. The subsequent three-year service delivery plan included a target to improve CAMHS by providing a range of therapeutic interventions in the most appropriate settings.

Also in 2002, the Northern Ireland Executive published a consultation report, 'Investing for Health', which highlighted mental health as a priority for action and noted growing concern about high rates of mental health problems in children and young people. Giving children the best start in life, safeguarding and protecting their needs and developing child and adolescent mental health services were all identified as crucially important (Northern Ireland Executive, 2002). However, whilst recognising that the mental health of children and young people was crucial, the subsequent action plan for 2003–2008, 'Promoting Mental Health', did not give CAMHS a high profile. The publication of *Building on Progress* coincided with the commencement of the Regional Review of Mental Health and Learning Disability in 2002, which was later to include the Child and Adolescent Mental Health Expert Working Committee (McDougall & Davren, 2006).

Every Child Matters

In 2003, the Green Paper *Every Child Matters* was published. This was the government's cross-departmental agenda for the transformation of children's services. It aimed to support each and every child to be healthy, stay safe, enjoy and achieve, make a positive contribution and achieve economic wellbeing (Department for Education and Skills, 2003). The Scottish Needs Assessment Report on

Child and Adolescent Mental Health (the SNAP report) was also published in 2003 by what was then the Public Health Institute of Scotland and is now NHS Scotland. The SNAP report made a number of important strategic recommendations. As well as a strong focus on involving children and their families or carers in the planning and delivery of CAMHS, a number of target areas for development were identified. These related to the need to mainstream CAMHS by focusing on mental health promotion and emotional wellbeing, early identification and prevention of mental health problems and disorders, research, and strengthening local, regional and national specialist CAMHS (Public Health Institute for Scotland, 2003).

In 2003 an initial budget of £24 million was allocated by the Scottish Executive's National Programme for Improving Mental Health and Wellbeing. This was to be used by local services to achieve four key aims: to raise public awareness and promote positive mental health; to eliminate stigma and discrimination; to reduce suicide rates, particularly amongst young men; and to support recovery from mental illness. Published alongside the SNAP report was the Scottish Executive's consultation document, 'An Integrated Strategy for the Early Years' (Scottish Executive, 2003), which aimed to influence policy at a structural level and drew together existing policies in relation to child care, health visitor services, pre-school education and parenting skills.

2004 was an eventful year for children's services. The *National Service Framework (NSF) for Children, Young People and Maternity Services* was published in England which set new standards and defined service models for children across all NHS and social care settings. A dedicated chapter on mental health and psychological wellbeing was included which included markers of good practice and further guidance on comprehensive CAMHS (DH, 2004). The following year saw the publication of an equivalent National Service Framework in Wales which also focused on children, young people and maternity services and included a module on mental health and psychological wellbeing.

Building on *Every Child Matters*, the Children Act 2004 received royal assent which paved the way for the introduction of Local Safeguarding Children's Boards and Children's Trust arrangements. At the same time the NSF for Children was published in England the National CAMHS Support Service (NCSS) was launched. NCSS comprised a team of regional development workers charged with the responsibility for helping local CAMHS partnerships achieve delivery of the comprehensive CAMHS target. The team also assisted local CAMHS partnerships to review their progress against the delivery of NSF priority areas and facilitate networking, multi-agency co-operation and the sharing of local good practice in CAMHS.

Also published in 2004 was the *Child Poverty Review* (HM Treasury, 2004) which examined the welfare reform and public service changes required to improve life chances for poor children. Linking poor mental health with truancy, substance misuse, unemployment and offending, the review promised to extend mental health services for children.

The role of mental health in schools was given a higher profile with the government's announcement of the Social and Emotional Aspects of Learning (SEAL)

programme in 2005. This was a comprehensive, whole-school approach to promote children's emotional health and wellbeing and by doing so enhance their
learning and chances of educational success. At the same time in 2005 the Scottish
Executive built on their SNAP report published two years earlier by identifying
standards for good care and supporting local planning and guidance (Scottish
Executive, 2005).

Northern Ireland's Department of Health, Social Services and Public Safety published a twenty-year vision for health and wellbeing in 2005. This recognised that
one of the most effective ways to improve the health and wellbeing of the nation was
to invest early with children and their parents.

Following concern that children in some areas of England were unable to access
comprehensive CAMHS, the government published additional indicators in 2005.
Three 'proxies' were developed to bring about service improvements: these were
access to 24-hour emergency services; access for 16 and 17 year olds; and better
services for children and young people with learning disabilities. Nearly a decade on
there remain gaps in access for children and young people across England and the
wider UK.

2008 was also a busy year for CAMHS. The *Children's Plan* was published and
this was closely followed by the Treasury's *Think Family Agenda*. Rehearsing many
of the strategic objectives set out in previous policy, the Children's Plan promised
greater support for families and a review of the education for children in primary
schools. Aiming to break the generational cycle of difficulties, the 'Think Family'
initiative highlighted the need for agencies and services to support whole families,
not just the child or adult who required help.

New Horizons was the English government's shared vision for mental health (DH,
2009a) which also took a lifespan approach. This was to help break the cycles that
combine to produce poor outcomes for children, such as social exclusion, domestic
violence and substance misuse, and was published alongside the government's child
health strategy, *Healthy Children, Brighter Futures* (DH, 2009b).

A recommendation in the Children's Plan was for the government to undertake a
national review of child and adolescent mental health services. 'Children in Mind'
was the final report of an independent review of CAMHS which made 20 recommendations for the government to consider. Top of the list was to implement a National
Advisory Council for Children's Mental Health and Psychological Wellbeing which
was established by the government in the spring of 2009.

THE FUTURE OF CAMHS POLICY AND STRATEGY?

The twenty-first century has witnessed a number of treatments imported from the
USA to the UK. These included Multi Systemic Therapy; Multidimensional Treatment Foster Care; and the Nurse Family Partnerships all of which the current government are funding. Common to all is a highly prescriptive, manualised approach
with a strong element of supervision and the monitoring of treatment fidelity.

Children's behaviour continues to play a leading role in the development of government policy. Following the summer riots of 2011 the moral panic that Duncan (2005) described in relation to teenage pregnancies was rekindled. A sense that British children were outside the control of their parents was played out in the media coverage that followed, with various links being made to breakdowns in morality, education and respect. Aiello and Parianti (2012) took a psychosocial perspective on the riots, identifying poor emotional recognition, a lack of self control and difficulties with social identity, and also suggesting that socially excluded young people may have looted shops to 'belong' and confirm they were not part of the society they had come to resent. This of course increased their social exclusion. Durkin (2012) sought to explore whether the behaviour of young people in the UK riots justified a label of 'sickness' or a psychiatric diagnosis which could be treated by mental health professionals. The research highlighted the implications of labelling behaviour as 'sick' and the importance of understanding behaviour in its wider context. Following the riots the British prime minister announced that more help must be given to the most troubled families, yet it remains to be seen how this will be reflected in policy.

Since the turn of the twenty-first century, our understanding of child and adolescent mental health problems has increasingly been assisted by modern science. Neuro-imagery, molecular genetic studies and other technologies have increased our knowledge about foetal and infant brain development and the effects of early deprivation on children. The pace of these developments will increase more and more rapidly every year.

The global context in which children and young people are living affects their mental health and life chances and brings new challenges, for better and for worse. The education and employment opportunities that are open to young people are rapidly transforming. In the US, 1 in 4 people today is working for a company they have been employed by for less than a year. According to the former US Secretary of Education, Richard Riley, the top 10 'in demand' jobs in 2010 did not exist in 2004. Globalisation also brings risks. Cyber-bullying, internet pornography and human trafficking are twenty-first-century phenomena that bring new risks and challenges for children.

CONCLUSION

As we pause and look back over time we might conclude that the development of services for children and young people with mental health problems has not been a strategic process. Rather than being based on evidence of what works and the needs of people who use them, interventions have often been designed around clinicians and services rather than children, families and local communities. Focusing less on causes and more on effects, different governments have attempted to address the mental health problems of childhood that undoubtedly lead to poor outcomes in adulthood. It is difficult to predict the direction that future child mental health policy may take but it will be essential that an 'invest to save' approach is adopted if we are to improve the mental health and life chances of our children.

Reflective Exercise

1. Do you consider that sufficient attention is taken of the early signs of mental health issues in children and young people?
2. To what extent do you think the voice of young people is 'heard' in the context of mental health care?
3. How could mental health be made an acceptable topic for consideration in the social and educational settings that young people inhabit?

BIBLIOGRAPHY

Abbott, P. & Wallace, C. (1998) Health visiting, social work, nursing and midwifery: a history. In P. Abbott & L. Meerabeau (eds), *The Sociology of the Caring Professions*. London: UCL Press.

Adler, L. & Chua, H. (2002) Management of ADHD in adults, *Journal of Clinical Psychiatry*, 63 (12): 29–35.

Aiello, G. & Pariante, C. (2012) Citizen, interrupted: the 2011 English riots from a psychosocial perspective, *Epidemiology and Psychiatric Sciences* (August), doi: 10.1017/S2045796012000364.

Ainsworth, M. (1962) *Deprivation of Maternal Care: A Reassessment of its Effects*. Geneva: WHO.

Black, D. (1993) A brief history of child and adolescent psychiatry. In D. Black & D. Cottrell (eds), *Seminars in Child and Adolescent Psychiatry*. London: Gaskell.

Bowlby, J. (1951) *Maternal Care and Mental Health*. Geneva: WHO.

Butler-Sloss, E. (1987) *Report of the Inquiry into Child Abuse in Cleveland*. London: HMSO.

Cameron, K. (1949) A psychiatric inpatient department for children, *Journal of Mental Science*, 95: 560–566.

Care Services Improvement Partnership (2008) *Right Time, Right Place: Learning from National Service Framework Development Initiatives: Children and Young People's Emotional Health and Well-being and Mental Health. 2005–2007*. London: HMSO.

Cottrell, D. & Kraam, A. (2005) Growing up? A history of CAMHS (1987–2005), *Child and Adolescent Mental Health*, 1093: 111–117.

Croates, S. (2004) John Bowlby and Margaret Mahler: their lives and theories, *Journal of the American Psychoanalytical Association* 52: 571–601.

Department for Education and Skills (2003) *Every Child Matters*. London: HMSO.

Department of Health (1956) *The Jameson Report: Report of the Working Party on the Field, Training and Recruitment of Health Visitors*. London: HMSO.

Department of Health (1998) *Quality Protects: Transforming Children's Services*. London: HMSO.

Department of Health (1999) *Review of the Mental Health Act 1983: Report of the Expert Committee*. London: HMSO.

Department of Health (2000) *Lost in Care: Report of the Tribunal of Inquiry into the Abuse of Children in Care in the Former County Council Areas of Gwynedd and Clwyd since 1974*. London: HMSO.

Department of Health (2004) *National Service Framework for Children, Young People and Maternity Services*. London: HMSO.

Department of Health (2009a) *New Horizons: A Shared Vision for Mental Health*. London: HMSO.

Department of Health (2009b) *Healthy Lives: Brighter Futures: The Strategy for Children's and Young People's Health*. London: HMSO.

Department of Health (2012) *No Health Without Mental Health: Implementation Framework*. London: HMSO.

Department of Health, Social Services and Public Safety (2001) *Northern Ireland Health and Social Wellbeing Survey 2001*. Belfast: DHSSPS.

Department of Health, Social Services and Public Safety (2003) *Promoting Mental Health: Strategy and Action Plan 2003–2008*. Belfast: Health Promotion Agency.

Department of Health, Social Services and Public Safety (2005) *A Healthier Future: A Twenty Year Vision for Health and Well-being in Northern Ireland: 2005–2025*. Belfast: DHSSPS.

Dourmashkin, R. (1997) What caused the 1918–30 epidemic of encephalitis lethargica?, *Journal of the Royal Society of Medicine*, 90 (9): 515–520.

Duncan, S. (2005) What's the problem?: teenage parents: a critical review. *Families and Social Capital ESRC Research Group Working Paper No. 15*. Bradford: University of Bradford.

Evans, B., Rahman, S. & Jones, E. (2008) Managing the unmanageable: inter-war child psychiatry at the Maudsley Hospital, London, *History of Psychiatry*, 19 (76): 454–475.

Gelder, M. (1991) Adolf Meyer and his influence on British psychiatry. In G. Berrios and H. Freeman (eds), *150 Years of British Psychiatry 1841–1991*. London: Gaskell.

Gingell, K. (2001) The forgotten children: children admitted to a county asylum between 1854 and 1900, *Psychiatric Bulletin*, November.

Green, H., McGinnity, A., Meltzer, H. et al. (2005) *Mental Health of Children and Young People in Great Britain 2004*. London: Palgrave.

Hersov, L. (1998) Preface. In J. Green and B. Jacobs (eds), *In-patient Child Psychiatry: Modern Practice, Research and the Future*. London: Routledge.

HM Treasury (2004) *Child Poverty Review*. London: HMSO.

Kerfoot, M. & Williams, R. (2005) Setting the scene: perspectives on the history of and policy for child and adolescent mental health services in the UK. In R. Williams & M. Kerfoot (2005) *Child and Adolescent Mental Health Services: Strategy, Planning, Delivery and Evaluation*. Oxford: Oxford University Press.

Levy, A. & Kahan, B. (1991) *The Pindown Experience and the Protection of Children: Report of the Staffordshire Childcare Inquiry*. Staffordshire County Council.

London School of Economics and Political Science (2012) *How Mental Illness Loses Out in the NHS: A Report for the Centre for Economic Performance's Mental Health Policy Group*. London: LSE.

McDougall, T. & Davren, M. (2006) The bigger picture: CAMHS nursing and the strategic context. In T. McDougall (ed.), *Child and Adolescent Mental Health Nursing*. London: Blackwell.

Maughan, B. & Kim-Cohen, J. (2005) Continuities between childhood and adult life, *British Journal of Psychiatry*, 187: 301–303.

Martin, A. & Volkmar, F. (2012) *Lewis' Child and Adolescent Psychiatry*. London: Lippincott Williams and Wilkins.

Munro-Davies, H.G. (1949) Visits to children in hospital, *Spectator*, 18 March.

National Assembly for Wales (2001) *Child and Adolescent Mental Health Services: Everybody's Business*. Cardiff: National Assembly for Wales.

NHS Executive (1995) *Priorities and Planning Guidance for the NHS, 1997/98*. London: HMSO.

NHS Health Advisory Service (1985) *Bridge Over Troubled Waters*. London: HMSO.

NHS Health Advisory Service (1995) *Together We Stand: The Commissioning, Role and Management of Child and Adolescent Mental Health Services*. London: HMSO.

Parry-Jones, W. (1998) Historical themes. In J. Green and B. Jacobs (eds), *In-patient Child Psychiatry: Modern Practice, Research and the Future*. London: Routledge.

Public Health Institute of Scotland (2003) *Scottish Needs Assessment Report on Child and Adolescent Mental Health*. Glasgow: PHIS

Rafalovich, A. (2001) The conceptual history of attention deficit hyperactivity disorder: idiocy, imbecility, encephalitis and the child deviant, *Deviant Behaviour*, 22 (2): 93–115.

Richards, M. & Abbott, R. (2009) *Childhood Mental Health and Life Chances in Post-War Britain*. London: Sainsbury Centre for Mental Health.

Roth, A. & Fonagy, P. (2005) *What Works for Whom? A Critical Review of Treatments for Children and Adolescents* (2nd edn). London: Guilford.

Rutter, M. (1981) *Maternal Deprivation Reassessed* (2nd edn). Harmondsworth: Penguin.

Rutter, M., Bishop, D., Pine, D. et al. (2009) *Child and Adolescent Psychiatry* (4th edn). London: Blackwell.

Sainsbury Centre for Mental Health (2009) *The Chance of a Lifetime: Preventing Early Conduct Problems and Reducing Crime*. London: SCMH.

Scottish Executive (2003*) An Integrated Strategy for the Early Years*. Edinburgh: Scottish Executive.

Scottish Executive (2005) *The Mental Health of Children and Young People: A Framework for Promotion, Prevention and Care*. Edinburgh: Scottish Executive.

Thom, D. (1992) Wishes, anxieties, play and gestures. In R. Cooter (ed.), *In the Name of the Child: Health and Welfare, 1880–1940*. London: Routledge.

Walk, A. (1964) The pre history of child psychiatry, *British Journal of Psychiatry*, 110: 754–767.

Wardle, C. (1991) Historical influences on services for children and adolescents before 1900. In G. Berrios & H. Freeman (eds), *150 Years of British Psychiatry, 1841–1991*. London: Gaskell. pp. 279–293.

Wender, P. (1995) *Attention Deficit/Hyperactivity Disorder in Adults*. New York: Oxford University Press.

While, A. (1987) The early history of health visiting: a review of the role of central government (1830–1914), *Child Care Health and Development*, 13: 127–136.

Wolkind, S. (1991) The components of affectionless psychopathy in institutionalised children, *Journal of Child Psychology and Psychiatry* 15: 215–220.

11 DUAL DIAGNOSIS

Cheryl Kipping

Chapter Overview

Whilst substance misuse is a challenge for those without a mental health problem, this chapter convincingly demonstrates the very real concern it creates for policy makers when addressing those who do have a mental health problem. The concern generated has seen a wealth of policy, services and structures explicitly created to meet this need.

There is a clear argument made in this chapter on how the knowledge and ability of all mental health nurses to engage with this agenda is essential. The author by means of a novel method has managed to corral the relevant policies to inform the issues raised.

The area of dual diagnosis however is not totally driven by the clean empirical approach and there can be obstacles to engaging with the client group due to a lack of understanding, information, or perhaps prejudice. The level of education required to meaningfully engage and offer care and treatment can be argued to be absent from the preparation of all health and social care professionals.

INTRODUCTION

Policies to inform service provision for people with a dual diagnosis, namely the co-existence of mental health and substance misuse disorders, can be traced back to the late 1990s. At that time several mental health and drug policies identified dual diagnosis as requiring attention but few provided guidance on what should be done.

People with a dual diagnosis are a very diverse group. A quadrant model has been used to illustrate this (see Figure 11.1). The horizontal axis represents the severity of mental illness and the vertical axis substance misuse. Depending on the severity of

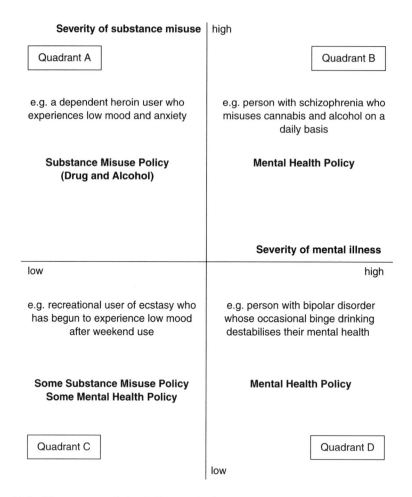

Figure 11.1 The scope of dual diagnosis (adapted from DH, 2002a)

each condition, a person's location can be 'plotted' on the figure. A range of policy guidance, some with a mental health focus, some with a substance misuse focus, and some solely focused on dual diagnosis, has shaped service provision for different sub-groups of people with a dual diagnosis.

A key reason for needing dual diagnosis policy is to overcome the conceptualisation of mental health and substance misuse as separate. Mental health and substance misuse impact on each other so working on one in isolation from the other is unlikely to be effective. However, in the United Kingdom mental health and substance misuse services are separate, often delivered by different providers (NHS and non-NHS), and even when both are provided by the same organisation (usually NHS Trusts) they are separate parts of the organisation and supported by different funding streams. Historically, substance misuse has also been viewed as a clinical specialty. Undergraduate and pre-registration training (regardless of discipline) have given little attention to substance misuse, resulting in many health-care staff being unprepared for such work. Together these have contributed to the view that people with a dual diagnosis should be referred to the 'other' service for treatment of the co-existing condition.

Taking this approach can further compound the challenges of addressing dual diagnosis because mental health and substance misuse services have different treatment philosophies. Substance misuse services usually require people to be motivated to address their use and approach services for help. Many people with mental health problems do not view their substance use as problematic so are unlikely to access substance misuse services. People with mental health problems can be compelled to receive treatment against their will if necessary (under the provision of the Mental Health Act 1983 – amended 2007), but such arrangements do not exist for substance misuse treatment.

This context has produced a situation where people have been 'bounced' between services, received care for only one aspect of their dual diagnosis, or fallen between services and not received treatment at all.

It is against this background that dual diagnosis policy has been developed. Five key policies can be identified that focus solely on dual diagnosis. Other policies that have shaped service provision can be grouped using the quadrant model. For people with severe mental illness and substance misuse problems (i.e. those in quadrants B and D) service provision is largely guided by mental health policy. For people with severe substance misuse problems and mental health problems (i.e. those in quadrant A) it is primarily informed by substance misuse policy. Any treatment accessed by people in quadrant C is likely to be provided by primary care services. As such, there are no specific mental health or substance misuse policies that focus on this group, however, some policies focused on other quadrants have implications for primary care. Inevitably policies focused on one quadrant will have aspects that are of relevance to others.

Policy should be informed by evidence but the evidence regarding effective service configurations and treatments for people with a dual diagnosis is limited (NICE, 2011a; Hunt et al., 2013). Practice developments have largely been based on expert consensus, and the treatment of each condition alone. Other factors that have influenced policy development include long-standing funding arrangements, service models and treatments (what is already in place and the way things have previously been done), as well as political expediency.

The range of policies that inform the treatment of people with dual diagnosis is broad so parameters have been set for this chapter. Dual diagnosis crosses the lifespan and may be encountered in a variety of clinical settings across primary, secondary and tertiary care. The policies included here focus on working-age adults in secondary mental health and substance misuse services. These differ in their remits (from solely England to the entire UK), however the focus here is on England. An 'additional reading' list is included at the end of the chapter highlighting policies specific to other age groups, the criminal justice system, where there are large numbers of people with dual diagnosis, and focusing on countries other than England.

In this chapter 'policy' is defined broadly and includes national strategies, policies, and good practice guidance aimed at improving the care and treatment of people with a dual diagnosis.

In the next section policies focused solely on dual diagnosis are described. The remainder of the chapter is informed by the quadrant model (Figure 11.1). An overview of mental health policies that have influenced the treatment of people in quadrants B and D is provided first. This is followed by a consideration of substance misuse policies, the main influence on the treatment of people located in quadrant A. Having identified the key policies and their recommendations a summary of common themes is presented. Attention is then given to the drivers that can promote policy implementation before reflecting on the extent to which the vision set out in the policy guidance is a reality.

DUAL DIAGNOSIS

The first dual diagnosis-specific guidance to be published was the Health Advisory Service's (HAS) *Substance Misuse and Mental Health Co-morbidity (Dual Diagnosis) Standards* (HAS, 2001). These were targeted at mental health services but included some standards for substance misuse services. The standards relate to four areas: commissioning, planning and integration; inter- and intra-agency organisational issues; organisation of care; and service delivery. They include requirements for a co-ordinated approach to commissioning mental health and substance misuse services to ensure adequate dual diagnosis funding, liaison between mental health and substance misuse services, the development of a local strategy, provision for dual diagnosis as part of mainstream mental health services, substance misuse to be considered in mental health assessments, risk assessment and management to include risks associated with substance misuse, policies to deal with substance misuse on hospital premises, and staff training. Standards for substance misuse services included substance misuse services to respond to dual diagnosis and staff training.

The *Mental Health Policy Implementation Guide: Dual Diagnosis Good Practice Guide* (DH, 2002a) (hereafter referred to as the *Dual Diagnosis Good Practice Guide*) was one of several policy implementation guides developed to expand on and support the implementation of the *National Service Framework for Mental Health* (NSFMH) (DH, 1999a). The NSFMH highlighted some of the challenges associated with dual diagnosis but it was the *Dual Diagnosis Good Practice Guide* that provided guidance on how to address these. Although it focused on people with severe mental illness it set out principles for considering the needs of anyone that might be considered to have a dual diagnosis.

Implementation of the guidance at local level was the responsibility of Local Implementation Teams (LITs) (groups set up to implement the NSFMH), in partnership with Drug Action Team (DATs) (groups responsible for the implementation of drug policy).

The guide identified strategic and practice requirements. These included the following:

- Project teams, comprised of key stakeholders (e.g. commissioners, managers, clinicians, mental health, substance misuse), should be set up to develop a local strategy based on a needs assessment and an agreed local definition of dual diagnosis. This should incorporate care pathways.
- A lead commissioner should be identified for dual diagnosis.
- Substance misuse should be considered usual rather than exceptional in people with severe mental health problems.
- Treatment for people with severe mental health and substance misuse problems should be delivered within mental health services ('mainstreaming') as part of an integrated treatment model (i.e. mental health and substance misuse problems addressed at the same time, in one setting, by one team). This should prevent people being shunted between services or dropping out of care.
- Substance misuse services should provide specialist advice and support to mental health services (recognising the knowledge and skills deficits for working with substance misuse in mental health).
- Mental health providers should designate a lead clinician for dual diagnosis.
- A training strategy should be developed to address the needs of all staff in contact with people with a dual diagnosis, qualified and unqualified, and all disciplines. Basic training should be available for all staff and advanced training and supervision for those with a greater role in working with this group (e.g. assertive outreach teams).
- Specialist dual diagnosis teams should work on an outreach/consultancy model (i.e. supporting mental health services rather than taking on the treatment of people with a dual diagnosis themselves).
- Substance misuse and risks associated with use should be considered in all mental health assessments.
- Treatment should be staged according to the person's readiness to change and engagement with services – a longitudinal and optimistic perspective is needed.
- A harm reduction approach should be adopted: the client should not be prematurely pushed towards abstinence.
- People with severe mental health problems and substance misuse should be subject to the Care Programme Approach (CPA).

Alongside the *Dual Diagnosis Good Practice Guide* (DH, 2002a) guidance on the assessment and management of dual diagnosis in inpatient and day hospital settings was developed (DH, 2006a). Although inpatient care provides a unique opportunity for working with this group, it also presents challenges, in particular the use of illicit drugs on wards, which can compromise safety.

The guidance identified factors to consider when developing local policies to promote drug-free wards and manage use when it does occur, for example, searching (people and premises), restricting visitors, involving the police, information sharing/confidentiality arrangements, procedures for the disposal of substances, reviewing care and treatment, providing information for service users and carers on local policies, and the consequences of contravening these. It also re-iterated recommendations from the *Dual Diagnosis Good Practice Guide* (DH, 2002a) and emphasised that the assessment and management of substance use were core components of mental health work.

Although the need for staff training was widely recognised and some guidance had identified topics for inclusion, a statement of dual diagnosis competencies did not exist until 'Closing the Gap', the dual diagnosis capabilities framework, was developed (Hughes, 2006). This identified 17 capabilities across three domains: values (e.g. recognising the legitimacy of working with people with dual diagnosis, therapeutic optimism), utilising knowledge and skills (e.g. engagement, education and health promotion, risk assessment and management), and practice development (e.g. identifying own learning needs, seeking supervision). Capabilities are identified at three levels: core, generalist, and specialist. Core capabilities are required by workers that encounter dual diagnosis but addressing this is not a key aspect of their work (e.g. police, housing support workers). Generalist capabilities are required by post-qualification staff who work with dual diagnosis regularly (e.g. mental health nurses, social workers, psychologists, psychiatrists, occupational therapists). Specialist capabilities are required by people who have responsibility for developing the dual diagnosis knowledge and skills of others.

The framework can be used to inform training, monitor staff development, and guide recruitment (informing job descriptions and person specifications).

The National Institute for Health and Clinical Excellence (NICE) produced the most recent dual diagnosis guidance: *Psychosis with Co-existing Substance Misuse: Assessment and Management of Adults and Young People* (NICE, 2011a). Recommendations are included for primary care, secondary mental health care, substance misuse services, inpatient mental health services, and staffed accommodation.

Preventing exclusion and promoting appropriate care pathways are strong themes. The guidance states that people with psychosis and substance misuse should not be excluded from mental health care because of their substance misuse, from substance misuse services because of their psychosis, or from staffed accommodation because of psychosis or substance misuse. Anyone with suspected psychosis and substance misuse should be referred to secondary mental health care for assessment. For most adults treatment for both conditions should be provided in secondary mental health care, using the CPA. Consideration should be given to seeking specialist advice and initiating joint work when the person has complex substance misuse problems or is ready for change and can benefit from the specialist interventions provided by substance misuse services. It is recommended that mental health and substance misuse services develop local protocols setting out responsibilities and processes for assessment, referral, treatment and shared care. The importance of staff competence is highlighted for secondary mental health care and substance misuse staff.

Looking more specifically at working individually with service users, the guidance emphasises the importance of engagement, building respectful, non-judgemental relationships, and being hopeful and optimistic. Recognising the ambivalence many people have towards substance misuse, a motivational approach is recommended. Assessment is a further theme: including substance misuse assessment as part of mental health assessment; assessing people with substance misuse problems for psychosis; and regularly assessing and reviewing risks (associated with substance use, mental health, and safeguarding children and vulnerable adults).

In relation to treatment, offering information so that people can make informed decisions is emphasised, as is tailoring the sequencing of treatment, taking account of the relative severity of the person's psychosis and substance misuse, and their readiness for change. Given the paucity of evidence for specific treatments for co-existing psychosis and substance misuse it is recommended that treatment for each condition should be offered in line with other NICE guidance (e.g. NICE, 2006, 2007a, 2007b, 2009, 2010a, 2011b).

Recognising the challenges posed by illicit substance use in inpatient services, the guidance recommends that policies and procedures to promote a substance-free therapeutic environment are developed.

Working with families and carers is another theme: involving them in care provision, addressing their needs, and making information available.

MENTAL HEALTH

Many mental health policies provide guidance on working with dual diagnosis, in particular for people in quadrants B and D in Figure 11.1.

Dual diagnosis was a recurring theme in the NSFMH (DH, 1999a). As well as identifying the challenges encountered when working with this group, it stated that their needs should be met within existing mental health and drug and alcohol services and that specific measures to promote engagement may be needed. The importance of assessing substance misuse as part of mental health assessment, and considering how specialist input could be accessed, were further themes. The increased risk of suicide associated with substance misuse was identified as another key consideration.

The *NHS Plan* (2000) built on the NSFMH and required assertive outreach (AO) teams to be developed for people with severe mental illness at risk of losing contact with services. Often this would be people with a dual diagnosis. More detailed guidance on AO teams was published subsequently (DH, 2001a). This included that staff should have skills in assessing and managing dual diagnosis and access to specialist help to support this work.

A review of progress against NSFMH standards (DH, 2004), including the *Dual Diagnosis Good Practice Guide* (DH, 2002a) requirements, reported 'modest' progress, with just 17% of LITs having a dual diagnosis strategy. Dual diagnosis was described as 'the most challenging clinical problem that we face' (2004: 1) and a priority for further action, with the following to be a focus:

- Assertive outreach teams and dedicated services for dual diagnosis.
- Better collaboration between drug and alcohol and mental health teams.

- Training for mental health staff in the assessment and clinical management of substance misuse.
- Intensive efforts to prevent drug misuse in people with severe mental illness.
- Prevention of drug misuse in in-patient units (2004: 73).

A review of the CPA (DH, 2008) identified people with a dual diagnosis as a 'key group' whose needs had not always been effectively met within CPA. Criteria to inform decisions about who should be subject to CPA were identified, many of which were characteristic of people with a dual diagnosis. The review stated that the 'default' position was that people with a dual diagnosis should be managed within the CPA.

By 2009 the ten year period covered by the NSFMH had ended and a new mental health policy framework was required. *New Horizons* (DH, 2009a) reiterated what had become familiar dual diagnosis themes: the importance of joint work between mental health and substance misuse services, the need for training and clinical leadership. This guidance was quickly superseded by the new government's own mental health strategy, *No Health Without Mental Health* (DH, 2011). This has been followed by an *Implementation Framework* (Centre for Mental Health et al., 2012). These documents identify the importance of services being available for people with a dual diagnosis, co-ordination between substance misuse and mental health services, and improvements in commissioning.

Several mental health policies have focused on the identification and management of risk. Dual diagnosis is a recurring theme. In comparison with people with mental illness alone, people using substances have increased risks in a range of domains, most notably suicide and homicide. The *National Confidential Inquiry Reports into Suicide and Homicide by People with Mental Illness (NCISH)*, which collate national data on suicides and homicides committed by people in contact with mental health services in the year before the incident, highlight these links (DH, 1999b, 2001b; Appleby et al., 2006, 2009, 2010, 2011, 2012, 2013).

In the most recent report over half of patient suicides had a history of alcohol and/or drug misuse (England 54%, Wales 56%, Northern Ireland 68% and Scotland 69%): 15% had a 'dual diagnosis', where this was defined narrowly as a person with severe mental illness and alcohol and/or drug misuse. About a quarter of patient homicides had a 'dual diagnosis' (Scotland 18%, Wales 21%, England 24%, Northern Ireland 29%) and over 85% a history of alcohol and/or drug misuse (Wales 85%, England 90%, Scotland 95% and Northern Ireland 100%).

The early NCISH reports (DH, 1999b, 2001b) resulted in the production of 'Twelve Points to a Safer Service', recommendations to promote safer mental health care. These included staff training in the management of risk, a strategy for dual diagnosis covering training on the management of substance use, joint work with substance misuse services, and staff with a specific responsibility to develop local services.

These recommendations were reiterated in the *National Suicide Prevention Strategy for England* (DH, 2002b) and further developed in the *Preventing Suicide Toolkits* (NIMHE, 2003; NPSA, 2009): a strategy should exist for the comprehensive care of people with a dual diagnosis; staff who provide care to people at risk of suicide are given approved training in the clinical management of cases of dual diagnosis; and statistics for co-morbidity/suicide are collected and used to inform resource allocation. Although the most recent suicide prevention strategy (HM Government/ DH, 2012) does not make specific recommendations it does highlight the association between alcohol and/or drug misuse and suicide.

Further dual diagnosis recommendations were made in the 2006 NCISH report, covering the need for staff training in substance misuse, joint work with drug and alcohol teams, local clinical leadership, and use of CPA for people with severe mental illness and substance misuse (Appleby et al., 2006).

The most recent NCISH report (Appleby et al., 2013) recommends that services for dual diagnosis patients should be maintained and that specialist services and risk management for patients misusing alcohol and/or drugs should be strengthened.

SUBSTANCE MISUSE POLICY

The focus of this chapter now shifts to substance misuse policies. These have shaped service provision for people in quadrant A. Drug and alcohol policies and funding streams are separate. Policies are wide ranging. As well as treatment they encompass law enforcement, licensing, policing, advertising, and public information campaigns. Only policy related to treatment will be considered here.

Over 70% of people accessing substance misuse services have mental health problems (most commonly anxiety, depression, and personality disorders) (e.g. Weaver et al., 2002; Delgadillo et al., 2012).

Drug policy

The link between drug use and mental health problems, and the need to respond to dual diagnosis, have long been recognised in national drug policies (e.g. DH, 1996, 1998; Home Office, 2002, 2008; HM Govt/Home Office, 2010) but early policies provided little guidance on action to be taken.

Following the advent of the National Treatment Agency (NTA), a special health authority, with responsibility for ensuring that national drug policy was delivered at a local level, more specific guidance was produced. Drug Action Teams (DATs) have responsibility for overseeing the development and delivery of drug treatment in each local area. DATs reported to the NTA.

The NTA published a variety of guidance to inform drug treatment. *Models of Care (MoC) for Treatment of Adult Drug Misusers* (NTA, 2002) and a *MoC Update* (NTA, 2006) have been particularly influential. These provided guidance on commissioning and delivering drug treatment and were likened to a NSF for the drug field. MoC (NTA, 2002) included a dual diagnosis section that drew heavily on the HAS (2001) standards and *Dual Diagnosis Good Practice Guide* (DH, 2002a). Recommendations included the need for each local area to identify the appropriate approach and service configurations to meet the needs of people with dual diagnosis, staff training (to include the recognition and care of people with mental illness), and collaborative work with mental health services. The *MoC Update* (NTA, 2006) described a four-tiered drug treatment framework and identified the need for drug assessment to include a consideration of mental health problems and risks, and care plans to address mental health needs. Collaboration with mental health services and the development of mental health liaison roles were promoted.

The most recent drugs strategy (HM Govt/Home Office, 2010), along with the government's more general policies on health and social care (DH, 2010; Health and Social Care Act 2012), are producing changes in drug treatment that could have significant implications for drug users with mental health problems.

Rather than focusing on reducing the harms associated with use, the strategy emphasises 'full recovery' ('getting off drugs for good': 2010: 18). Payment to services will be contingent on a full recovery being achieved. The link between mental illness and substance misuse is acknowledged and the importance of addressing mental health as part of a 'whole systems' approach to building 'recovery capital', the resources needed for recovery, is noted. Improved mental health is also identified as a drug treatment outcome.

The need to identify and address mental health needs is picked up in subsequent guidance (NTA, 2012). This states that mental health services should lead care provision for people with severe mental health problems. Drug services need some ability to treat people with mild to moderate mental health problems, and IAPT (Increasing Access to Psychological Therapies) services have a role in providing psychological interventions for people with anxiety and depression who are stable (e.g. on opioid substitutes), in line with best practice guidance (IAPT, Drugscope, NTA, 2012).

New arrangements for the funding and organisation of drug treatment were introduced in April 2013. The NTA was subsumed under Public Health England. Local authorities are responsible for commissioning drug and alcohol services from a public health grant. In line with the government focus on commissioning for outcomes, 'payment by results' is being piloted. Service funding is contingent on achieving positive outcomes, such as the number of people attaining 'full recovery'.

More specific clinical practice guidance has also influenced the treatment of dual diagnosis in drug services. *Drug Misuse and Dependence: Guidelines on Clinical Management* (DH England and the devolved administrations, 2007) included a mental health section that noted 'evidence of much unmet need' (p. 87). This endorsed the DH (2002a) guidance, highlighting the importance of mental health and risk assessment as integral to drug assessment, communication between services, and staff competence. It also noted that inadequate management of mental health may affect drug treatment outcomes. Suicide was identified as a cause of drug-related deaths.

Two NICE guidelines relate to drug misuse (NICE, 2007a, 2007b). Although opioid use is the focus, cannabis, stimulant and benzodiazepine use are given some attention. The guidelines identify the importance of considering psychological and psychiatric needs as part of assessment (NICE, 2007a, 2007b) and suggest that treatment for co-morbid anxiety and depression should be available (in line with other NICE guidance: NICE, 2007c, 2007d) (NICE, 2007a). Inpatient and residential treatment options are identified as appropriate for people with 'significant' co-morbid mental health problems seeking detoxification and abstinence (NICE 2007a, 2007b).

Alcohol policy

Despite alcohol problems being more common than drug problems, alcohol policy has been slower to develop. Alcohol strategies have consistently highlighted the association between alcohol and mental health problems (Prime Minister's Strategy Unit, 2004; DH et al., 2007; HM Govt/Home Office, 2012), but as with the drug strategies these have been short on recommendations.

The first *Alcohol Harm Reduction Strategy* (Prime Minister's Strategy Unit, 2004) drew attention to the DH (2002a) *Dual Diagnosis Good Practice Guide*, highlighted the importance of early identification of alcohol problems and for medical and nurse training to include a focus on alcohol. Provision was made for further work to better understand need (the Alcohol Needs Assessment Research Project (ANARP) – DH, 2005) and draw together evidence on the most effective treatments (*Alcohol Effectiveness Review*: Raistrick et al., 2006). ANARP (DH, 2005) identified a large gap between the need for, and access to, alcohol treatment, noting that people with a dual diagnosis were particularly poorly served by alcohol services.

The *Alcohol Effectiveness Review* (Raistrick et al., 2006) dedicated a chapter to dual diagnosis ('psychiatric co-morbidity'). It noted that co-morbidity was so common that it should be considered the norm and that staff in alcohol services needed to be competent to deliver integrated treatment (i.e. addressing mental health and alcohol problems). Recognising that services have not always worked effectively together the review suggested that the quadrant model (Figure 11.1) could be used as a framework to inform the construction of services and pathways to ensure that people with a dual diagnosis are not excluded from treatment and not moved from one agency to another.

The *Alcohol Harm Reduction Strategy* (Prime Minister's Strategy Unit, 2004) also tasked the NTA with developing a Models of Care framework for alcohol. Care pathways were to be part of this. At the local level DATs were encouraged to take responsibility for alcohol, becoming DAATs (Drug and Alcohol Action Teams).

Models of Care for the Treatment of Alcohol Misuse (MoCAM) (DH/NTA, 2006) provided guidance on the commissioning and provision of local alcohol treatment systems, setting out a four-tiered treatment framework. The complex needs associated with dual diagnosis were highlighted and reference was made to the *Dual Diagnosis Good Practice Guide* (DH, 2002a). Attention was drawn to the need for alcohol assessments to include a consideration of mental health problems and risks, and collaboration with mental health services was promoted.

The development of liaison roles with psychiatric services was also suggested. Following MoCAM, alcohol treatment pathway guidance was published (DH, 2009b). This included an example of a pathway for people in alcohol treatment with mental health problems.

Safe, Sensible, Social: The Next Steps in the National Alcohol Strategy (DH et al., 2007) built on the 2004 strategy. It re-iterated similar messages and required each local area to develop an alcohol harm reduction strategy (including health-related harm).

Key objectives of the most recent *Alcohol Strategy* (HM Govt/Home Office, 2012) include ensuring that everyone is aware of the risks of excessive alcohol consumption and can make informed choices about drinking, and that support for behaviour change is available, particularly for the most vulnerable.

NICE has published public health guidance and clinical guidelines on *Alcohol Use Disorders* (NICE, 2010a, 2010b, 2011b). The public health guidance (NICE, 2010b) recommends that alcohol screening is integral to health and social care practice and particularly for those at increased risk of harm from alcohol, such as people with mental health problems.

The harmful drinking and alcohol dependence guideline (NICE, 2011b) identified the importance of mental health assessment being part of a comprehensive alcohol assessment. For people requiring assisted alcohol withdrawal, 'significant' psychiatric morbidity is identified as an indication that inpatient (rather than community) detoxification is needed. The guidance also recommends that people with co-morbid alcohol problems and anxiety or depression should address the alcohol problem first as this can lead to a significant improvement in mental health. Abstinence is identified as the preferred treatment goal for people with psychiatric co-morbidity, but if the person wants to work towards moderation alcohol treatment should not be refused and a harm reduction approach should be considered.

THE ROLE OF NURSES

Although the policies described are relevant to all health-care professionals, nurses have a key role to play in improving service provision for people with a dual diagnosis. It is they who are most commonly at the 'front-line' of care delivery. The *Chief Nursing Officer's Review of Mental Health Nursing* (DH, 2006b) highlights this, stating that mental health nurses in all settings should be able to respond to the needs of people with a dual diagnosis. In order to do this they need training on dual diagnosis issues and access to specialist advice to support their work.

SUMMARY OF THEMES

Having considered many policies from a variety of perspectives you will have noticed that there are many common themes. These are summarised below:

- Substance misuse problems are common in people with mental health problems and should be considered usual rather than exceptional.
- Mental health problems are common in people with substance misuse problems and should be considered the norm.
- Local strategies are needed for addressing the needs of people with a dual diagnosis.
- Commissioners need to consider the needs of people with a dual diagnosis and ensure there is a coordinated approach to service planning.
- The needs of people with a dual diagnosis should be met in existing services, usually within an integrated treatment model (mental health and substance misuse problems being addressed at the same time, in the same setting, by one team).

  o Liaison and joint work between mental health and substance misuse services is needed

    - for the development of local protocols and care pathways.
    - for the provision of specialist advice.
    - for the delivery of joint care (where appropriate).

- Staff training is needed in the assessment and management of substance misuse, and associated risks (mental health staff).
- Staff training is needed in the assessment and management of mental health, and associated risks (substance misuse staff).
- Assertive Outreach teams should be a focus for the care of people with severe mental illness and substance use that are difficult to engage with services.
- Assessment of substance misuse should be part of mental health assessment.
- Assessment of mental health needs should be part of substance misuse assessment.
- Risk assessment and management should consider the increased risks associated with dual diagnosis.
- Engaging people with a dual diagnosis can be challenging. A flexible and assertive approach may be required.
- Treatment should be staged according to the relative severity of the person's mental illness and substance misuse and their readiness to change. A longitudinal and optimistic approach is required, with realistic goals, often focused on harm-reduction, rather than abstinence.
- People with severe mental illness and substance misuse problems should have care provided within the CPA framework.
- Policies are needed to prevent substance use on inpatient wards.
- Local clinical leadership and specialist roles are needed to support the development and delivery of care provision for this group.
- People with a dual diagnosis should receive treatment in line with the relevant NICE guidance (i.e. for each individual condition).

FROM GUIDANCE TO IMPLEMENTATION

While policies may provide helpful guidance, unless systems are in place to promote compliance they may not be implemented. This section provides an overview of the drivers that can support policy implementation.

When the NSFMH was current LITs were asked to report to the DH annual progress on dual diagnosis standards derived from the DH (2002a) guidance. In 2006/7 an in-depth review was conducted (CSIP, 2007). Findings from these processes resulted in standards being highlighted and further recommendations being made (DH, 2004; CSIP, 2007).

Financial considerations are an important driver. For several years the NHS mental health contract suggested that a dual diagnosis measure be included. In 2009/10 the CQUIN (Commissioning for Quality and Innovation) payment framework was introduced. This enables commissioners to allocate a proportion of income to the achievement of quality goals. Failing to meet these results in income being lost. In some parts of the country dual diagnosis standards have been CQUIN targets.

Another financial driver is the National Health Service Litigation Authority (NHSLA) Standards (NHSLA, 2012, 2013). The NHSLA is like an insurance scheme for Trusts. Trusts pay in and the NHSLA pays out if a successful claim is made. A Trust's 'premium' is based on how robustly it demonstrates compliance with NHSLA standards. One standard relates to dual diagnosis.

There are also NHSLA standards to determine whether NICE and NCISH guidance are being met. As noted both have made recommendations about the treatment of people with a dual diagnosis.

Another body that can influence policy implementation is the Care Quality Commission (CQC). The CQC regulates care services. A failure to meet quality and safety standards could result in cancellation of a service's registration. One standard relates to responding to illicit drug use and supply on premises. An organisation's approach to dual diagnosis work may also inform the assessment of more general standards.

The CQC also conducts surveys. The community mental health survey asks service users whether they have been asked about their use of alcohol and non-prescription drugs. The staff survey has included a question on whether staff have had training, learning or development in how to assess and treat service users with a dual diagnosis.

FROM VISION TO REALITY

The former National Director of Mental Health stated 'It is everyone's business to provide good quality services for people with mental health and substance misuse difficulties' (CSIP, 2007: 2). So to what extent has this vision, along with the more detailed policy guidance described in this chapter, become a reality?

Over the years since the Dual Diagnosis Good Practice Guide (DH, 2002a) was published progress has been rather 'stop-start'. There is no doubt that this key guidance has been very influential. Many policies have reiterated its recommendations and other related themes and there has been value in this because each new piece of guidance refocuses attention on the issues.

There is evidence that dual diagnosis is being addressed in some areas and this is making a difference. Drawing on NCISH data, While et al. (2012) found that areas that had dual diagnosis policies had lower rates of suicide than those that did not. As this chapter suggests, however, progress has been patchy and significant challenges remain.

A journal debate that considered whether 'mainstreaming' was working (Hughes, 2009) identified three main obstacles: change being largely dependent on key individuals championing dual diagnosis; a lack of role legitimacy (staff not seeing dual diagnosis as part of their role); and difficulty in providing adequate opportunities for staff to develop and apply the knowledge, skills and attitudes needed for the work. These factors remain important.

The key challenge to improving services for people with a dual diagnosis continues to be the separation of mental health and substance misuse. At every level, national, regional and local strategic bodies, commissioning arrangements and services are separate, and each has differing priorities. For example, in the substance misuse sector a focus on drugs, rather than alcohol, and meeting the needs of class A drug users in particular, has militated against the needs of people with severe mental health problems, who most commonly misuse alcohol and cannabis, being met. The requirement for people to be motivated to address their use, and a lack of provision for an assertive approach to engaging people in substance misuse treatment, have further compounded this. In the mental health sector, a focus on meeting the needs of people with severe mental illness has resulted in people with so-called mild to moderate mental health problems that are misusing substances being excluded, particularly if they do not readily engage in treatment. Unhelpful, and often impossible, attempts to identify which problem is 'primary' have also promoted exclusion.

Reductions in public sector funding over recent years have also had a significant impact. Many dual diagnosis specialist posts have been lost. These typically delivered training, promoted joint work and liaison between mental health and substance misuse services, and supported service users to navigate local care pathways. AO teams, tasked with working with people with complex dual diagnosis needs who were difficult to engage in services, have been disbanded in many areas. Changes to the composition of the substance misuse treatment sector, because of the need to drive down costs and government policy to open NHS services to competition, have resulted in fewer NHS and more voluntary/independent sector providers. This has reduced mental health expertise in the sector (e.g. mental health nurses, psychiatrists, psychologists), potentially limiting the extent to which mental health problems can be addressed within substance misuse services.

More generally, reductions in the capacity of mental health and substance misuse services have resulted in a focus on 'core business'. Opportunities for working flexibly with people with a dual diagnosis may be limited, staff feel over-stretched, and there is a greater likelihood that dual diagnosis work will be seen as an added burden. Reduced capacity may also result in increased disputes between mental health and substance misuse services about where the needs of people with a dual diagnosis can most appropriately be met. Pressures in services also impact on attendance at training and keeping updated with new clinical guidance that could enhance practice.

Ongoing uncertainty associated with reduced funding, competition between providers, and changes to commissioning, have resulted in a tendency for people to look inwards rather than working with partners to develop and sustain strategic dual diagnosis initiatives.

The disbanding of regional and national bodies that promoted dual diagnosis service improvement has made it difficult for people to share good practice and learn from each other. NIMHE had a dual diagnosis workstream which kept dual diagnosis on the national agenda and developed guidance and tools to support dual diagnosis work.

This may all sound gloomy, and the challenges cannot be underestimated. There are, however, some positives. Many health and social care professionals are passionate about improving dual diagnosis service provision in line with policy guidance and are finding innovative ways forward. Nationally there are about 12 dual diagnosis consultant nurses who take a leading role in developing dual diagnosis initiatives. Some other dual diagnosis roles have also been preserved in recognition of the benefits they bring. In areas where no specialist dual diagnosis roles exist, other methods for focusing on dual diagnosis have been developed, for example local link worker roles (e.g. Edwards, 2011).

In moving forward top-down and bottom-up approaches are needed. The top-down approach will probably be driven by concerns with CQUINs and NHSLA assessments. These are important drivers for change and have promoted a greater focus on dual diagnosis. The bottom-up approach will most likely be influenced by front-line staff who recognise the importance of addressing mental health and substance misuse in an integrated way and work in flexible ways or 'go the extra mile' to ensure that the often diverse and complex needs of people with a dual diagnosis are met.

Changes to commissioning for both mental health and substance misuse may provide new opportunities. The development of NICE quality standards that will inform commissioning will promote best practice. The government's recognition of the importance of a whole-systems approach to recovery from substance misuse may prove important for people with a dual diagnosis, and guidance to promote the provision of psychological interventions for people with common mental health problems and substance use in IAPT services will increase service capacity.

We live in changing times, but one certainty is that dual diagnosis will not go away. Ultimately the test of whether good dual diagnosis care is being provided is when service users tell us that they have not been excluded from services because of their mental health or substance misuse problem, that they have been treated with respect and not felt judged, and that staff have been knowledgeable about their mental health and substance misuse, and have worked collaboratively with them to help them achieve their goals.

Reflective Exercise

1. Reflecting on your experiences of working with people with dual diagnosis, to what extent do you think service provision has been in line with the policy guidance described in this chapter?
2. In your role, what can you do to promote better dual diagnosis care/treatment?
3. Do you think there has been a reluctance to engage with this client group and if so how has this been made known?

BIBLIOGRAPHY

Appleby, L., Kapur, N., Shaw, J. et al. (2006) Avoidable Deaths: Five Year Report of the National Confidential Inquiry into Suicide and Homicide by People with Mental Illness. Manchester: University of Manchester.

Appleby, L., Kapur, N., Shaw, J. et al. (2009) *National Confidential Inquiry into Suicide and Homicide by People with Mental Illness: Annual Report England and Wales.* Available at www.medicine.manchester.ac.uk/cmhr/centreforsuicideprevention/nci/reports/

Appleby, L., Kapur, N., Shaw, J. et al. (2010) *National Confidential Inquiry into Suicide and Homicide by People with Mental Illness: Annual Report England and Wales.* Available at www.medicine.manchester.ac.uk/cmhr/centreforsuicideprevention/nci/reports/

Appleby, L., Kapur, N., Shaw, J. et al. (2011) *National Confidential Inquiry into Suicide and Homicide by People with Mental Illness: Annual Report England, Wales and Scotland.* Available at www.medicine.manchester.ac.uk/cmhr/centreforsuicideprevention/nci/reports/

Appleby, L., Kapur, N., Shaw, J. et al. (2012) *National Confidential Inquiry into Suicide and Homicide by People with Mental Illness: Annual Report England, Wales, Scotland and Northern Ireland.* Available at: www.medicine.manchester.ac.uk/cmhr/centreforsuicideprevention/nci/reports/

Appleby, L., Kapur, N., Shaw J. et al. (2013) National Confidential Inquiry into Suicide and Homicide by People with Mental Illness: Annual Report England, Northern Ireland, Scotland and Wales. Available at www.bmh.manchester.ac.uk/cmhr/centreforsuicideprevention/nci/reports/NCIAnnualReport2013V2.pdf

Care Services Improvement Partnership (2007) *Mental Health NSF Autumn Assessment 2007: Dual Diagnosis Themed Review.* Leeds: CSIP.

Centre for Mental Health, Department of Health, Mind, et al. (2012) *No Health Without Mental Health: Implementation Framework.* Available at www.dh.gov.uk/health/files/2012/07/No-Health-Without-Mental-Health-Implementation-Framework-Report-accessible-version.pdf

Delgadillo, J., Godfrey, C., Gilbody, S. & Payne, S. (2012) Depression, anxiety, comorbid substance use: association patterns in outpatient addictions treatment, *Mental Health and Substance Use,* 1–17. DOI: 10.1080/17523281.2012.660981

Department of Health (1996) *The Task Force to Review Services for Drug Misusers: Report of an Independent Review of Drug Treatment Services in England.* Wetherby: DH.

Department of Health (1998) *Tackling Drugs to Build a Better Britain.* London: HMSO.

Department of Health (1999a) *National Service Framework for Mental Health: Modern Standards and Service Models.* London: DH.

Department of Health (1999b) *Safer Services: Report of the National Confidential Inquiry into Suicide and Homicide by People with Mental Illness.* London: DH.

Department of Health (2000) *The NHS Plan: A Plan for Investment, A Plan for Reform.* London: HMSO.

Department of Health (2001a) *Mental Health Policy Implementation Guide.* London: HMSO.

Department of Health (2001b) *Safety First: Five Year Report of the National Confidential Inquiry into Suicide and Homicide by People with Mental Illness.* London: DH.

Department of Health (2002a) *Mental Health Policy Implementation Guide: Dual Diagnosis Good Practice Guide.* London: DH.

Department of Health (2002b) *National Suicide Prevention Strategy for England.* London: DH.

Department of Health (2004) *The National Service Framework – Five Years On.* London: DH.

Department of Health (2005) Alcohol Needs Assessment Research Project (ANARP): The 2004 National Alcohol Needs Assessment for England. London: DH.

Department of Health (2006a) *Dual Diagnosis in Mental Health Inpatient and Day Hospital Settings.* London: DH.

Department of Health (2006b) *From Values to Action: The Chief Nursing Officer's Review of Mental Health Nursing.* London: DH.

Department of Health (2008) *Refocusing the CPA: Policy and Positive Practice Guidance.* London: DH.

Department of Health (2009a) *New Horizons: A Shared Vision for Mental Health.* London: DH.

Department of Health (2009b) *Local Routes: Guidance for Developing Alcohol Treatment Pathways.* London: DH.

Department of Health (2010) *Equity and Excellence: Liberating the NHS.* Norwich: HMSO.

Department of Health (2011) *No Health Without Mental Health: A Cross-Government Mental Health Outcomes Strategy for People of All Ages.* London: DH.

Department of Health (England) and the devolved administrations (2007) *Drug Misuse and Dependence: UK Guidelines on Clinical Management.* London: DH (England), the Scottish Government, Welsh Assembly Government and Northern Ireland Executive.

Department of Health, Home Office, Department of Education and Skills, Department of Culture, Media and Sport (2007) *Safe, Sensible, Social: The Next Steps in the National Alcohol Strategy.* London: DH.

Department of Health/National Treatment Agency (2006) *Models of Care for Alcohol Misusers.* London: DoH.

Edwards R. (2011) The development of dual diagnosis link workers in a mental health trust: reflections from clinical practice, *Advances in Dual Diagnosis*, 4 (2): 75–83.

Health Advisory Service (2001) *Substance Misuse and Mental Health Co-morbidity (dual diagnosis): Standards for Mental Health Services.* London: HAS.

Health and Social Care Act (2012) www.legislation.gov.uk

HM Government/Department of Health (2012) *Preventing Suicide in England: A Cross-government Outcomes Strategy to Save Lives.* London: DH.

HM Government/Home Office (2010) *Drug Strategy 2010: Reducing Demand, Restricting Supply, Building Recovery: Supporting people to live a drug-free life.* Available at www.homeoffice.gov.uk/publications/alcohol-drugs/drugs/drug-strategy/drug-strategy-2010

HM Government/Home Office (2012) *The Government's Alcohol Strategy.* Norwich: HMSO.

Home Office (2002) *Tackling Crack: A National Crack Plan.* London: Home Office.

Home Office (2008) *Drugs: Protecting Families and Communities – The 2008 Drug Strategy.* London: Home Office.

Hughes, L. (2006) Closing the gap: a capability framework for working effectively with combined mental health and substance use problems (dual diagnosis), Centre for Clinical and Workforce Innovation, University of Lincoln, Mansfield.

Hughes, L. (2009) Debate: Is mainstreaming working?, *Advances in Dual Diagnosis*, 2 (3): 36–37.

Hunt, G.E., Siegfried, N., Morley, K. et al. (2013) Psychosocial interventions for people with both severe mental illness and substance misuse (review), *Cochrane Database of Systematic Reviews*, 10: CDOO1088.

Increasing Access to Psychological Therapies, Drugscope, NTA (2012) *IAPT Positive Practice Guide for Working with People Who Use Drugs and Alcohol.* Available at www.iapt.nhs.uk/silo/files/iaptdrugandalcoholpositivepracticeguide.pdf

Mental Health Act 1983 (amended 2007) Available at www.legislation.gov.uk/all?title=Mental%20health%20act%20

National Health Service Litigation Authority (2012) *National Health Service Litigation Authority Standards for NHS Trusts Providing Acute, Community or Mental Health and Learning Disability Services and Non-NHS Providers of NHS Care.* Available at www.nhsla.com/riskmanagement

National Health Service Litigation Authority (2013) *NHSLA Risk Management Standards 2013-14 for NHS Trusts providing Acute, Community, or Mental Health and Learning Disability Services and Non-NHS Providers of NHS Care*. Available at www.nhsla.com/safety/Documents/NHS%20LA%20Risk%20Management%20Standards%202013-14.pdf

National Institute for Health and Clinical Excellence (NICE) (2006) *Bipolar Disorder: The Management of Bipolar Disorder in Adults, Children and Adolescents, in Primary and Secondary Care*, NICE clinical guideline 38. London: NICE.

National Institute for Health and Clinical Excellence (NICE) (2007a) *Drug Misuse: Psychosocial Interventions*, NICE clinical guideline 51. London: NICE.

National Institute for Health and Clinical Excellence (NICE) (2007b) *Drug Misuse: Opiate Detoxification, NICE clinical guideline 52*. London: NICE.

National Institute for Health and Clinical Excellence (NICE) (2007c) *Anxiety: Management of Anxiety Disorder (panic disorder, with or without agoraphobia, and generalized anxiety disorder) in Adults in Primary, Secondary and Community Care*, NICE clinical guideline 22 (amended). London: NICE.

National Institute for Health and Clinical Excellence (NICE) (2007d) *Depression: Management of Depression in Primary and Secondary Care, NICE clinical guideline 23 (amended)*. London: NICE.

National Institute for Health and Clinical Excellence (NICE) (2009) Schizophrenia: Core Interventions in the Treatment and Management of Schizophrenia in Adults in Primary and Secondary Care, NICE clinical guideline 82. London: NICE.

National Institute for Health and Clinical Excellence (NICE) (2010a) *Alcohol Use Disorders: Diagnosis and Clinical Management of Alcohol-Related Physical Complications*, NICE clinical guideline 100. London: NICE.

National Institute for Health and Clinical Excellence (NICE) (2010b) *Alcohol Use Disorders: Preventing Harmful Drinking*, public health guidance 24. London: NICE.

National Institute for Health and Clinical Excellence (NICE) (2011a) *Psychosis with Co-existing Substance Misuse*, NICE clinical guideline 120. London: NICE.

National Institute for Health and Clinical Excellence (NICE) (2011b) Alcohol Use Disorders: Diagnosis, Assessment and Management of Harmful Drinking and Alcohol Dependence, NICE clinical guideline 115. London: NICE.

National Institute for Mental Health in England (2003) Preventing Suicide: A Toolkit for Mental Health Services. Leeds: NIMHE.

National Patient Safety Agency (2009) *Preventing Suicide: A Toolkit for Mental Health Services*. Available at www.nrls.npsa.nhs.uk/resources/?EntryId45=65297

National Treatment Agency (2002) *Models of Care for Treatment of Adult Drug Misusers*. London: NTA.

National Treatment Agency (2006) *Models of Care for Treatment of Adult Drug Misusers: Update*. London: NTA.

National Treatment Agency (2012) *Medications in Recovery: Re-orienting Drug Dependence Treatment*. Available at www.nta.nhs.uk/uploads/medications-in-recovery-main-report[0].pdf

Prime Minister's Strategy Unit (2004) *Alcohol Harm Reduction Strategy for England*. London: Prime Minister's Strategy Unit.

Raistrick, D., Heather, N. & Godfrey, C. (2006) *Review of the Effectiveness of Treatment for Alcohol Problems National Treatment Agency*. London: HMSO.

Weaver, T., Charles, V., Madden, P. & Renton, A. (2002) Co-morbidity of Substance Misuse and Mental Illness Collaborative Study (COSMIC): A study of the prevalence and management of co-morbidity amongst adult substance misuse and mental health treatment populations, report submitted to the DH, Imperial College, London.

While, D., Bickley, H., Roscoe, A. et al. (2012) Implementation of mental health service recommendations in England and Wales and suicide rates, 1997–2006: A cross-sectional and before-and-after observational study, *The Lancet*. Available at www.lancet.com DOI:10.1016/S0140-6736(11)61712-1

ADDITIONAL READING

Older people

Royal College of Psychiatrists (2011) *Our Invisible Addicts*. London: RCP.

Young people

National Institute for Health and Clinical Excellence (NICE) (2007) *Community-based interventions to reduce substance misuse among vulnerable and disadvantaged children and young people*, Public Health Guidance 4. London: NICE.

Royal College of GPs, Alcohol Concern, Drugscope, Royal College of Psychiatrists (2012) *Practice Standards for Young People with Substance Misuse Problems*. London: Royal College of Psychiatrists Centre for Quality Improvement.

Criminal justice

Bradley, K. (2009) *The Bradley Report: Lord Bradley's Review of People with Mental Health Problems or Learning Disabilities in the Criminal Justice System*. London: DH.

Department of Health (2009) *A Guide for the Management of Dual Diagnosis for Prisons*. London: DH.

Policies in other countries

Scottish Advisory Committee on Drug Misuse and the Scottish Advisory Committee on Alcohol Misuse (2003) *Mind the Gaps: Meeting the Needs of People with Co-occurring Substance Misuse and Mental Health Problems*. Edinburgh: Scottish Executive.

Welsh Assembly Government (2007) *A Service Framework to Meet the Needs of People with a Co-occurring Substance Misuse and Mental Health Problem*. Available at http://wales.gov.uk/topics/housingandcommunity/safety/publications/cooccuring/?lang=en

12 POLICY INTO ACTION?

Cris Allen

Chapter Overview

This chapter takes an unusual view and perhaps an unusual method to ask a fairly usual question. Namely, 'why doesn't policy become practice'? The author sweeps through a journal that he is well acquainted with and a horizon he is familiar scanning (in a previous role) and provides some answers. His overview captures what was a very busy period in the formation of policy and which he refers to as a 'blizzard'. Undoubtedly I would share his view that this blizzard also involved more than a flurry of consultations!

The prevalence of policy in mental health and its attempt to shape, nudge, lever, and indeed in some cases incentivise change shows just how important the process is considered by those in power and those attempting to wrest power for a specific purpose or cause. Of course this process carries on, and it is one of the central tenets of this book that an understanding of those processes will inform and explain how services and practice are configured.

INTRODUCTION

When I first worked in a psychiatric hospital in 1975 as a porter and subsequently began training as a mental health nurse I can't recall ever being subject to any protocol, procedure, strategy or guidance, or being informed about the presence or importance of any national or local policies.

This now seems implausible in our policy-laden world.

Other contributors to this book will doubtless have defined 'policy'. However, my aged *Oxford Dictionary* informs me that it is 'prudent conduct, sagacity, course or general plan of action (to be) adopted by government, party, person etc, craftiness'.

'Craftiness'? On reflection this is a characteristic that has been increasingly deployed when it comes to the development of national policies and in their implementation in practice within NHS organisations in England.

In this chapter I will take a very broad interpretation of the term 'policy' and, coupled with some shameless 'craftiness', I will refer to imperatives, strategies, guidance, protocols, procedures and legislation as 'policy'.

The last decade or more has witnessed an outpouring of high-level policy that has had some form of impact on people who work in mental health services and those who use them. Sometimes this has been of great benefit to people and sometimes it has been nothing more than an encumbrance. Some policies that have had the best of intentions to really make a difference to the excluded and marginalised have completely failed to have the desired effect at a local level. But where does one begin, in terms or providing some form of chronological narrative about it all?

I should, therefore, explain how I intend to develop such a narrative or commentary on the success or failure of recent policy. I have searched through almost all the issues of the journal *Mental Health Practice* (MHP) from May 2000 to 2010 in order to trace announcements about the publication or issue of new policy (or news, reports, analyses, updates and articles relating to their implementation and their success or their failure). In doing this a large number of policy subject areas, or themes, emerged.

The four most frequently occurring themes were, perhaps unsurprisingly, related to the prevention and management of violence, acute inpatient mental health wards, people from black and minority ethnic backgrounds with mental illness and the reform of the Mental Health Act (1983). These themes form much of the content of this chapter, and by way of a caveat, they don't make for particularly comfortable reading and are England-centric.

However, 1999 is the probable place to start. That was the year that saw the publication of the most significant and successful policy contribution to England's mental health services. *The National Service Framework* – commonly described as the NSF – addressed the mental health needs of adults up to 65 years old. It sets out national standards and national service models and the national underpinning programmes to support its implementation.

One of the effects of the NSF was to give wider attention to, and a focus on, mental health and unleash an unprecedented cascade of further policy material, which in some instances brought significant and welcome changes to services. Some people criticised the NSF's lack of attention to acute inpatient mental health wards.

In May 2000, *MHP* (Vol: 3. No: 8.) contained an article about my appointment to the role of Mental Health Adviser at the Royal College of Nursing (RCN). This stated that a 'key issue likely to repeatedly turn up in Mr Allen's in-tray is the government's plans to reform mental health legislation in England and Wales and Scotland'. Furthermore, it said that Mr Allen would 'have to keep an eye on a whole raft of political and policy changes as well'.

True indeed.

This issue of the journal also included some commentary about the little that had been done to improve mental health services for people from black and minority ethnic backgrounds, evidenced by a snapshot survey from the mental health organisation MIND.

By September 2000 (*MHP*, Vol: 4. No: 1.) the raft of political and policy changes was well afloat with the unveiling of the *NHS Plan*. This presented, amongst other things, a long list of developments to strengthen mental health services. It included access to new crisis resolution services 24-hours a day, an expansion of assertive outreach teams and the introduction of 1,000 graduates trained in 'brief therapy' to assist general practitioners in the treatment of common mental health problems, with a further 500 graduates to work in accident and emergency departments and within NHS Direct to respond to people who needed immediate help.

I don't recall that the cadre of graduates ever materialised in primary care – although some graduates were recruited much later on, to the Improving Access to Psychological Therapies (IAPT) programme – nor did I ever spot a 'graduate worker' in an accident and emergency department.

In November 2000 (*MHP*, Vol: 4. No: 3.) the news section contained an article about the 60 people who killed themselves in England's acute inpatient wards every year and the government's target to reduce this to zero by 2002. In my role as RCN adviser I was quoted as supporting the practical measure of removing fixtures and fittings – or ligatures as we came to know them – but also pointed out that nurses on some wards were so overstretched they were unable to continually observe all the patients identified as being at risk of suicide.

In February 2001, *MHP* (Vol: 4. No: 5.) reported the recent unveiling of the government's plans to reform mental health legislation in England and Wales, captured in the White Paper, *Reforming the Mental Health Act*. Among its key proposals were those to extend compulsory treatment beyond hospital settings and the compulsory treatment of patients who may be a risk to others as a result of mental disorder. There was an analysis written by me of the good – and less good – aspects of the White Paper, the stance that the RCN and its mental health nurse members had taken during the consultation period, and the concerns that they still had.

One of the challenges I experienced whilst I was in my job was that despite my own best efforts and those of colleagues, engaging mental health nurses in influencing policy developments was always somewhat disappointing. Opportunities were lost when the full force of 50,000 nurses across the UK could not be galvanised to shape, or scupper, ill-conceived policy or legislative change. This was also true when, a few years later, I returned to the NHS. Getting nurses to engage in the interpretation of national policy into something that made sense to them and the people who used services at the local care-face could be as painful as banging one's head against the wall.

Jumping, rather clumsily, ahead to December 2009, *MHP* (Vol: 13. No: 4.) reported that the Mental Health Alliance (MHA) claimed that 4,000 people were, by then, subject to Community Treatment Orders (CTO) – to which a Department of Health (DH) spokesperson responded, 'the uptake of CTOs suggests that mental health professionals are finding them a useful resource'. I wonder whether the people constrained by CTOs agreed, and whether all the mental health nurses who hadn't leant their weight to the lobbying activity in 2001 thought CTOs proved to be a 'useful resource'. Furthermore, was this merely the result of the continual reduction in bed numbers, which left clinicians with little choice but to anchor people to services through CTOs but keep them, at all costs, out of the dwindling number of acute beds?

March 2001 (*MHP*, Vol: 4. No: 6.) was the month in which Professor Kevin Gournay described the likely outcomes of a major United Kingdom Central Council for Nursing, Midwifery and Health Visiting (UKCC) exercise that sought to improve the way NHS staff managed violence and aggression in mental health units.

Professor Louis Appleby told *MHP* in April 2001 (Vol: 4. No: 6.) that 'we are planning to ensure the status, rewards and therapeutic activity of inpatient care receives a much-needed boost'.

In the following month (Vol: 4. No: 8.), the editor of *MHP* offered 'two cheers', for the previously heralded 'boost', in his editorial for the way in which the £30m injection for inpatient services was, in part, being given to trusts 'which had evidently failed to ensure their units were kept up to a reasonable standard in recent years'. The DH stated that many wards were in a poor condition and in need of refurbishment and decoration while some even failed to meet patients' basic requirements for safety, privacy and dignity. Coinciding with this the 120-page *Mental Health Policy Implementation Guide: Adult Acute Inpatient Care Provision* was issued by the DH.

A 'crackdown on violence towards staff' was promised in July (*MHP*, Vol: 4. No: 10.) when the UKCC revealed the results of a survey of inpatient services in 40 NHS trusts across the UK. It found that many had ineffective policies while three had none at all, and that only a minority of the 800 nurses who took part in the survey had received training in dealing with violent patients and that refresher courses were rarely available. The UKCC was to use the results to develop a template for training nurses and to provide a 'kite-mark' system for trainers to promote good practice. It was also reported that the then Secretary of State for Health, Alan Milburn, had signalled that national guidance designed to protect NHS staff from violent or abusive patients would be issued later in 2001.

Over the page lay a feature about Dr Joanna Bennett and her campaign for a public inquiry to be held into the death of her brother, David 'Rocky' Bennett, who had died in October 1998 after being restrained by up to five nursing staff at a medium secure unit. The inquest had taken place in May and the jury had returned a verdict of accidental death, 'aggravated by neglect'. The coroner also set out six recommendations, one of which focused on the need for staff in inpatient units to be proactive in tackling racial abuse by, and against, patients. Dr Bennett said 'it's about time we did something about this type of blatant racism'.

In October (Vol: 5. No: 2.) *MHP*'s news pages covered the report issued by the Workforce Action Team (WAT), which had been set up as one for the NSF's five underpinning programmes to address matters that might otherwise hinder the implementation of the NSF and the *NHS Plan*.

One of its proposals was for the recruitment of more workers – in addition to, not in place of, anything that already exists, it stated – who could provide service users with practical help and support. This would be achieved by creating a large workforce of Support, Time, Recovery (STR) workers, who would contribute to the skills-mix solutions required to deliver the NSF.

My recollection of this 'policy initiative' is that a flurry of activity took place in mental health services to re-badge a multitude of health-care support workers as STR workers, without much additional recruitment of a cohort of truly new people, designated as STR workers.

Much later, in March 2005 (Vol: 8. No: 6.), *MHP* would report the DH's claim that the target of 3,000 STR workers had been met. Not without some 'craftiness' I would suggest – and anyway, where are all those STR workers now? Re-badged back into the roles from which they came, I suspect.

The report also stated that the WAT viewed the workforce as 'our most valuable asset', one which should be supported, nurtured and educated. This is likely to have a resoundingly hollow ring for mental health nurses who currently struggle to acquire much in the way of support, nurture or continuing professional education.

The October 2001 issue of *MHP* (Vol: 5. No: 2.) also highlighted the UKCC's report, *The Recognition, Prevention and Therapeutic Management of Violence*, which set out ten overarching recommendations along with proposals for the content of training courses and trust policies.

In December (Vol: 5. No: 4.) *MHP* reported that Professor Louis Appleby had told a seminar for nurse consultants that it was one of the most optimistic times to work in the mental health field, and that 'nurse consultants are an excellent example of how the shape of the workforce should not only reflect the needs of the patients ... but also develop the potential of our best staff'.

More recently NHS trusts' enthusiasm, if it ever really existed, has diminished and the growth of nurse consultant posts has either stalled or gone into a tailspin, with several being made redundant.

Also in December a renewed focus was placed on acute inpatient wards, when the Sainsbury Centre for Mental Health (SCMH), in collaboration with the RCN and other organisations, launched the Acute Solutions Programme, designed to address the host of user concerns about acute inpatient wards, which had been highlighted in the SCMH's Acute Problems report in 1998. Further evidence that inpatient units remained a difficult nut to crack emerged in February 2002 (Vol: 5. No: 5.) when *MHP* reported that the Mental Health Act Commission's (MHAC) annual report had suggested that shortages of experienced and qualified staff were continuing to blight the quality of care provided to inpatients.

At the official launch of the *Mental Health Policy Implementation Guide: Adult Acute Inpatient Care Provision* Professor Louis Appleby said that the nation's inpatient units represented a 'shameful underworld'. In response the SCMH's director of policy stated that 'inpatient care has become a backwater in policy and profile terms. Without clear plans and targets of the type developed for other parts of the mental health care system it will remain the poor relation and its state of functioning continue to affect the system as a whole'.

The news pages in September's *MHP* (Vol: 6. No: 1.) stated 'protest planned over legislation reforms', which reported the planned action by 2,000 protesters to march to the DH's London HQ to voice their opposition to the draft mental health bill, which had been unveiled in June. The protest was being coordinated by the MHA, which represented over 50 organisations, including the RCN.

Furthermore, *MHP* reported that after a two-year inquiry into the care and treatment of African and Caribbean adults with mental health problems, the SCMH had found little to praise about services, and recommended that any changes should be black-led if they were to succeed. This was the stark conclusion of their report *Breaking the Circles of Fear: A Review of the Relationship between Mental Health Services and African and Caribbean Communities.*

The Commission for Health Improvement (CHI) – one of a succession of regulatory authorities – reported that an 'institutional culture pervades' aspects of the services provided by the Berkshire Healthcare NHS Trust, where service users had to choose their meals one week in advance and eat their last meal of the day at 4.30pm.

Ironically, institutionalised practice was echoed in December's *MHP* (Vol: 6. No: 4.) in Justine Heyden's analysis of the changes that had arisen from asylum care to the present day. She implied that nothing had changed, with locked doors and defensive practice prevailing.

In February 2003 (Vol: 6. No: 5.) I wrote a résumé in *MHP* of the policy initiatives that had emerged in the previous year and provided a forecast for the future.

> The forecast for this year suggests there will be little let up in the policy blizzard that affected the UK in 2002. England and Scotland are likely to experience heavy deluges with little respite. Wales is expected to be quieter with fewer policy flurries and occasional settled periods. In Northern Ireland several fronts will vie for supremacy, giving rise to considerable high pressure but possibly little precipitation. The overall outlook, therefore, is that the generation and implementation of policy affecting mental health nurses will remain at, or near, the higher than normal averages we witnessed last year. In England, even those with a keen interest in policy issues can be forgiven for not being able to cite, chapter and verse, all the policy implementation guidance and consultation documents that emerged last year.

The policy blizzard was certainly fatiguing me by then – and people working in mental health services.

In April (*MHP*, Vol: 6. No: 7.) it was reported that 'mental health services are pervaded by institutional racism and are failing to ensure that black people receive a standard of care that is comparable with their white counterparts'. This was the grim conclusion of a long-awaited publication from the National Institute for Mental Health in England (NIMHE), entitled *Inside-Outside*.

Innes Garcia, in the same issue, described a SCMH research study that would seek to establish the true burden of administrative work for mental health staff and whether all the paperwork was really necessary.

Wasn't the incipient creep of administrative burden in part due to the policy and governance blizzards that had begun to encircle mental health services and their staff?

In July's *MHP* (Vol: 6. No 10.) it was, very sadly, reported that a healthcare assistant had been killed at Springfield hospital. Alan Milburn's pledges of 2001 had obviously failed this individual.

That issue of MHP also contained an article that described how managers in mental health services were subject to stress, resulting from 'change, change, change': 'Much of the pressure felt by those working in mental health services can be attributed to the rapid and frequent changes that have been initiated in recent years, at all levels', it stated.

In October (Vol: 7. No 2.) *MHP* reported that a mental health nurse had been stabbed in the stomach and arms by a patient who was subsequently charged with attempted murder.

By November (*MHP*, Vol: 7. No: 3.) there was more bad news, with a CHI report on Rowan ward in Manchester Mental Health and Social Care NHS Trust. This found that 'poor management' allowed 'old fashioned and regimented nursing care to flourish'. The ward had 'a poor institutionalised environment, low staffing levels, high use of bank and agency staff, little staff development, poor supervision – and a closed inward-looking culture'. And in addition, 'The care received by vulnerable older people was unacceptable'.

This added dismally to the catalogue of substandard inpatient care that seemed to continue unabated, with each report further undermining the morale of many good nurses and other staff.

Another recurring theme reappeared in the same issue. The SCMH warned that people from African Caribbean backgrounds did not seek help from mental health services because they feared 'heavy handed treatment, injury and even death'. It had made this statement after a jury reached a decision of unlawful killing in the case of Roger Sylvester, a black Londoner with a history of mental health problems who died in hospital in 1999 after being taken there by police officers who had restrained him. Health Minister Rosie Winterton launched a consultation paper, entitled 'Delivering Race Equality: A framework for action', in an attempt to improve mental health services for black and minority ethnic communities.

MHP reported on the MHAC's tenth biennial report, which noted that many wards were acknowledged to be 'substandard, frightening and even dangerous'. It also urged the government to draw up 'a robust code of practice to bolster the forthcoming changes to the mental health legislation in England and Wales. The introduction of the draft bill itself was to be delayed, to undergo 'pre-legislative scrutiny', a move welcomed by organisations in the field.

March 2004 saw *MHP* (Vol: 7. No: 6.) reporting the recent release of the 'long-awaited' independent inquiry report into the death of David 'Rocky' Bennett. The report found that 'institutional racism is the cause of mental health services' inability to meet the needs of black and minority ethnic patients'. The report made 22 recommendations in all, including one calling for a national system for training in control and restraint. John Reid, then Secretary of State for Health, said 'I accept that there is discrimination in the NHS, both direct and indirect. There is no place for racism or discrimination. It is unacceptable, it contradicts the basic value of equality that is the cornerstone of the health services'.

The, not so merry, month of May (*MHP*, Vol: 7. No: 8.) brought no better news: 'Most mental health units remain bleak environments for staff and patients alike – despite the flood of policy initiatives that has been promulgated by the government in recent years'. That was the conclusion of 'Behind Closed Doors', a report issued jointly by Rethink, Sane and the Jayne Zito Trust, along with the National Association of Psychiatric Inpatient Units. It acknowledged some 'excellent inpatient services with dedicated professional staff', but feedback from service users had suggested that acute care was 'neither safe nor therapeutic'.

The report also pointed out that around 650 national strategies, guidelines, frameworks and protocols had been issued by the government over the previous five years, but claimed that these had led to 'little progress at the clinical frontline'.

Policy enthusiasts – and policy cynics – may wish to read the last paragraph again and reflect momentarily on the eye-popping figure it contains.

In June (*MHP*, Vol: 7. No: 9.) the National Institute for Clinical Excellence (NICE) released information about its forthcoming 'short-term management of disturbed (violent) behaviour in adult psychiatric inpatient settings guideline'. *MHP* said that it took into account the findings from the Bennett inquiry and that service providers should draw up policies that made it clear who would be trained and how often they would receive this training. The techniques on offer needed to be specified. Training programmes and any auditing of the content had to be in accordance with the principles then being developed by NIMHE and the, then recently established, Counter Fraud and Security Management Service.

The publication of the re-drafted mental health Bill for England and Wales had done little to placate the groups representing service users and professionals who had given an earlier version the thumbs-down, reported *MHP* in October (Vol: 8. No: 2.). Opposition came from the MHA, which by then represented over 60 organisations.

Chris Hart, in his *MHP* column in December (Vol: 8. No: 4.), reported on a recent nurse consultants' conference and a survey which revealed they were having a positive impact on the professions and on services but the dramatic increase in new posts that had been evident a few years previously had since slowed alarmingly.

In February 2005, *MHP* (Vol: 8. No: 5.) provided news of an update report on mental health services by Professor Louis Appleby. He stated 'in reviewing the impact of the NSF I have been struck most of all by the huge amount of activity it has generated, the benefits of which are now becoming apparent. An impressive range of policy initiatives has been triggered in an area of health care that was previously neglected'. He highlighted that suicide rates were at their lowest level, most service users said their experience of mental health care had been positive, staff numbers had increased, and modern treatments were widespread. Specialist community teams had been set up across the country offering home treatment, early intervention, or intensive support for complex needs.

The long-awaited NICE Guideline 25 – *Violence: The short-term management of disturbed/violent behaviour in psychiatric inpatient settings and emergency departments* – was formally launched.

It had taken three years to develop the guideline.

In March (Vol: 8. No: 6.), it was reported in *MHP* that the unit where healthcare assistant Eshan Chattun was killed in 2003 had undergone a £750,000 upgrade.

Stable doors and bolting horses came to mind.

The Scrutiny Committee found the Mental Health Bill to be 'fatally flawed' in May (*MHP*, Vol: 8. No: 8.).

We learnt, yet again, from *MHP* in June (Vol: 8. No: 9.) that inpatient wards were unsatisfactory. Ward staffing levels had to be covered by national standards according to 'Acute Care 2004', a report setting out the findings of the first national survey of acute inpatient mental health wards. SCMCH said the report, commissioned by NIMHE, was based on a survey of 50 NHS trusts and 300 wards in England. It found an over-reliance on bank and agency staff and that as a result of the creation of new community teams many wards reported increasingly severe mental health problems and high levels of need.

The Healthcare Commission's *National Audit of Violence* findings were published in July. An analysis article by Daniel Allen in *MHP* (Vol: 8. No: 10.) summarised these thus: 'Bored, drunk, drug-taking patients in overcrowded, unsafe environments with too few properly trained staff. Result? Violence'.

In February 2006 (Vol: 9. No: 5.) *MHP* announced that patients were becoming stranded in specialist units run by the independent sector that were many miles from their home, according to the MHAC's biennial report for 2003–2005. This painted a bleak picture of many inpatient wards, with over half of all wards being full or having more patients than beds, while staffing shortages and unpleasant ward environments undermined the therapeutic purpose of an admission.

The MHA remained exercised about the draft mental health bill, claiming it must be radically overhauled if it was to promote, rather than damage, race equality. In its submission to the government's consultation paper on the Race Equality Impact Assessment of the mental health bill, the MHA warned that the draft bill would be likely to have a disproportionate impact on black people if it were enacted.

In March (*MHP*, Vol: 9. No: 6.) an article on nursing establishments in acute inpatient units claimed that despite the recent raft of policy and professional guidance on the need to improve inpatient care, alongside the recognition that adequate and appropriate staffing levels were essential, there had been no guidance relating to nationally agreed standards for minimum staffing in such units.

The debates over minimum staffing levels continue to rumble on.

We learnt in June (*MHP*, Vol: 9. No: 9.) that mental health services were being singled out for cuts by NHS trusts and local councils in response to the mounting financial crisis in the health and social care fields, according to the mental health charity Rethink. In its report, 'A Cut too Far', it said it had found evidence of more than £30m of cuts in more than 30 areas of England. This total was almost double the government's estimate of £16m in cuts.

These figures now look like pocket-money when compared with the financial cuts the NHS has more recently been instructed to make.

Yet another examination of acute inpatient wards was heralded in July (*MHP*, Vol: 9. No: 10.). Mounting criticism had prompted the government to ask the Healthcare Commission to examine the issues. The Commission was to investigate ways of improving the safety and physical environment of violent and disturbed patients – as well as the working conditions of nurses.

Using talking therapies made financial sense, we were informed in the same month. The Depression Report, produced by Lord Professor Richard Layard from the London School of Economics, called for the implementation of a proper psychological therapy service in every part of the country by 2013. Such a service would pay for itself in the reduced expenditure on incapacity benefits from people being able to go back to work, it claimed. The report was widely backed by various organisations.

Innes Garcia, having finished the SCMH research into administrative burden, concluded that clinical staffing levels needed to take into account the administrative workload – it was a subject area that had been brushed under the carpet for too long.

In September (*MHP*, Vol: 10. No: 1.) it was reported that a study – *With Safety in Mind: Patient Safety in Mental Health Services* – by the National Patient Safety Agency (NPSA), had sparked calls for 'zero tolerance' of violence and abuse in inpatient mental health units after figures showed the prevalence of incidents that resulted in death or serious harm to patients. The analysis by the NPSA of 45,000 incidents reported over two years revealed that most caused little harm to patients, but 2% of the cases resulted in severe harm or death and the agency said mental health services must redouble their efforts to ensure the safety of patients. Campaign groups were also concerned about the level of sexual abuse revealed by the report: 122 of the incidents reported to the agency involved allegations of rape, exposure, sexual advances or touching – with staff members among the alleged perpetrators.

Chris Hart was in robust form in November's *MHP* (Vol: 10. No: 3.), writing in his opinion piece

> ... now is the time for a debate about what we want from our health services in particular. We've had almost ten years of a government so paranoid and bent on social control it's often left me wondering if the bureaucrats like Milburnakov and Reidski didn't just come here under assumed identities to run the NHS. Targets, checklists and dozens of contradictory priorities have characterised mismanagement on an epic scale. All this and the race to a commercialised service has been hidden under the cloak of modernisation.

As 2006 (*MHP*, Vol: 10. No: 4.) came to a close, the MHA lobbied parliament in a bid to persuade MPs that the latest version of the mental health bill was 'not fit for purpose'.

In February 2007 (*MHP*, Vol: 10. No: 5.) the SCMH said that the number of mental health nurses in England must increase by 20,000 by the end of the decade if the government's plans to improve services were to be fully implemented. The SCMH report entitled, 'Delivering the Government's Mental Health Policies: Services, Staffing and Costs' recognised that substantial resources had been channelled into improving mental health care in recent years but stated that the total spending needed to rise by a further 50% in real terms.

March (*MHP*, Vol: 10. No: 6.) saw campaigners welcoming news that the House of Lords had voted by 216 to 128 in favour of the amendment to bring in exclusions to the definition of mental disorder in the mental health bill.

Health Minister Rosie Winterton called for a 'rapid improvement' in the way mental health services respond to people with black and minority ethnic backgrounds. Launching *Positive Steps: A Practical Guide to Delivering Race Equality in Mental Healthcare*, a resource pack aimed at healthcare professionals, she said that the action plan had been backed with new resources, including 500 community development workers.

There's nothing like yet another resource pack as a solution to rectify an issue that had been shouted from the rooftops for many a year but never properly addressed.

April's *MHP* (Vol: 10. No: 7.) reported that the MHA had said that ministers must place clear limits on the use of CTOs after a report commissioned by the DH found there was no evidence that these were effective. MHA chair Andy Bell said 'we hope that the government will now seek to end the controversy of the past nine years and create fair, workable and evidence-based legislation that is fit for the next 30 years'.

However, in May (*MHP*, Vol: 10. No: 8.) controversy over the bill showed no sign of abating with campaigners again denouncing it as dangerous and restrictive. As it received its second reading in the House of Commons the MHA said the proposals were causing widespread concern among health and social care professionals, those with mental illness and their families. Added to this Black Mental Health UK called for race equality principles to be added to the face of the bill.

There was some rather better news in June (*MHP*, Vol: 10. No: 9.) with a report that AIMS – accreditation of acute inpatient mental health services – was helping to drive up standards and improve safety in acute psychiatric wards.

Three cheers for AIMS.

In July (*MHP*, Vol: 10. No: 10.), however, there was less good news concerning the split that had occurred in the MHA after eight years. Eight organisations, including the RCN, had broken away to form the Mental Health Coalition and had welcomed the changes made to the mental health bill. But by September (*MHP*, Vol: 11. No: 1.) there were mixed reactions to the 'improved' mental health bill, although some organisations representing mental health professionals welcomed the 'significant improvements' that had paved the way for the bill to be given the green light by MPs.

Also in September the redoubtable Chris Hart shared more of his frank opinions: 'We now have a health service so tightly micro-managed that targets, checklists, standards and policies dominate the landscape like a nuclear power station built in the middle of a nature reserve' and 'The pace of the "modernisation" agenda has rendered history redundant. Anything more than a year or two old is not just forgotten, it is regarded as simply irrelevant'.

In November (Vol: 11. No: 3.) *MHP* brought news of a SCMH report, commissioned by the DH as part of its Delivering Race Equality programme, which highlighted that only two thirds of staff in mental health services had received training in race equality awareness. The programme required all mental health staff to receive training in cultural competence, a recommendation coming from the inquiry into the death of David 'Rocky' Bennett.

The last issue of 2007 (*MHP*, Vol: 11. No: 4.) contained an article explaining the proposals for a new, single 'super regulator', with Alan Johnson, then Secretary of State for Health, saying 'the Care Quality Commission will ensure that all patients receive a safe and quality service, no matter what part of the system they are accessing and at which point'.

Including at Winterbourne View and Mid-Staffordshire NHS Foundation Trust for example Mr Johnson and those who succeeded you?

MHP told its readers in February 2008 (Vol: 11. No: 5.) that the NHS in England could save millions of pounds a year if crisis resolution and home treatment teams (CRHT) were employed in a more systematic fashion, according to a National Audit Office (NAO) report. *Helping People Through Mental Health Crisis: The Role of Crisis Resolution and Home Treatment Services,* found that in almost half (47%) of the hospital admissions it had examined there had been no CRHT input.

A classic example of 'whole-systems', 'joined-up working', policy in practice?

An analysis article on the third annual Count Me In census warned that it made gloomy reading, reporting precious little progress in treating everyone with a mental health problem equally. It said 'thirty-one-thousand patients, 257 healthcare providers and one clear message: people from some black and minority ethnic groups are three times more likely than average to be admitted as mental health patients. Delivering Race Equality, a five-year action plan was launched three years ago. With two to go, time is running out'.

There was also the first of Geoff Brennan's 'Voices' columns, which prompted the editor of *MHP* to write in his editorial: 'Geoff Brennan vents his frustration at those doom-mongers who never seem to have a positive word to say about acute inpatient services. By my reckoning, he lists 13 national initiatives that are helping to make an impact on an area of practice that has been sadly neglected in recent years. Even if the initiatives aren't quite "reasons to be cheerful", they should make us feel reasonably upbeat'.

However, this did not quite chime with the news in the March *MHP* (Vol: 11. No: 6.), in which we were informed that many mental health units were 'tougher and scarier' places than they had been ten years previously, according to the MHAC. In its twelfth biennial report for 2005–2007, entitled *Risk, Rights, Recovery*, the commission referred to the 'compassion and care' that was in evidence in mental health services, with its inspectors witnessing staff wielding their 'extraordinary power' over patients in a 'heartening way': 'The busy acute wards that we visit appear to be tougher and scarier than we saw a decade ago. Something needs to be done about this. It is scandalous that we are forcing vulnerable people onto mental health wards that are frightening and dangerous places'. Bed occupancy was high and staffing levels were not always adequate, the report also noted.

It's almost as though the authors of such reports simply copied and pasted slabs of gloom from one report into the next, so familiar had the tale become and the lack of any substantial remedies.

In April (Vol: 11. No: 7.) *MHP* produced a deeper analysis of the MHAC's report by Daniel Allen, in which he presented some of the most disturbing incidents witnessed by the commissioners over a six-month period. The incidents included: a dying man being nursed in the dining room of an older people's unit while other patients ate their lunch; a male staff member using his mobile phone to photograph a female patient naked in a bathroom; a staff member laughing off a vulnerable woman's allegations of sexual abuse by predatory male patients; and three staff members restraining a patient by holding a towel across his mouth and pulling it from behind, making it difficult for him to breathe. Allen wrote, 'each of the incidents make a mockery of the notion that mental health has been "modernised", and offers a more lasting impression of inpatient units than the Commission's assertion that, despite the failings, many services display an "immense amount" of compassion and care'.

June (*MHP*, Vol: 11. No: 9.) yielded some better news as Marion Janner welcomed a DH announcement that her Star Wards initiative was to receive financial support: 'Since its launch more than 200 wards have joined the Star Wards initiative, which aims to enable mental health inpatients to make the best use of their time in hospitals by sharing and publicising best practice' Ms Janner said.

Funny how an initiative from a person who used services has had a far more beneficial impact than many national policies and stands like a beacon above the otherwise woeful narrative on inpatient care.

In July (*MHP*, Vol: 11. No: 10.) *A New Vision for Mental Health* – a discussion paper by a coalition representing seven organisations in the field – said traditional ways of measuring outcomes, such as 'symptom reduction' were now outmoded: 'The effectiveness of any intervention, service or support for those suffering mental distress must be evaluated according to much broader quality of life dimensions, which are identified by service users as important to them', it declared. The paper called on the government to undertake a 'radical rethink' of its mental health policy and argued that the demise of the ten-year NSF in 2009 represented an ideal opportunity to create a 'new era' for service users. It urged mental health professionals to stop seeing themselves as 'experts' and to become 'coaches' or 'partners' when working with service users.

The next three paragraphs hop forward from 2008 through 2009, 2010 and 2011, in order to chronicle events that followed the publication of *A New Vision for Mental Health*.

This discussion paper perhaps influenced the development of *New Horizons*, the government's vision for mental health services for the next ten years, which was subsequently published, for consultation, in 2009 (*MHP*, Vol: 13. No: 1.), as the life of the NSF ended. *New Horizons* was widely welcomed but Malcolm Rae – a well regarded leader in mental health nursing – said it did not give enough attention to acute care and he urged nurses to respond to the consultation and emphasise the importance of this.

However, the editor of *MHP* wrote, later and with caution, in February 2010 (Vol: 13. No: 5.), 'the government's ten-year strategy *New Horizons* sets out an ambitious programme of action to improve the mental health of the nation and develop better services. It includes 120 action points, ranging from new initiatives, such as the imminent publication of a public mental health framework. Its success will rest on how widely its principles are accepted and acted on across government departments'. He then went on to say 'The DH is planning to increase funding for front line NHS services in line with inflation in 2011/12 and 2012/13. But paradoxically it also expects efficiency savings of £15–£20 billion a year, £10b of which will come from "efficient, integrated and people centred community and mental health services". Mental health services are often at the back of the queue when the cash is being doled out, and now it looks like they will be in the firing line when the cuts come'.

And so, indeed, this has come to pass.

In October 2010 (Vol: 14. No: 2.) *MHP* reported that the new coalition government had abandoned *New Horizons* – 'the DH is to make radical changes to its mental health strategy by replacing targets with "clear outcome measures" and by focusing on how these can be delivered. Paul Burstow, Care Services Minister, criticised the previous government's policies and its *New Horizons* strategy saying its policies were big on principles but short on details and that its good intentions had foundered because of poor delivery'.

The coalition published its replacement, *No Health Without Mental Health: A Cross-Government Mental Health Outcomes Strategy for People of All Ages*, in February 2011, and this was reported on, and commented on, by *MHP* in March 2011 (Vol: 14. No: 6.).

Some would say this was equally big on principles but short on details and at risk of failing on delivery due to a new health and social care system that the coalition government subsequently implemented despite almost universal opposition, coupled with its savage financial cuts across the NHS.

Secretary of State for Health Andrew Lansley – the architect of the Health and Social Care Act – and Care Minister Paul Burstow were both sacked in the coalition government's first reshuffle in September 2012.

I shall now return, briefly, to 2008 for the remaining highlights – or lowlights – of that year.

MHP reported in September 2008 (Vol: 12. No: 1.) that only eight NHS trusts in England were providing an 'excellent' standard of service in acute inpatient units. This was according to a study conducted by the Healthcare Commission, entitled *Pathway to Recovery: A review of acute inpatient mental health services*. The study described the gulf separating the best performing trusts from those whose provision was said to be 'weak'. One trust in nine scored 'weak' on the criteria relating to safety, showing that in these trusts there was considerable room for improvement in ensuring the safety of service users, visitors and staff.

In October (*MHP*, Vol: 12. No: 2.) acute inpatient units were told to adopt a 'just do it' style in a new NIMHE publication, *More Than Just Staffing Numbers: A Workbook for Acute Care Workforce Redesign and Development*. Its central theme was that it was futile to try to answer the thorny question of what constituted adequate staffing levels on acute wards: 'There is a need to craft local solutions to local situations'. A sister publication, *Laying the Foundations for Better Acute Mental*

Health Care: A Service Redesign and Capital Investment Workbook, acknowledged that nine years after the publication of the NSF there was 'still some way to go nationally' before the 'whole system approach' to acute care it had envisaged was realised.

'Just do it' could have been interpreted as 'it's your fault'.

The *MHP* editorial in February 2009 (Vol: 12. No: 5.) thundered 'what are you going to do to improve mental health care for people from black and minority ethnic groups? I only ask because no one else seems to be able to change the current dire situation, which was highlighted in the Healthcare Commission's latest audit of mental health and learning disability services. It showed that there has been no improvement in the experiences of service users from BME backgrounds since its first such survey in 2005' and 'The government's Delivering Race Equality programme is laudable, but three years into its five-year plan it has yet to prove its worth'.

The editor was equally forthright in October (*MHP*, Vol: 13. No: 2.) when his editorial addressed another theme that has peppered this chapter, the management of violence.

> Control and restraint has been a major feature of the nursing landscape over the past two decades. Before its introduction in the 1980s nurses and other staff tended to muddle through by overpowering combative patients as best they could. The introduction of control and restraint heralded the prospect of safer wards and fewer injuries to staff and patients but over the years there have continued to be injuries and some patients have regrettably died while being restrained by staff using the techniques they have been taught.

The editorial went on to preface an *MHP* article by Patterson et al. that called for an explicit government commitment to the principles of 'restraint reduction' – and a mandatory national scheme of accreditation of all training.

Anyone not heard that last item before?

In March 2010 (Vol: 13. No: 6.) the editor of *MHP* was moved to return to his editorial subject of February 2009.

> Reading the CQC's fifth Count Me In census it is easy to believe that we are all stuck in a time loop. Because it seems that no amount of effort can make a substantial difference to the lot of people from black and minority ethnic communities when it comes to mental health care. People from BME backgrounds are three times more likely than average to be detained under the MHA, despite the DH's Delivering Race Equality action plan, which was published in 2005. It would be unfair to suggest that nothing has been achieved, but you could be forgiven for thinking that rather than five years having passed, the same year has been repeated five times over.

One could argue that of the four main themes in this chapter only the reform of the Mental Health Act has made it over the finishing line – albeit without pleasing everybody. The remaining three themes (the prevention and management of violence, acute inpatient mental health wards and people from black and minority ethnic backgrounds with mental illness) have wallowed in myriad attempts to bring lasting improvement, although of course many examples of good practice, innovation and improvement can be found.

As I complete this chapter in 2013 the RCN has been commissioned by the DH to lead a project that will consider and revise existing guidance on the use of physical interventions.

So at least the prevention and management of violence has secured another ride on the policy merry-go-round.

Chris Hart can have the last word:

What is clear is that much of the change initiated at government and service level doesn't permeate into nurses' day-to-day work. Given that nurses have the most contact with patients, this is a significant barrier to change. Before we spend another decade in futile pursuit of an unattainable nirvana, we need to answer the question about what change we really want and what is happening in the clinical workplace that leaves it so divorced from policymakers. Knowing what we want to change and how to achieve it are quite separate things. (*MHP*, October 2008. Vol: 12. No: 2.).

Reflective Exercise

1. Do you consider it hard to implement policy into practice?
2. What (if you do) are the obstacles to such implementation?
3. How much is power a dynamic in this process of change?
4. What means are used to prevent implementation and why?

INDEX

Figures and Tables are indicated by page numbers in bold.